Small Cell Lung Cancer: A New Era Is Beginning?

Small Cell Lung Cancer: A New Era Is Beginning?

Editors

Alessandro Morabito
Christian Rolfo

MDPI • Basel • Beijing • Wuhan • Barcelona • Belgrade • Manchester • Tokyo • Cluj • Tianjin

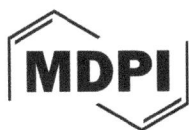

Editors
Alessandro Morabito
Istituto Nazionale Tumori
Italy

Christian Rolfo
University of Maryland School of Medicine
USA

Editorial Office
MDPI
St. Alban-Anlage 66
4052 Basel, Switzerland

This is a reprint of articles from the Special Issue published online in the open access journal *Cancers* (ISSN 2072-6694) (available at: https://www.mdpi.com/journal/cancers/special_issues/Small_Cell_Lung_Cancer).

For citation purposes, cite each article independently as indicated on the article page online and as indicated below:

LastName, A.A.; LastName, B.B.; LastName, C.C. Article Title. *Journal Name* **Year**, *Volume Number*, Page Range.

ISBN 978-3-0365-2301-9 (Hbk)
ISBN 978-3-0365-2302-6 (PDF)

© 2021 by the authors. Articles in this book are Open Access and distributed under the Creative Commons Attribution (CC BY) license, which allows users to download, copy and build upon published articles, as long as the author and publisher are properly credited, which ensures maximum dissemination and a wider impact of our publications.

The book as a whole is distributed by MDPI under the terms and conditions of the Creative Commons license CC BY-NC-ND.

Contents

About the Editors vii

Alessandro Morabito and Christian Rolfo
Small Cell Lung Cancer: A New Era Is Beginning?
Reprinted from: *Cancers* **2021**, *13*, 2646, doi:10.3390/cancers13112646 1

Hsiao-Ling Chen, Yu-Kang Tu, Hsiu-Mei Chang, Tai-Huang Lee, Kuan-Li Wu, Yu-Chen Tsai, Mei-Hsuan Lee, Chih-Jen Yang, Jen-Yu Hung and Inn-Wen Chong
Systematic Review and Network Meta-Analysis of Immune Checkpoint Inhibitors in Combination with Chemotherapy as a First-Line Therapy for Extensive-Stage Small Cell Carcinoma
Reprinted from: *Cancers* **2020**, *12*, 3629, doi:10.3390/cancers12123629 5

Antonella De Luca, Marianna Gallo, Claudia Esposito, Alessandro Morabito and Nicola Normanno
Promising Role of Circulating Tumor Cells in the Management of SCLC
Reprinted from: *Cancers* **2021**, *13*, 2029, doi:10.3390/cancers13092029 23

Valeria Denninghoff, Alessandro Russo, Diego de Miguel-Pérez, Umberto Malapelle, Amin Benyounes, Allison Gittens, Andres Felipe Cardona and Christian Rolfo
Small Cell Lung Cancer: State of the Art of the Molecular and Genetic Landscape and Novel Perspective
Reprinted from: *Cancers* **2021**, *13*, 1723, doi:10.3390/cancers13071723 39

Diego Cortinovis, Paolo Bidoli, Stefania Canova, Francesca Colonese, Maria Gemelli, Maria Luisa Lavitrano, Giuseppe Luigi Banna, Stephen V. Liu and Alessandro Morabito
Novel Cytotoxic Chemotherapies in Small Cell Lung Carcinoma
Reprinted from: *Cancers* **2021**, *13*, 1152, doi:10.3390/cancers13051152 51

Chiara Lazzari, Aurora Mirabile, Alessandra Bulotta, Maria Grazia Viganó, Francesca Rita Ogliari, Stefania Ippati, Italo Dell'Oca, Mariacarmela Santarpia, Vincenza Lorusso, Martin Reck and Vanesa Gregorc
History of Extensive Disease Small Cell Lung Cancer Treatment: Time to Raise the Bar? A Review of the Literature
Reprinted from: *Cancers* **2021**, *13*, 998, doi:10.3390/cancers13050998 69

Maria Gabriela Raso, Neus Bota-Rabassedas and Ignacio I. Wistuba
Pathology and Classification of SCLC
Reprinted from: *Cancers* **2021**, *13*, 820, doi:10.3390/cancers13040820 83

Erik H. Knelson, Shetal A. Patel and Jacob M. Sands
PARP Inhibitors in Small-Cell Lung Cancer: Rational Combinations to Improve Responses
Reprinted from: *Cancers* **2021**, *13*, 727, doi:10.3390/cancers13040727 95

Selina K. Wong and Wade T. Iams
Front Line Applications and Future Directions of Immunotherapy in Small-Cell Lung Cancer
Reprinted from: *Cancers* **2021**, *13*, 506, doi:10.3390/cancers13030506 111

Nicola Martucci, Alessandro Morabito, Antonello La Rocca, Giuseppe De Luca,
Rossella De Cecio, Gerardo Botti, Giuseppe Totaro, Paolo Muto, Carmine Picone,
Giovanna Esposito, Nicola Normanno and Carmine La Manna
Surgery in Small-Cell Lung Cancer
Reprinted from: *Cancers* **2021**, *13*, 390, doi:10.3390/cancers13030390 . . . . **127**

About the Editors

Alessandro Morabito graduated from Medicine and Surgery in 1991 and he completed his specialized training in Oncology in 1995. He was on the Scientific Board of the "Centro Elaborazione Dati Clinici in Oncologia del Mezzogiorno" within a finalized project of the National Research Council from 1993 to 1995. In 1998 he had a Fellowship, FIRC, at Georgetown University in Washington D.C (USA) and in 2010 he received a Masters Degree in Health Management, University Federico II of Napoli. In July 2020 he received the Scientific National Qualification for Associate Professor in Oncology. Dr. Alessandro Morabito was named Deputy Head at the Clinical Trials Unit of INT-IRCCS Foundation G.Pascale of Naples in 2005 and he is currently Director of Thoracic Medical Oncology of INT-IRCCS Foundation G.Pascale of Naples since 2010. He has been Principal Investigator of more than 60 Clinical Trials on Lung Cancer and principal investigator of Investigational Grant AIRC IG 2013 N.14425. He has been a speaker or moderator at more than 400 Oncologic Scientific Conferences and a peer reviewer for approximately 20 International Oncological Journals. He is co-author of more than 220 publications, with more than 2000 points of impact factor, a citation index of 22.176, and H index of 34.

Christian Rolfo is the Associate Director of Clinical Research at the Center for Thoracic Oncology, Tisch Cancer Institute in the Mount Sinai System. In addition, he is Professor of Medicine at the Division of Hematology and Oncology at Icahn School of Medicine, Mount Sinai, New York, NY, USA. From April 2018 to May 2021 he was serving as Director of Thoracic Medical Oncology and Director of Early Clinical Trials at the University of Maryland Marlene and Stewart Greenebaum Comprehensive Cancer Center (UMGCCC), in Baltimore, Maryland, USA. In addition, he was appointed Professor of Medicine at the Division of Oncology at Maryland University, School of Medicine. Prof. Rolfo is a Medical Oncologist focused on Thoracic Oncology, Drug Development, and Translational Oncology. From 2012 to March 2018 he was working as Director of the Phase I - Early Clinical Trials Unit, Director of the Clinical Trials Management Program at Antwerp University Hospital, and Senior Staff member of Thoracic Oncology Cluster at Antwerp University Hospital in Belgium. In addition, he is Professor of Oncology at Antwerp University in the Center for Oncological Research (CORE) in Antwerp, Belgium. Professor Rolfo graduated with a degree in medicine from the National University of Córdoba, Argentina, in 1996; he then studied at the University of Milan and the National Cancer Institute of Milan, Italy, receiving European Oncology Board certification in 2003, followed by Spanish Board Certification in Medical Oncology in 2007. He obtained a PhD and Doctor Europaeus in Clinical and Experimental Oncology Research cum laude from the University of Palermo, Italy, in 2009 under the direction of Professor Rosell, and a Master of Business Health Administration from the Polytechnic University of Valencia, Spain, in 2010. He worked as clinical researcher in the Spanish Lung Cancer Group in Mallorca, Spain, for 8 years. He is actively working on drug development and Lung Cancer and Mesothelioma treatment. His research is focused in molecular oncology and Immunotherapy in Thoracic Oncology and in a pan-tumoral approach, using new techniques in liquid biopsies, specifically in exosome isolation and circulating free tumor DNA. His group identified ALK translocation in exosomes in NSCLC patients, which showed, for the first time, the videos of labeled EVs uptake by living lung cancer cells. He is currently working in the identification of new biomarkers involved in immunotherapy and TKI drug-resistance. In drug development, Prof. Rolfo contributed to the development of several compounds including Erlotinib, pharmacokinetics of Olaparib, Entrectinib, among several other drugs in early phases. Prof. Rolfo served as an expert member of the Commission for Medicinal Products for Human Use and First in Human Drugs Commission at the Federal Agency of Health and Medicinal Products from Belgium and external expert for the European Agency of Medicine (EMA). Professor Rolfo is the Chair of the educational committee at the International Association for the Study of Lung Cancer (IASLC) and the president of the International Society of Liquid Biopsy (ISLB). He is the Editor in Chief of Critical Review in Oncology Hematology. He has an H index 41 and more than 250 publications.

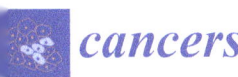

Editorial

Small Cell Lung Cancer: A New Era Is Beginning?

Alessandro Morabito [1,*] and Christian Rolfo [2,*]

1 Medical Oncology, Thoracic Department, Istituto Nazionale Tumori "Fondazione G. Pascale"-IRCCS, 80131 Napoli, Italy
2 Center for Thoracic Oncology, Tisch Cancer Institute, Mount Sinai System & Icahn School of Medicine, Mount Sinai, New York, NY 10128, USA
* Correspondence: a.morabito@istitutotumori.na.it (A.M.); christian.rolfo@mssm.edu (C.R.)

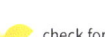

Citation: Morabito, A.; Rolfo, C. Small Cell Lung Cancer: A New Era Is Beginning? Cancers 2021, 13, 2646. https://doi.org/10.3390/cancers13112646

Received: 24 May 2021
Accepted: 26 May 2021
Published: 28 May 2021

Publisher's Note: MDPI stays neutral with regard to jurisdictional claims in published maps and institutional affiliations.

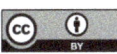

Copyright: © 2021 by the authors. Licensee MDPI, Basel, Switzerland. This article is an open access article distributed under the terms and conditions of the Creative Commons Attribution (CC BY) license (https://creativecommons.org/licenses/by/4.0/).

Small cell lung cancer (SCLC) accounts for about 15% of all lung cancers and it is the most aggressive one. Treatment of SCLC has always represented a significant challenge for oncologists. Attempts to improve the results of first-line treatment have all failed for decades, emphasizing the need for novel therapeutic strategies and the development of validated biomarkers [1]. This scenario has only begun to change recently thanks to the overall survival advantage reached with the addition of immune checkpoint inhibitors (ICI) to first-line chemotherapy, the availability of new effective agents in pretreated patients, and improvements in the knowledge of the biology of SCLC. This Special Issue includes nine articles (one original article and eight reviews), mainly focused on the major progress in SCLC treatment, presented by international leaders in the field of thoracic oncology. The review by Raso MG et al. highlighted current pathological concepts, including classification, immunohistochemistry features, and differential diagnosis [2]. Moreover, they summarized the knowledge of the immune tumor microenvironment, tumor heterogeneity, and genetic variations of SCLC. However, the current classification of SCLC as a single entity hinders effective targeted therapies against this heterogeneous neoplasm. Recent comprehensive genomic analyses have improved our understanding of the diverse biological processes that occur in this tumor type, suggesting that a new era of molecular-driven treatment decisions is finally foreseeable for SCLC patients. A new classification based on RNA expression in mouse-derived SCLC lines has been proposed [3]. This classification identifies four main subdivisions based on the level of expressions of ASCL1 (achaete-scute homolog 1), classified as SCLC-A; NEUROD1 (neurogenic differentiation factor one), classified as SCLC-N; POU2F3 (pou class 2 homeobox 3), classified as SCLC-P; and YAP1 (yes-associated protein 1), classified as SCLC-Y. These findings highlight the heterogeneity of SCLC, with the identification of unique subtypes that could allow the deployment of targeted treatments. For patients with limited stage (LS)-SCLC, the review by Martucci N. et al. summarized the main results observed with surgery, as part of a multimodality treatment [4]. In particular, they showed that several prospective, retrospective, and population-based studies have demonstrated the feasibility of a multimodality approach, including surgery in addition to chemotherapy and radiotherapy in selected patients with stage I SCLC. For patients with extended stage (ES)-SCLC, the review by Lazzari C et al. summarized the main progress of recent years, mainly due to the introduction of immune checkpoint inhibitors, and they discussed the future directions of the clinical research [5]. Currently, the combinations of platinum and etoposide, plus atezolizumab or durvalumab, have been approved for the first-line treatment of ES-SCLC; however, there is no head-to-head comparison of these regimens with different ICIs. A systematic review and a network meta-analysis presented by Chen HL et al. firstly proposed a ranking for progression-free survival, overall survival, objective response rate, and grade 3–4 adverse events for the different combinations of ICIs and chemotherapy for ES-SCLC first-line treatment [6]. In particular, they showed that nivolumab was associated with the best ranking for overall survival, followed by atezolizumab, durvalumab, pembrolizumab, and ipilimumab, but it had also the highest probability of grade 3–4 adverse events. Of course, additional randomized phase III studies are needed to verify these conclusions. Other immunotherapy strategies are also currently being explored, including chimeric antigen receptor (CAR) T cells, tumor vaccines, antibody-drug conjugates (ADCs), and immunomodulators [7]. Moreover, preclinical studies have highlighted a consistent and complex cross-talk between immune cells and angiogenic molecules; on these bases, several clinical trials are currently ongoing to evaluate the efficacy of immunotherapy plus antiangiogenic agents in SCLC patients [8]. In the second-line setting, lurbinectedin, an oncogenic transcription inhibitor analogue of trabectedin, received accelerated approval by the FDA in early 2020 after demonstrating a favorable response rate and a duration of response in an open-label phase II trial [9]. Among the new agents in development, PARP inhibitors represent a therapeutic class that has become an important treatment option for multiple tumor types, although their single agent activity in SCLC is limited [10]. Combining PARP inhibitors with agents that damage DNA and inhibit DNA damage response (DDR), as well as enhancing antitumor immunity down-stream of DNA damage, represent rational therapeutic strategies with preclinical and early trial data to support specific combinations. Finally, the high aggressiveness of SCLC and the lack of active treatments underlie the need for the identification of biomarkers that can aid in the development of personalized medicine in SCLC. Non-invasive biomarkers in peripheral blood, including circulating tumor cells (CTCs) or cell free DNA (cfDNA), can offer the opportunity to achieve prognostic and/or predictive information to study mechanisms of resistance and discover novel targets for therapeutic approaches, thus overcoming the frequent inadequate amounts of tumor samples [11]. A European pooled analysis of 367 individual patients' data confirmed that higher pre-treatment CTC counts are a negative independent prognostic factor in SCLC when considered as a continuous variable or as dichotomized counts of ≥ 15 or ≥ 50 [12]. Therefore, incorporating CTC counts as a continuous variable could improve clinical–pathological prognostic models. In addition, the analysis of the molecular profile of CTCs and the generation of CTC-derived xenografts (CDXs) are encouraging deeper knowledge of SCLC biology, with the major finding that SCLC is a highly heterogeneous disease. In conclusion, is a new era beginning for SCLC? We believe so. We hope that the current lack of targetable oncogenic drivers for SCLC will be overcome by the application of novel technologies of molecular analysis, the identification of different molecular subtypes, and the definition of molecular markers which are predictive of a response to new targeted agents, thus allowing significant advances in the knowledge of SCLC and a better customization of the treatments for each patient.

Funding: This research received no external funding.

Conflicts of Interest: The authors declare the following conflicts of interest: A.M. received honoraria from Roche, AstraZeneca, Boehringer, MSD, BMS, Pfizer, Takeda, Lilly, Novartis. C.R. received honoraria as a speaker: MSD, Roche, Astra Zeneca, Advisory board: Inivata, ArcherDx, MD Serono, Novartis, Boston Pharmaceuticals, BMS, Research Grant: Lung Cancer Research Foundation-Pfizer Grant 2019 American Cancer Society Research Collaboration non remunerated: Guardant Health.

References

1. Morabito, A.; Carillio, G.; Daniele, G.; Piccirillo, M.C.; Montanino, A.; Costanzo, R.; Sandomenico, C.; Giordano, P.; Normanno, N.; Perrone, F.; et al. Treatment of small cell lung cancer. *Crit. Rev. Oncol. Hematol.* **2014**, *91*, 257–270. [CrossRef] [PubMed]
2. Raso, M.G.; Bota-rabassedas, N.; Wistuba, I.I. Pathology and classification of SCLC. *Cancers* **2021**, *13*, 820. [CrossRef] [PubMed]
3. Denninghoff, V.; Russo, A.; de Miguel-Pérez, D.; Malapelle, U.; Benyounes, A.; Gittens, A.; Cardona, A.F.; Rolfo, C. Small cell lung cancer: State of the art of the molecular and genetic landscape and novel perspectives. *Cancers* **2021**, *13*, 1723. [CrossRef]
4. Martucci, N.; Morabito, A.; La Rocca, A.; De Luca, G.; De Cecio, R.; Botti, G.; Totaro, G.; Muto, P.; Picone, C.; Esposito, G.; et al. Surgery in small-cell lung cancer. *Cancers* **2021**, *13*, 390. [CrossRef]
5. Lazzari, C.; Mirabile, A.; Bulotta, A.; Viganò, M.G.; Ogliari, F.R.; Ippati, S.; Dell Oca, I.; Santarpia, M.; Lorusso, V.; Reck, M.; et al. History of extensive disease small cell lung cancer treatment: Time to raise the bar? A review of the literature. *Cancers* **2021**, *13*, 998. [CrossRef] [PubMed]

Chen, H.L.; Tu, Y.K.; Chang, H.M.; Lee, T.H.; Wu, K.L.; Tsai, Y.C.; Lee, M.H.; Yang, C.J.; Hung, J.Y.; Chong, I.W. Systematic review and network meta-analysis of immune checkpoint inhibitors in combination with chemotherapy as a first-line therapy for extensive-stage small cell carcinoma. *Cancers* **2020**, *12*, 3629. [CrossRef] [PubMed]

Esposito, G.; Palumbo, G.; Carillio, G.; Manzo, A.; Montanino, A.; Sforza, V.; Costanzo, R.; Sandomenico, C.; La Manna, C.; Martucci, N.; et al. Immunotherapy in small cell lung cancer. *Cancers* **2020**, *12*, 2522. [CrossRef] [PubMed]

Montanino, A.; Manzo, A.; Carillio, G.; Palumbo, G.; Esposito, G.; Sforza, V.; Costanzo, R.; Sandomenico, C.; Botti, G.; Piccirillo, M.C.; et al. Angiogenesis Inhibitors in Small Cell Lung Cancer. *Front. Oncol.* **2021**, *11*, 1872.

Cortinovis, D.; Bidoli, P.; Canova, S.; Colonese, F.; Gemelli, M.; Lavitrano, M.L.; Banna, G.L.; Liu, S.V.; Morabito, A. Novel cytotoxic chemotherapies in small cell lung carcinoma. *Cancers* **2021**, *13*, 1152. [CrossRef] [PubMed]

Knelson, E.H.; Patel, S.A.; Sands, J.M. PARP inhibitors in small-cell lung cancer: Rational combinations to improve responses. *Cancers* **2021**, *13*, 727. [CrossRef] [PubMed]

De Luca, A.; Gallo, M.; Esposito, C.; Morabito, A.; Normanno, N. Promising role of circulating tumor cells in the management of SCLC. *Cancers* **2021**, *13*, 2029. [CrossRef] [PubMed]

Foy, V.; Lindsay, C.R.; Carmel, A.; Fernandez-Gutierrez, F.; Krebs, M.G.; Priest, L.; Carter, M.; Groen, H.J.M.; Hiltermann, T.J.N.; de Luca, A.; et al. EPAC-lung: European pooled analysis of the prognostic value of circulating tumour cells in small cell lung cancer. *Transl. Lung Cancer Res.* **2021**, *10*, 1653–1665. [CrossRef] [PubMed]

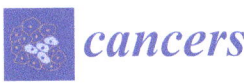

Article

Systematic Review and Network Meta-Analysis of Immune Checkpoint Inhibitors in Combination with Chemotherapy as a First-Line Therapy for Extensive-Stage Small Cell Carcinoma

Hsiao-Ling Chen [1], Yu-Kang Tu [2,3], Hsiu-Mei Chang [1], Tai-Huang Lee [4], Kuan-Li Wu [5], Yu-Chen Tsai [5], Mei-Hsuan Lee [5,*], Chih-Jen Yang [5,6,7,8,*], Jen-Yu Hung [4,5,7] and Inn-Wen Chong [6,7,8,9]

[1] Department of Pharmacy, Kaohsiung Municipal Ta-Tung Hospital, Kaohsiung 80145, Taiwan; hlchen369@gmail.com (H.-L.C.); 880504@kmhk.org.tw (H.-M.C.)
[2] Institute of Epidemiology and Preventive Medicine, National Taiwan University, Taipei 100225, Taiwan; yukangtu@ntu.edu.tw
[3] Department of Medical Research, National Taiwan University Hospital, Taipei 100225, Taiwan
[4] Department of Internal Medicine Kaohsiung Municipal Ta-Tung Hospital, Kaohsiung Medical University, Kaohsiung 88145, Taiwan; weatlee@gmail.com (T.-H.L.); jenyuhung@gmail.com (J.-Y.H.)
[5] Division of Pulmonary and Critical Care Medicine, Department of Internal Medicine, Kaohsiung Medical University Hospital, Kaohsiung Medical University, Kaohsiung 88708, Taiwan; 980448kmuh@gmail.com (K.-L.W.); 1010362kmuh@gmail.com (Y.-C.T.)
[6] Department of General Medicine, Kaohsiung Medical University Hospital, Kaohsiung Medical University, Kaohsiung 88708, Taiwan; chong@kmu.edu.tw
[7] Faculty of Medicine, College of Medicine, Kaohsiung Medical University, Kaohsiung 88708, Taiwan
[8] Respiratory Therapy, College of Medicine, Kaohsiung Medical University, Kaohsiung 88708, Taiwan
[9] Department of Biological Science & Technology, National Chiao Tung University, Hsinchu 300, Taiwan
* Correspondence: mhsuan99@gmail.com (M.-H.L.); chjeya@cc.kmu.edu.tw (C.-J.Y.); Tel.: +886-7-320-8159 (C.-J.Y.); Fax: +886-7-316-1210 (C.-J.Y.)

Received: 29 October 2020; Accepted: 1 December 2020; Published: 3 December 2020

Simple Summary: Patients with extensive-stage small cell lung cancer (ED-SCLC) have a very short survival time even if they receive standard chemotherapy. Currently, the combination of chemotherapy plus immune checkpoint inhibitors (ICIs) as the first line treatment had superior survival than chemotherapy alone in randomized control trials. However, there is a lack of head-to-head comparisons for these combination regimens. We conducted a systematic review and network meta-analysis to provide a treatment ranking of ICIs for ED-SCLC. In summary, the probability of nivolumab was associated with the best ranking for overall survival, followed by atezolizumab, durvalumab, pembrolizumab, and ipilimumab. The ranking of progression free survival from the best to the worst was as follows: nivolumab, pembrolizumab, atezolizumab, durvalumab, and ipilimumab. However, nivolumab had the highest probability of grade 3–4 adverse events in our study. Further head-to head large-scale phase III randomized controlled studies are needed to verify our conclusions.

Abstract: Patients with extensive-stage small cell lung cancer (ED-SCLC) have a very short survival time even if they receive standard cytotoxic chemotherapy with etoposide and platinum (EP). Several randomized controlled trials have shown that patients with ED-SCLC who received a combination of EP plus immune checkpoint inhibitors (ICIs) had superior survival compared with those who received EP alone. We conducted a systematic review and network meta-analysis to provide a ranking of ICIs for our primary endpoints in terms of overall survival (OS), progression free survival (PFS), and objective response rate (ORR), as well as our secondary endpoint in terms of adverse events. The fractional polynomial model was used to evaluate the adjusted hazard ratios for the survival indicators (OS and PFS). Treatment rank was estimated using the surface under the cumulative ranking curve (SUCRA), as well as the probability of being best (Prbest) reference. EP plus nivolumab, atezolizumab or durvalumab had significant benefits compared with EP alone in terms of OS (Hazard Ratio HR = 0.67, 95% Confidence Interval CI = 0.46–0.98 for nivolumab, HR = 0.70, 95% CI = 0.54–0.91 for atezolizumab, HR = 0.73, 95% CI = 0.59–0.90 for durvalumab) but no significant differences were observed for pembrolizumab or ipilimumab. The probability of nivolumab being ranked first among all treatment arms was highest (SCURA = 78.7%, Prbest = 46.7%). All EP plus ICI combinations had a longer PFS compared with EP alone (HR = 0.65, 95% CI = 0.46–0.92 for nivolumab, HR = 0.77, 95% CI = 0.61–0.96 for atezolizumab, HR = 0.78, 95% CI = 0.65–0.94 for durvalumab, HR = 0.75, 95% CI = 0.61–0.92 for pembrolizumab), and nivolumab was ranked first in terms of PFS (SCURA = 85.0%, Prbest = 66.8%). In addition, nivolumab had the highest probability of grade 3–4 adverse events (SUCRA = 84.8%) in our study. We found that nivolumab had the best PFS and OS in all combinations of ICIs and EP, but nivolumab also had the highest probability of grade 3–4 adverse events in our network meta-analysis. Further head-to head large-scale phase III randomized controlled studies are needed to verify our conclusions.

Keywords: immune checkpoint inhibitors; extensive-stage small cell lung cancer; nivolumab; ipilimumab; pembrolizumab; atezolizumab; durvalumab; chemotherapy

1. Introduction

Small cell lung cancer (SCLC) accounts for 10–15% of all lung cancer cases and is known for its aggressive behavior, rapid doubling time, growth, and early spread to distant sites. The most common risk factor for SCLC is smoking tobacco, and up to 98% of patients with SCLC have a history of smoking. SCLC is characterized by multiple genetic alterations, reflecting its genomic instability [1,2]. The majority of SCLCs express alterations in chromosome 3p and mutations in *RB1, TP53, RASSF1, MYC, FGFR1,* and *PTEN* [3,4]. In addition to these genomic alterations, there are also malfunctions in specific regulatory pathways. Long term exposure to tobacco smoke causes an increase in the tumor mutation burden (TMB) and SCLC is associated with a higher expression of DNA damage response (DDR) pathway mediators [5]. Early detection of SCLC is very challenging due to the lack of specific symptoms and the rapid tumor growth, making current approaches to screening ineffective for diagnosing patients at early disease stages [6–8]. Around 70% of cases present with extensive-stage SCLC at diagnosis (ED-SCLC); the remaining 30% of patients have limited-stage SCLC (LD-SCLC) [8]. First-line standard chemotherapy is a combination of etoposide with platinum (EP) [6,7]. In ED-SCLC, chemotherapy is the mainstay treatment in the first-line setting. The median overall survival (OS) rates range from 15 to 20 months for LS-SCLC and 8 to 13 months for ED-SCLC. The five-year survival rate is 20% to 25% for LS-SCLC, but only about 2% for ED-SCLC, and there is an average OS period of only two to four months for untreated ED-SCLC patients [6]. SCLC is usually sensitive to the initial chemotherapy treatment; however, most patients develop recurrent disease, often with metastasis to additional sites after the initial treatment. Currently, radiation therapy to the chest and prophylactic cranial irradiation are applied to destroy undetectable cancer cells and decrease the risk of recurrence. Topotecan is a standard second-line treatment choice but its efficacy is very limited [6]. There is no standard of care beyond second-line therapy. Systemic therapy for SCLC patients has not changed substantially in several decades [2,6]. Consequently, there is an urgent medical need to bring new treatment options to SCLC patients.

SCLC is a tumor with one of the highest rates of somatic mutations and this characteristic can result in a higher likelihood of identifying tumor-specific neoantigens that may ultimately trigger an adaptive immune response that is capable of detecting and eradicating tumor cells [1,2]. Preclinical data has demonstrated that treatment with antibodies specific for anti-cytotoxic T lymphocyte associated antigen 4 (CTLA-4) can restore an immune response through the increased accumulation and survival of memory T cells and depletion of regulatory T cells (Tregs). The use of monoclonal antibodies (mAbs) to block either programmed cell death 1 (PD-1) or anti-programmed cell death ligand 1 (PD-L1) prevents the downregulation of T cell effector function, allowing T cells to mediate tumor cell death. Several phase III trials reported that immune checkpoint inhibitors (ICIs) in combination with chemotherapy had clinical benefit in terms of progression free survival (PFS) and OS when used as a salvage therapy for advanced non-small cell lung cancer compared with those patients who received chemotherapy alone [9–12]. Since then, several trials have been designed to combine chemotherapy with ICIs, including anti-CTLA4, anti-PD-1 or anti-PD-L1, as a first line therapy for ED-SCLC [13–18]. Except for anti-CTLA4, ICIs plus chemotherapy provided a better survival benefit for newly diagnosed ED-SCLC. However, there is a lack of head-to-head comparisons for these combination regimens in the treatment of ED-SCLC. As ICIs are very expensive and ED-SCLC patients have a short survival time, we urgently need to know which ICI plus EP is most effective and reliable. Therefore, we used PFS, OS, objective response rate (ORR) and grade 3–4 adverse drug reactions as the major outcomes in a network meta-analysis of current randomized phase II and phase III trials which reported on ICI plus EP treatment to evaluate their clinical efficacy.

2. Results

2.1. Literature Search

A total of 393 studies were identified following electronic searches, and eight studies were identified from American Society of Clinical Oncology (ASCO) and European Medical Oncology (ESMO). After the exclusion of duplicate studies, 211 papers underwent title/abstract screening. Of those, 82 were excluded due to being incomplete randomized controlled trials (RCTs) and 93 were excluded on the basis of the title/abstract review, leaving 36 studies that underwent a full text review. At the end of the review process, six met the inclusion criteria and underwent qualitative synthesis and quantitative meta-analysis. A Preferred Reporting Items for Systematic Reviews and Meta-Analyses (PRISMA) flow diagram is presented in Figure 1 and the reasons for exclusion are provided in Table S1.

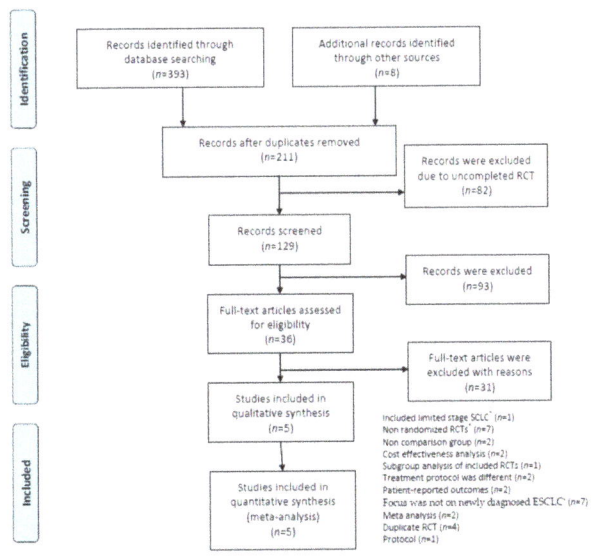

Figure 1. PRIMSA flow diagram.

Study Characteristics and Quality Evaluation

The characteristics of the included studies are provided in Table 1. All six trials were phase II or III and were completed between 2013 and 2020 for newly diagnosed ED-SCLC patients who had not received previous treatment. Except for CA184-041 [16], the control group of all included trials was chemotherapy with etoposide plus platinum (EP) agents. There were two study arms in four of the trials which compared chemotherapy plus ICIs, such as ipilimumab [17], nivolumab [14], pembrolizumab [18], or atezolizumab [13], to chemotherapy alone, while there were three study arms in the CASPIAN [15] and CA184-041 trials. However, the groups with durvalumab, tremelimumab and EP in the CASPIAN trial did not meet the predefined statistical significance threshold at the time of the interim analysis and therefore the result was not presented in the final report. Besides, the group with the concurrent regimen in CA184-041 [16], a phase II trial for ipilimumab, was not regarded as a treatment arm in CA184-156 [17], a phase III trial for ipilimumab, due to there being no improvement in efficacy. The percentage of patients aged ≥ 65 years across the trials ranged from 23.1% to 52.3%, and the percentage of males ranged from 44.4% to 78.4%. The percentage of brain or CNS metastases ranged from 8.68% to 12.14% across all included trials. Response evaluation criteria in solid tumors version 1.1 (RECIST) was used to assess tumor shrinkage (objective response) and disease progression in four of the trials. The other two trials for ipilimumab (CA184-041 and CA184-156) assessed the tumor burden using the modified World Health Organization (mWHO) criteria, as well as the immune-related (IR) response criteria. In conclusion, CA-184-041 [16] was excluded from our analysis due to heterogeneity in the chemotherapy regimen. Furthermore, data from CA184-156 was not included in the network comparisons for PFS and ORR because different criteria were used for cancer progression and treatment response.

The results of the quality assessment are presented in Figure S1. Detailed information about EA5161 was determined from the protocol in ClinicalTrials.gov because limited data was provided in the report from the 2020 annual meeting of the American Society of Clinical Oncology. Both CASPIAN and EA5161 were open label studies; therefore, a high risk of bias was declared for blinding. Besides, unclear assessments were presented and resulted from a lack of detailed information about the random sequence generation and allocation process.

Table 1. Characteristics of the included studies.

Trial Name	ICI-Based Treatment	Year	Phase	Age ≥ 65 (%)	Males (%)	Brain or CNS* Meta (%)	Experimental Arm 1 (Number)	Experimental Arm 2 (Number)	Control Arm (Number)	Criteria for Progression or Response	Criteria for AE*
PD-1 inhibitors											
Keynote-604 [18]	pembrolizumab	2020	3	52.3%	64.9%	12.14%	(n = 228) Induction: 4 × 21 days cycle Pembrolizumab + EP* maintenance* pembrolizumab every 3 weeks		(n = 225) EP alone 4 × 21 days cycle	RECIST* version 1.1	CTCAE*
EA5161 [14]	nivolumab	2020	2	unknown median Age = 65	44.4%	11.25%	(n = 80) induction: 4 × 21 days cycle Nivolumab + EP maintenance* nivolumab every 2 weeks		(n = 80) EP alone 4 × 21 days cycle	RECIST version 1.1	CTCAE
PD-L1 inhibitors											
IMpower133 [13]	atezolizumab	2018	3	46.2%	64.8%	8.68%	(n = 201) induction: 4 × 21 days cycle atezolizumab + EP maintenance* atezolizumab every 3 weeks		(n = 202) EP alone 4×21 days cycle	RECIST version 1.1	CTCAE
CASPIAN [15]	durvalumab	2019	3	39.7%	69.6%	10.24%	(n = 268) induction: 4 × 21 days cycle durvalumab + EP Maintenance* durvalumab every 4 weeks	(n = 268) induction: 4 × 21 days cycle durvalumab + EP + tremelimumab Maintenance* durvalumab every 4 weeks	(n = 269) EP alone 4 × 21 days cycle	RECIST version 1.1	CTCAE
CTLA4 inhibitors											
CA184-041	ipilimumab	2013	2	23.1%	78.4%	unknown	(n = 42)	(n = 42)	(n = 45)	1. mWHO*	CTCAE

Table 1. Cont.

Trial Name	ICI-Based Treatment	Year	Phase	Age ≥ 65 (%)	Males (%)	Brain or CNS * Meta (%)	Experimental Arm 1 (Number)	Experimental Arm 2 (Number)	Control Arm (Number)	Criteria for Progression or Response	Criteria for AE *
[16]							phase regmen 6 × 21 days cycle	concurrent regman 6 × 21 days cycle	paclitaxel + carboplatin 4 × 21 days cycle		
							paclitaxel + carboplatin at cycle 1-2	ipilimumab +paclitaxel +		2. irRC *	
							ipilimumab +paclitaxel + carboplatin at cycle 3-6	carboplatin at cycle 1-4			
								paclitaxel + carboplatin at cycle 5-6			
							maintenance *	maintenance *			
							ipilimumab every 12 weeks	ipilimumab every 12 weeks			
CA184-156	ipilimumab	2016	3	39.6%	56.9%	10.48%	(n = 478)		(n = 476)	1. mWHO	CTCAE
[17]							phase regmen: 6 × 21 days cycle		EP alone 4 × 21 days cycle	2. irRC	
							EP at cycle 1-2				
							ipilimumab + EP at cycle 3-6				
							maintenance *				
							Ipilimumab every 12 weeks				

* CNS: central nervous system, EP: etoposide and platinum, AE: adverse event, RECIST: Response evaluation criteria in solid tumors version, CTCAE: Common Terminology Criteria for Adverse Events, mWHO: modified World Health Organization criteria, irRC: immune-related response criteria.

2.2. Pooled Results for ICIs and Their Effect on Efficacy and Safety

Pooled results for the effect of different ICIs on OS, PFS and ORR as well as grade 3–4 adverse events are provided in Figures S2 and S3. Compared to chemotherapy alone, ICI plus chemotherapy significantly increased the OS and PFS but no significant effect was observed for ORR. On the other hand, ICI plus chemotherapy slightly increased the risk of grade 3–4 adverse events. With regards to the blockade of ICIs, anti-PD-1 agents (nivolumab and pembrolizumab) were associated with significant benefits in OS and PFS. A noticeable OS benefit was seen in the patients who received anti-PD-L1 agents (atezolizumab and durvalumab), but there were no significant effects in PFS and ORR. Only one RCT evaluated the efficacy of an anti-CTLA4 agent (ipilimumab), but there was no improvement in OS between the patients who received ipilimumab plus chemotherapy and those who received chemotherapy alone. In terms of safety, no statistical risks were reported among the patients who received ICIs plus chemotherapy, regardless of the subgroup of ICIs.

Efficacy and Safety Evaluation from the Network Meta-Analysis

The network constructions are presented in Figure 2. For OS and grade 3–4 adverse events, five ICIs plus chemotherapy and chemotherapy alone were included in the network meta-analysis. In terms of PFS and ORR, four ICIs plus chemotherapy and chemotherapy alone were included in the network meta-analysis. The effect sizes of the pairwise comparisons are summarized in Figure 3 and the surface under cumulative ranking curve (SUCRA) rankings are detailed in Figure 4. The probability of being the best treatment is shown in Figure 5 for all efficacy and safety indicators.

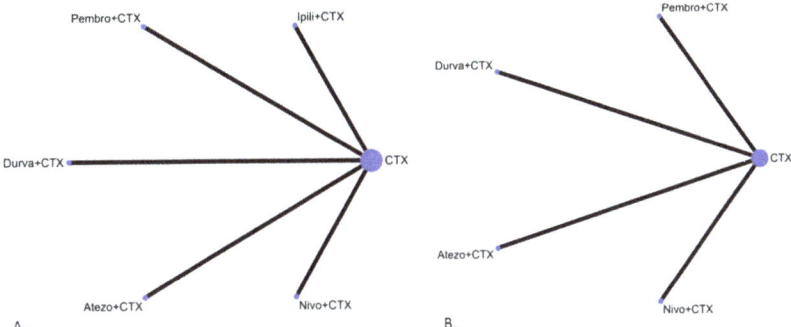

Figure 2. Network construction. (**A**) Network constructions for comparison in overall survival and grade 3–4 adverse events; (**B**) Network constructions for comparison in progression free survival and objective response ratio.

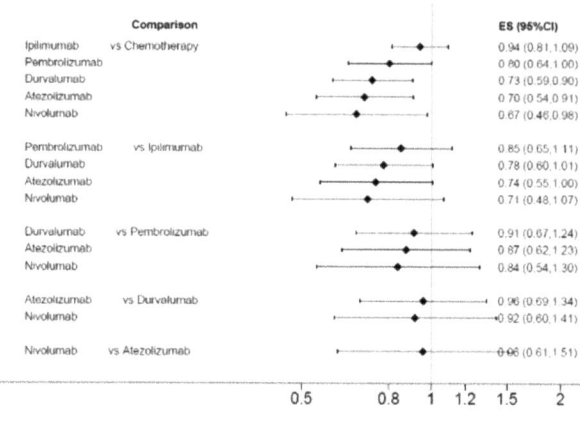

A.

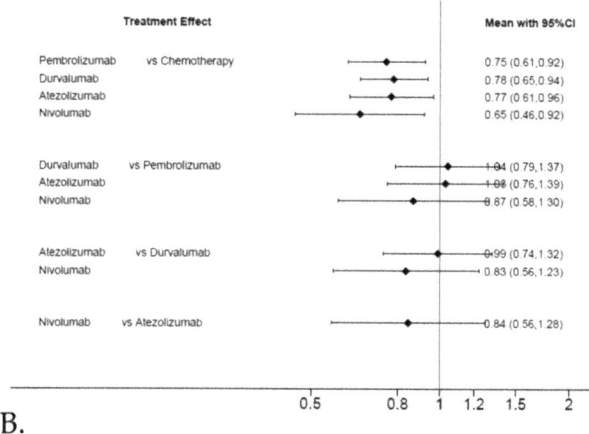

B.

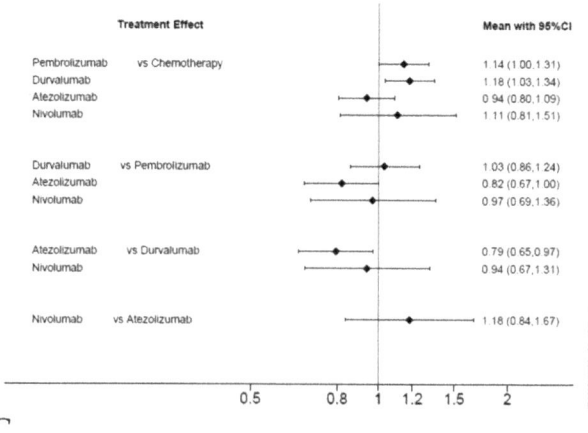

C.

Figure 3. *Cont.*

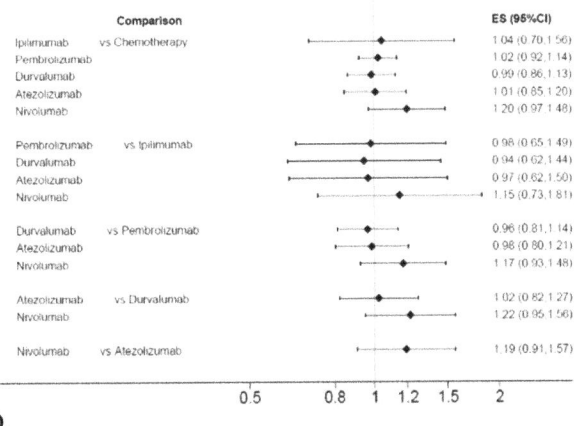

D.

Figure 3. Summary of effect sizes from pairwise comparisons. (**A**) Hazard Ratio for overall survival; (**B**) Hazard Ratio for progression free survival; (**C**) Response Ratio for objective response rate; (**D**) Risk Ratio for grade 3–4 adverse events.

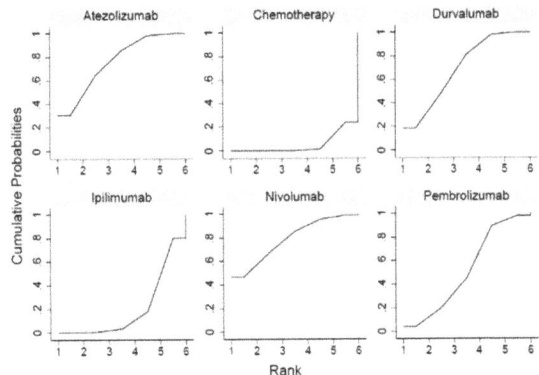

A.

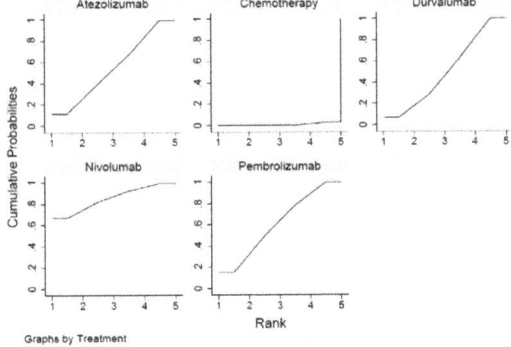

B.

Figure 4. *Cont.*

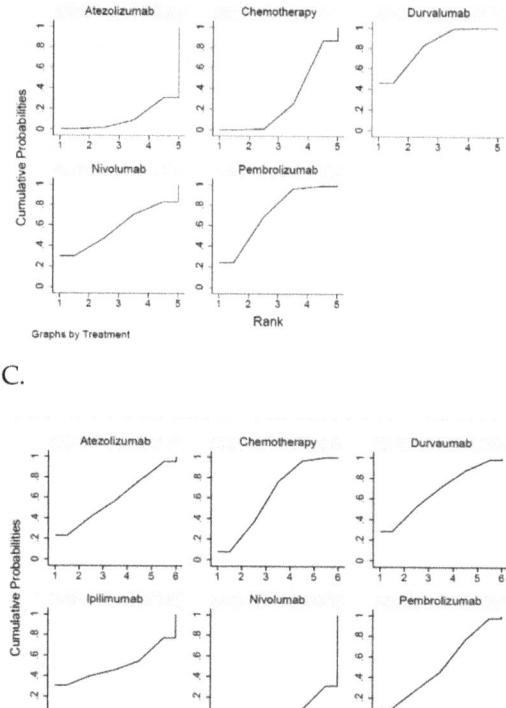

Figure 4. Cumulative ranking probability for different treatments. (**A**) Overall survival; (**B**) Progression free survival; (**C**) Objective response rate; (**D**) Grade 3–4 adverse events.

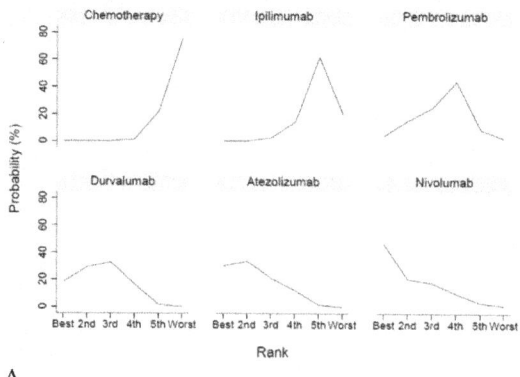

Figure 5. *Cont.*

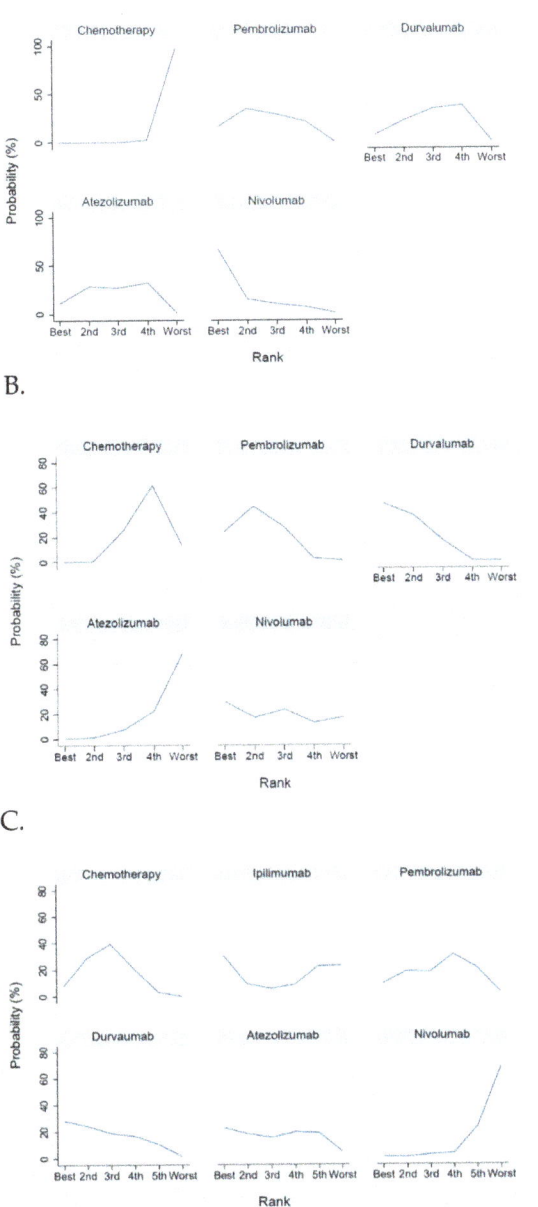

Figure 5. Probability to be the best treatment for different treatments. (**A**) Overall survival; (**B**) Progression free survival; (**C**) Objective response rate; (**D**) Grade 3–4 adverse events.

2.3. Efficacy and Safety Evaluation

In terms of pairwise comparisons for OS (Figure 3A), chemotherapy plus nivolumab, atezolizumab or durvalumab gave a significantly improved benefit compared with chemotherapy alone (HR = 0.67, 95% CI = 0.46–0.98 for nivolumab, HR = 0.70, 95% CI = 0.54–0.91 for atezolizumab, HR = 0.73, 95% CI

= 0.59–0.90 for durvalumab). However, the efficacy was shown to be similar between pembrolizumab or ipilimumab plus chemotherapy and chemotherapy alone (HR = 0.80, 95% CI = 0.64–1.00 for pembrolizumab, HR = 0.92, 95% CI = 0.80–1.09 for ipilimumab). Although no superior effects were indicated in pairwise comparisons between different ICIs, anti-PD-1 agents (pembrolizumab or nivolumab) and anti-PD-L1 agents (atezolizumab or durvalumab) had lower HRs compared with the anti-CTLA4 agent (ipilimumab). Regarding the treatment efficacy ranking, the probability showed that nivolumab was associated with the best ranking for OS (highest SCURA and Prbest value; SCURA = 78.6%, Prbest = 46.7%), followed by atezolizumab (SCURA = 75.7%), durvalumab (SCURA = 68.9%), pembrolizumab (SCURA = 51.3%), ipilimumab (SCURA = 20.4%) and chemotherapy alone (SCURA = 5.0%). Based on the results from subgroup analysis (Figure S4), ranking was similar to the overall subjects. Although durvalumab was not regarded as being a better ICI in OS, it was recommended as the best choice for females younger than 65 years old with brain metastasis at baseline.

In terms of PFS (Figure 3B), all ICIs included in our analysis improved PFS compared with chemotherapy alone (HR = 0.65, 95% CI = 0.46–0.92 for nivolumab, HR = 0.77, 95% CI = 0.61–0.96 for atezolizumab, HR = 0.78, 95% CI = 0.65–0.94 for durvalumab, HR = 0.75, 95% CI = 0.61–0.92 for pembrolizumab). Even though the different ICIs had a similar effect on PFS, treatment with nivolumab had a lower HR than the others. Additionally, the probability showed that nivolumab was associated with the best ranking for PFS (highest SUCRA and Prbest; SCURA = 85.0%, Prbest = 66.8%). As for the blockade of ICIs, anti-PD-1 agents (SCURA = 85.0% for nivolumab and 60.8% for pembrolizumab) were associated with better rankings than anti-PD-L1 agents (SCURA = 54.2% for atezolizumab and 49.5% for durvalumab). Chemotherapy alone had the lowest score (SCURA = 0.6%).

In terms of the objective response rate (Figure 3C), durvalumab was associated with a superior ranking compared with chemotherapy alone (response ratio = 1.18, 95% CI = 1.03–1.34) but no significant differences were observed between the other ICIs and chemotherapy alone. Based on pairwise comparisons between ICIs, no significant difference was observed between any comparable ICIs except for durvalumab, which produced a noticeable benefit over atezolizumab. Moreover, durvalumab was regarded to have a better objective response rate. Durvalumab had the highest SUCRA and Prbest scores (SCURA = 82.1%, Prbest = 46.2%), followed by pembrolizumab (SCURA = 71.8%) and nivolumab (SCURA = 57.4%). However, adding atezolizumab to chemotherapy treatment did not give a better ranking compared with chemotherapy alone, as the SCURA value of atezolizumab was the lowest (SUCRA = 28.3% for chemotherapy alone and SCURA = 10.4% for atezolizumab).

In terms of pairwise comparisons for grade 3–4 adverse events (Figure 3D), we found no significant differences in the risk of grade 3–4 adverse events between any two treatment arms. Although a higher risk was observed among nivolumab users, the risk ratios were close to one and there were no statistical differences. Based on the SUCRA value, a larger SUCRA value indicated a higher treatment risk. Nivolumab (SUCRA = 86.9%, Prbest = 61.3%) had the highest probability of grade 3–4 adverse events, followed by ipilimumab (SUCRA = 51.3%), pembrolizumab (SUCRA = 49.4%), atezolizumab (SUCRA = 42.3%), chemotherapy alone (SUCRA = 37.4%) and durvalumab (SUCRA = 32.7%). Finally, death events for the included RCTs are summarized in Table S2. Due to the limited data that was provided in the published RCTs, it was not possible to classify death events into any events leading to death, immune-mediated adverse events leading to death, or chemotherapy leading to death, so we did not conduct network meta-analyses for death events. The ranking of specific toxicities was similar to the ranking of overall adverse events, except for ipilimumab (Figure S5). Ipilimumab had a lower risk for anemia (ranking = five of six), neutropenia (ranking = six of six) and thrombocytopenia (ranking = six of six); however, ipilimumab had worse safety data for overall adverse events (ranking = two of six).

3. Discussion

ICI plus chemotherapy has been shown to be superior to traditional chemotherapy in both OS and PFS for patients with treatment naïve ED-SCLC in several trials [13–15,18]. Our network meta-analysis firstly proposed a ranking for PFS, OS, ORR and grade 3–4 adverse events for different combinations of ICI and chemotherapy for ED-SCLC treatment.

Add-on ICIs are a feasible way of improving the very short survival time of ED-SCLC patients who receive the standard EP regimen [13–15,18]. Although a response rate of 50% to 80% is achieved in first-line treatment with EP chemotherapy, progression occurs rapidly and there is only a 15–20% response to secondary topotecan chemotherapy [6,8]. Since SCLC has a very short survival time, new treatment strategies are urgently needed. The clinical efficacy of immunotherapies has been observed in patients with refractory or metastatic SCLC [12,19–23]. The phase II KEYNOTE-158 study [21] showed that the PFS of pembrolizumab for relapsed SCLC was 2.0 months, the median OS was 9.1 months, and the one-year PFS and OS were 16.8% and 40.2%, respectively. In a non-randomized cohort of patients with advanced SCLC treated in the CheckMate 032 study [19], the estimated two-year OS rate was 14% with nivolumab monotherapy and 26% with nivolumab plus ipilimumab. Nivolumab plus ipilimumab appeared to provide a greater clinical benefit than nivolumab monotherapy in SCLC patients with a high tumor mutation burden [5]. Furthermore, several trials were designed as a first line therapy for ED-SCLC.

A randomized phase II study (CA184-041) led by Reck et al. was designed to compare paclitaxel with carboplatin plus ipilimumab and paclitaxel with carboplatin alone, but the results did not reveal a significant difference in the ORR, PFS or OS between the treatments [16]. A randomized phase III trial (CA184-156) was further designed to compared ipilimumab and EP with EP alone, and the study showed a minimal increase in median PFS, but there was no significant change in median OS [17]. Recently, several phase II and III trials have been designed to evaluate the addition of PD-1 and PD-L1 inhibitors to EP, and they have demonstrated positive results [13–15,18]. Some traditional meta-analyses of the efficacy of ICIs plus EP have shown that a combination of EP plus ICIs gives superior PFS and OS compared with EP alone for the treatment of ED-SCLC [24,25]. However, the current network meta-analysis proposed not only the efficacies, but also showed the ranking of these ICIs plus chemotherapy combinations on PFS, OS, ORR and grade 3–4 adverse events in different combinations. Firstly, our study showed that all ICIs with EP combination regimens had superior PFS compared with EP treatment alone. All combinations of ICIs with EP enrolled in our network meta-analysis improved the PFS compared with chemotherapy alone. Among all ICI plus EP combinations, nivolumab plus EP had the lowest HR, and nivolumab plus EP ranked first in the treatment of ED-SCLC for PFS and could be regarded as the most reliable combination among all evaluated regimens. In addition, anti-PD-1 agents plus EP ranked better than anti-PD-L1 agents plus EP and EP alone in our analysis.

EP plus nivolumab, atezolizumab or durvalumab all had a significantly better ranking for OS compared with EP alone, but no significant benefits were observed for pembrolizumab or ipilimumab plus EP. Anti-PD-1 agents and anti-PD-L1 agents had lower HRs compared with the anti-CTLA4 agent. In fact, ipilimumab plus paclitaxel and carboplatin failed to demonstrate the efficacy of paclitaxel and carboplatin alone in a phase II trial and it also failed in a phase III study when compared with ipilimumab plus EP [16,17]. Furthermore, nivolumab was ranked as the most optimal ICI among all ICIs plus EP in the treatment arms, followed by atezolizumab, durvalumab, pembrolizumab, ipilimumab and EP alone.

Some previous trial results indicated that ICIs plus chemotherapy were better than chemotherapy alone in terms of ORR and disease control rate (DCR) [15,18]. However, some showed that there was no significant difference in the ORR and DCR between ICIs plus chemotherapy and chemotherapy alone [13,14]. In our analysis, ICIs with EP were compared with EP alone in terms of ORR and DCR. Durvalumab was determined to be the optimal treatment regimen with a better objective response rate, but no significant differences were presented between other ICIs and chemotherapy alone in our network meta-analysis. Interestingly, there was a discrepancy between the ranking of ORR benefit and OS/PFS benefit. This discrepancy may have been caused by measurement bias due to how tumor measurements were taken (in the setting of the subjectivity of RECIST) and also when these measurements were made [26].

Clinically, grade 3–4 adverse events always limit the application of effective combinations of ICIs and EP and grade 3–4 adverse events become the main concern [9,16]. Some previous analyses of these trials indicated that there were fewer serious hematology-related toxicities for the ICI plus chemotherapy group compared with the chemotherapy alone group, however, serious non-hematology-related toxicities were more common in patients receiving an ICI combined with chemotherapy, and there were significant increases in fatigue, rashes, diarrhea, and elevated aminotransferase enzymes [16,27]. In the current study, we found non-significant differences in the risk of grade 3–4 adverse events between any two treatment arms, but nivolumab plus EP had the highest risk. Among all ICIs, nivolumab plus EP had the highest probability of grade 3–4 adverse events as determined by the SUCRA ranking method.

Our meta-analysis had some limitations. First, heterogeneity was present among these included RCTs, such as the regimen for chemotherapy and criteria for treatment response or progression. Therefore, the CA184-041 phase II RCT was excluded from the quantitative synthesis. In addition, the EA5161 study is a small sample phase II trial assessing the effect of nivolumab on ED-SCLC. Although narrow CIs provided strong evidence in EA5161, further RCTs with large sample sizes are needed to confirm our findings. Therefore, our results only serve as a platform for future trials that attempt to introduce nivolumab as a first-line therapy for ES-SCLC in a large phase III RCT, not as direct evidence to promote nivolumab-based therapy as a frontline option at present.

4. Methods

This study was conducted in accordance with the Preferred Reporting Items for Systematic Reviews and Meta-Analyses (PRISMA) guidelines. A prospective protocol was created in advance and registered on the International Prospective Register of Systematic Reviews PROSPERO website (registration number: CRD42020215762) [27].

4.1. Search Strategy and Study Selection

A comprehensive literature search was performed of PubMed, Embase, Cochrane library ClinicalTrials.gov, the database of the American Society of Clinical Oncology (ASCO) and the dataset of European Medical Oncology (ESMO) from their conception until 30 September 2020 without a language limitation. Full details of the search strategy are presented in Tables S3 and S4 and the search keywords were as follows: small cell lung cancer (SCLC or small cell lung carcinoma), immune checkpoint inhibitors (ICIs) anti-CTLA4, anti-PD-1 or anti-PD-L1, and the specific names of drugs (ipilimumab, nivolumab, durvalumab, pembrolizumab, atezolizumab, lambrolizumab, avelumab or tremelimumab). In order to include more relevant studies, controlled vocabulary search terms for PubMed (MeSH) and Embase (Emtree) were used and additional references were sought from the reference lists of the retrieved studies. The inclusion criteria were as follows: (1) completed phase II–III randomized control trials (RCTs) involving adults with ED-SCLC; (2) the RCTs involved newly diagnosed untreated patients with ED-SCLC; (3) the RCTs investigated and compared the efficacy and safety of an ICI combined with chemotherapy with chemotherapy alone.

4.2. Data Extraction and Quality Assessment

Two independent reviewers (H.L. Chen and C.J. Yang) performed the data extraction and quality assessment. Any unresolved discrepancies in the data extraction or appraisal of the results were resolved by discussion with a third reviewer (M.S. Lee). The extracted information included trial details, such as trial name, year published, phase of trial, baseline characteristics, regimen and patient number, primary endpoints, secondary endpoints, and criteria for treatment response. Only grade 3–4 adverse events as defined by the Common Terminology Criteria for Adverse Events (CTCAE) were included for the safety analysis [28]. Quality assessment was performed using the Cochrane

Collaboration's Risk of Bias tool. Quality assessment was performed using Review Manager version 5.1 [29].

4.3. Data Synthesis and Statistical Analysis

Treatment efficacies were evaluated in terms of OS, PFS and ORR. The safety outcomes focused on grade 3–4 adverse events as determined by the CTCAE. A fractional polynomial model was used to evaluate the adjusted hazard ratios (HRs) for the survival indicators (OS and PFS). In terms of binomial indicators, response ratio was regarded as the effect size for the objective response rate and risk ratio was used for adverse events along with 95% confidence intervals (CIs).

We first generated the network graphs for different outcomes separately to determine which treatments were directly or indirectly comparable. After that, we performed a frequentist network meta-analysis to estimate the comparative effect of each pair of treatments included in the constructed network. Fixed-effect models were used, since in most cases the treatment of interest was evaluated in one trial and the number of included trials per comparison was too small to estimate between-study heterogeneity. Finally, treatment rank was estimated by a surface under cumulative ranking curve (SUCRA), as well as the probability of being best (Prbest). SUCRA was computed for a more precise estimation of the ranking probabilities and the larger the SUCRA value, the better the intervention. The Prbest value indicated that the treatment was the best choice in the top rank. All statistical analyses and network graph generation were performed using Stata 11.2 [30].

5. Conclusions

In summary, our network meta-analysis showed that EP plus all ICIs have longer PFS compared with chemotherapy alone, while nivolumab ranked first in the SUCRA ranking analysis. Furthermore, EP plus nivolumab, atezolizumab or durvalumab all provided significant improvements for OS compared with EP alone, and nivolumab also ranked first among all treatment arms. In addition, durvalumab plus EP showed a better objective response rate than the other ICIs plus EP. Finally, nivolumab had the highest probability of grade 3–4 adverse events according to the SUCRA ranking. Given the limited number of studies included in the meta-analysis, additional large-scale phase III RCT studies are needed to verify these conclusions.

Supplementary Materials: The following are available online at http://www.mdpi.com/2072-6694/12/12/3629/s1, Table S1. List of Excluded Papers with Reasons, Figure S1: Quality Assessment Using the Risk of Bias Tool (ROB Tool), Figure S2: Forest Plot and Pooled HR 95% CI for (A) Overall survival; (B) Progression free survival; (C) Objective response rate, Figure S3: Forest Plot and Pooled HR 95% CI for Grade 3–4 Adverse Events, Figure S4: League Table with NMA Estimates for Subgroup Analysis of Overall Survival, Figure S5: League Table with NMA Estimates for Specific Adverse Effects, Table S2: Summary of Death Events for the Included RCTs, Table S3: Search Strategy in PubMed, Table S4: Search Strategy in Embase.

Author Contributions: H.-L.C., C.-J.Y. and M.-H.L.: protocol development, data analysis, and manuscript writing. Y.-K.T.: data analysis. H.-M.C., T.-H.L., K.-L.W. and I.-W.C.: data interpretation. Y.-C.T. and J.-Y.H.: data extraction. All authors have read and agreed to the published version of the manuscript.

Funding: This research received no external funding.

Conflicts of Interest: The authors declare no conflict of interest.

References

1. Sabari, J.K.; Lok, B.H.; Laird, J.H.; Poirier, J.T.; Rudin, C.M. Unravelling the biology of sclc: Implications for therapy. *Nat. Rev. Clin. Oncol.* **2017**, *14*, 549–561. [CrossRef] [PubMed]
2. Subbiah, S.; Nam, A.; Garg, N.; Behal, A.; Kulkarni, P.; Salgia, R. Small cell lung cancer from traditional to innovative therapeutics: Building a comprehensive network to optimize clinical and translational research. *J. Clin. Med.* **2020**, *9*, 2433. [CrossRef] [PubMed]
3. George, J.; Lim, J.S.; Jang, S.J.; Cun, Y.; Ozretic, L.; Kong, G.; Leenders, F.; Lu, X.; Fernandez-Cuesta, L.; Bosco, G.; et al. Comprehensive genomic profiles of small cell lung cancer. *Nature* **2015**, *524*, 47–53. [CrossRef] [PubMed]

4. Peifer, M.; Fernandez-Cuesta, L.; Sos, M.L.; George, J.; Seidel, D.; Kasper, L.H.; Plenker, D.; Leenders, F.; Sun, R.; Zander, T.; et al. Integrative genome analyses identify key somatic driver mutations of small-cell lung cancer. *Nat. Genet.* **2012**, *44*, 1104–1110. [CrossRef]
5. Dong, Z.; Bing, X.; Yong, Y.; Peng, Y.; Sheng-Nan, L.; Qiang, L. Progress in immunotherapy for small cell lung cancer. *World J. Clin. Oncol.* **2020**, *11*, 370–377.
6. Oze, I.; Hotta, K.; Kiura, K.; Ochi, N.; Takigawa, N.; Fujiwara, Y.; Tabata, M.; Tanimoto, M. Twenty-seven years of phase iii trials for patients with extensive disease small-cell lung cancer: Disappointing results. *PLoS ONE* **2009**, *4*, e7835. [CrossRef]
7. Rudin, C.M.; Ismaila, N.; Hann, C.L.; Malhotra, N.; Movsas, B.; Norris, K.; Pietanza, M.C.; Ramalingam, S.S.; Turrisi, A.T., 3rd; Giaccone, G. Treatment of small-cell lung cancer: American society of clinical oncology endorsement of the american college of chest physicians guideline. *J. Clin. Oncol.* **2015**, *33*, 4106–4111. [CrossRef]
8. Nicholson, A.G.; Chansky, K.; Crowley, J.; Beyruti, R.; Kubota, K.; Turrisi, A.; Eberhardt, W.E.; van Meerbeeck, J.; Rami-Porta, R.; Goldstraw, P.; et al. The international association for the study of lung cancer lung cancer staging project: Proposals for the revision of the clinical and pathologic staging of small cell lung cancer in the forthcoming eighth edition of the tnm classification for lung cancer. *J. Thorac. Oncol.* **2016**, *11*, 300–311. [CrossRef]
9. Almutairi, A.R.; Alkhatib, N.; Martin, J.; Babiker, H.M.; Garland, L.L.; McBride, A.; Abraham, I. Comparative efficacy and safety of immunotherapies targeting the pd-1/pd-l1 pathway for previously treated advanced non-small cell lung cancer: A bayesian network meta-analysis. *Crit. Rev. Oncol. Hematol.* **2019**, *142*, 16–25. [CrossRef]
10. Ando, K.; Kishino, Y.; Homma, T.; Kusumoto, S.; Yamaoka, T.; Tanaka, A.; Ohmori, T.; Ohnishi, T.; Sagara, H. Nivolumab plus ipilimumab versus existing immunotherapies in patients with pd-l1-positive advanced non-small cell lung cancer: A systematic review and network meta-analysis. *Cancers* **2020**, *12*, 1905. [CrossRef]
11. Franek, J.; Cappelleri, J.C.; Larkin-Kaiser, K.A.; Wilner, K.D.; Sandin, R. Systematic review and network meta-analysis of first-line therapy for advanced egfr-positive non-small-cell lung cancer. *Future Oncol.* **2019**, *15*, 2857–2871. [CrossRef] [PubMed]
12. Calles, A.; Aguado, G.; Sandoval, C.; Alvarez, R. The role of immunotherapy in small cell lung cancer. *Clin. Transl. Oncol.* **2019**, *21*, 961–976. [CrossRef] [PubMed]
13. Horn, L.; Mansfield, A.S.; Szczesna, A.; Havel, L.; Krzakowski, M.; Hochmair, M.J.; Huemer, F.; Losonczy, G.; Johnson, M.L.; Nishio, M.; et al. First-line atezolizumab plus chemotherapy in extensive-stage small-cell lung cancer. *N. Engl. J. Med.* **2018**, *379*, 2220–2229. [CrossRef] [PubMed]
14. Leal, T.; Wang, Y.; Dowlati, A.; Chen, Y.; Ramesh, A.; Razaq, M.; Liu, J.; Joseph, C.; King, D.M.; Ahuja, H.G.; et al. Randomized phase II clinical trial of cisplatin/carboplatin and etoposide (CE) alone or in combination with nivolumab as frontline therapy for extensivestage small cell lung cancer (ESSCLC): ECOG-ACRIN EA5161. *J. Clin. Oncol.* **2020**, *38*, 9000. [CrossRef]
15. Paz-Ares, L.; Dvorkin, M.; Chen, Y.; Reinmuth, N.; Hotta, K.; Trukhin, D.; Statsenko, G.; Hochmair, M.J.; Ozguroglu, M.; Ji, J.H.; et al. Durvalumab plus platinum-etoposide versus platinum-etoposide in first-line treatment of extensive-stage small-cell lung cancer (caspian): A randomised, controlled, open-label, phase 3 trial. *Lancet* **2019**, *394*, 1929–1939. [CrossRef]
16. Reck, M.; Bondarenko, I.; Luft, A.; Serwatowski, P.; Barlesi, F.; Chacko, R.; Sebastian, M.; Lu, H.; Cuillerot, J.M.; Lynch, T.J. Ipilimumab in combination with paclitaxel and carboplatin as first-line therapy in extensive-disease-small-cell lung cancer: Results from a randomized, double-blind, multicenter phase 2 trial. *Ann. Oncol.* **2013**, *24*, 75–83. [CrossRef]
17. Reck, M.; Luft, A.; Szczesna, A.; Havel, L.; Kim, S.W.; Akerley, W.; Pietanza, M.C.; Wu, Y.L.; Zielinski, C.; Thomas, M.; et al. Phase iii randomized trial of ipilimumab plus etoposide and platinum versus placebo plus etoposide and platinum in extensive-stage small-cell lung cancer. *J. Clin. Oncol.* **2016**, *34*, 3740–3748. [CrossRef]
18. Rudin, C.M.; Awad, M.M.; Navarro, A.; Gottfried, M.; Peters, S.; Csoszi, T.; Cheema, P.K.; Rodriguez-Abreu, D.; Wollner, M.; Yang, J.C.; et al. Pembrolizumab or placebo plus etoposide and platinum as first-line therapy for extensive-stage small-cell lung cancer: Randomized, double-blind, phase iii keynote-604 study. *J. Clin. Oncol.* **2020**, *38*, 2369–2379. [CrossRef]

19. Antonia, S.J.; Lopez-Martin, J.A.; Bendell, J.; Ott, P.A.; Taylor, M.; Eder, J.P.; Jager, D.; Pietanza, M.C.; Le, D.T.; de Braud, F.; et al. Nivolumab alone and nivolumab plus ipilimumab in recurrent small-cell lung cancer (checkmate 032): A multicentre, open-label, phase 1/2 trial. *Lancet Oncol.* **2016**, *17*, 883–895. [CrossRef]
20. Iams, W.T.; Porter, J.; Horn, L. Immunotherapeutic approaches for small-cell lung cancer. *Nat. Rev. Clin. Oncol.* **2020**, *17*, 300–312. [CrossRef]
21. Chung, H.C.; Piha-Paul, S.A.; Lopez-Martin, J.; Schellens, J.H.M.; Kao, S.; Miller, W.H., Jr.; Delord, J.P.; Gao, B.; Planchard, D.; Gottfried, M.; et al. Pembrolizumab after two or more lines of previous therapy in patients with recurrent or metastatic sclc: Results from the keynote-028 and keynote-158 studies. *J. Thorac. Oncol.* **2020**, *15*, 618–627. [CrossRef] [PubMed]
22. Ma, X.; Wang, S.; Zhang, Y.; Wei, H.; Yu, J. Efficacy and safety of immune checkpoint inhibitors (icis) in extensive-stage small cell lung cancer (sclc). *J. Cancer Res. Clin. Oncol.* **2020**. [CrossRef] [PubMed]
23. Jones, G.S.; Elimian, K.; Baldwin, D.R.; Hubbard, R.B.; McKeever, T.M. A systematic review of survival following anti-cancer treatment for small cell lung cancer. *Lung Cancer* **2020**, *141*, 44–55. [CrossRef] [PubMed]
24. Facchinetti, F.; Di Maio, M.; Tiseo, M. Adding pd-1/pd-l1 inhibitors to chemotherapy for the first-line treatment of extensive stage small cell lung cancer (sclc): A meta-analysis of randomized trials. *Cancers* **2020**, *12*, 2645. [CrossRef]
25. Landre, T.; Chouahnia, A.K.; Des Guetz, G.; Assié, J.B.; Chouaid, C. 1799P Immune checkpoint inhibitor plus chemotherapy versus chemotherapy alone as first-line for extensive stage small cell lung cancer: A meta-analysis. *Ann. Oncol.* **2020**, *31* (Suppl. S4), S1041. [CrossRef]
26. Villaruz, L.C.; Socinski, M.A. The Clinical Viewpoint: Definitions, Limitations of RECIST, Practical Considerations of Measurement. *Clin. Cancer Res.* **2013**, *19*, 2629–2636. [CrossRef]
27. Systematic Review and Network Meta-Analysis of First-Line Therapy Combination of Immune Checkpoint Inhibitors and Chemotherapy for Extensive-Stage Small Cell Carcinoma (ID: CRD42020215762). Available online: https://www.crd.york.ac.uk/prospero/ (accessed on 26 November 2020).
28. U.S. Department of Health and Human Services. Common Terminology Criteria for Adverse Events (CTCAE) Version 5.0. Available online: https://ctep.cancer.gov/protocolDevelopment/electronicapplications/docs/ (accessed on 9 October 2020).
29. The Nordic Cochrane Centre, The Cochrane Collaboration. *Review Manager (RevMan)*; Version 5.3; The Nordic Cochrane Centre, The Cochrane Collaboration: Copenhagen, Denmark, 2014.
30. Stata Corp. *Stata Statistical Software: Release 12, Version*; StataCorp LP: College Station, TX, USA, 2011.

Publisher's Note: MDPI stays neutral with regard to jurisdictional claims in published maps and institutional affiliations.

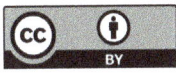

© 2020 by the authors. Licensee MDPI, Basel, Switzerland. This article is an open access article distributed under the terms and conditions of the Creative Commons Attribution (CC BY) license (http://creativecommons.org/licenses/by/4.0/).

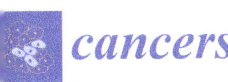

Review

Promising Role of Circulating Tumor Cells in the Management of SCLC

Antonella De Luca [1], Marianna Gallo [1], Claudia Esposito [1], Alessandro Morabito [2] and Nicola Normanno [1,*]

1. Cell Biology and Biotherapy Unit, Istituto Nazionale Tumori—IRCCS—Fondazione G. Pascale, 80131 Naples, Italy; a.deluca@istitutotumori.na.it (A.D.L.); marianna.gallo@istitutotumori.na.it (M.G.); claudia.esposito@istitutotumori.na.it (C.E.)
2. Thoracic Medical Oncology Unit, Istituto Nazionale Tumori—IRCCS—Fondazione G. Pascale, 80131 Naples, Italy; a.morabito@istitutotumori.na.it
* Correspondence: n.normanno@istitutotumori.na.it; Tel.: +39-081-5903-826

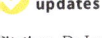

Citation: De Luca, A.; Gallo, M.; Esposito, C.; Morabito, A.; Normanno, N. Promising Role of Circulating Tumor Cells in the Management of SCLC. *Cancers* 2021, *13*, 2029. https://doi.org/10.3390/cancers 13092029

Academic Editor: Helmut H. Popper

Received: 2 March 2021
Accepted: 20 April 2021
Published: 22 April 2021

Publisher's Note: MDPI stays neutral with regard to jurisdictional claims in published maps and institutional affiliations.

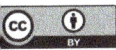

Copyright: © 2021 by the authors. Licensee MDPI, Basel, Switzerland. This article is an open access article distributed under the terms and conditions of the Creative Commons Attribution (CC BY) license (https:// creativecommons.org/licenses/by/ 4.0/).

Simple Summary: Despite the recent approval of immune-checkpoint inhibitors, therapeutic strategies for the treatment of small-cell lung cancer (SCLC) patients remained unchanged for decades. The aggressiveness of the disease and the lack of active treatments underlie the need for the identification of biomarkers that can drive therapeutic decisions. Here we discuss the potential role of circulating tumor cells in SCLC research as a promising tool for improving the clinical management of SCLC patients.

Abstract: Small cell lung cancer is an aggressive disease for which few therapeutic options are currently available. Although patients initially respond to therapy, they rapidly relapse. Up to today, no biomarkers for guiding treatment of SCLC patients have been identified. SCLC patients rarely undergo surgery and often the available tissue samples are inadequate for biomarker analysis. Circulating tumor cells (CTCs) are rare cells in the peripheral blood that might be used as surrogates of tissue samples. Different methodological approaches have been developed for studies of CTCs in SCLC. In addition to CTC count, which might provide prognostic and predictive information, genomic and transcriptomic analyses allow the characterization of molecular profiles of CTCs and permit the study of tumor heterogeneity. The employment of CTC-derived xenografts offers complementary information to genomic analyses and CTC enumeration about the mechanisms involved in the sensitivity/resistance to treatments. Using these approaches, CTC analysis is providing relevant information on SCLC biology that might aid in the development of personalized therapeutic strategies for SCLC patients.

Keywords: small-cell lung cancer; circulating tumor cells; chemotherapy; prognostic biomarker; targeted agents

1. Introduction

Small cell lung cancer (SCLC) is the most aggressive lung cancer subtype and represents about 13% of all new diagnosed lung cancers [1]. SCLC is a disease characterized by neuroendocrine features, a rapid tumor cell growth and the tendency to disseminate early. The majority of patients (about 70%) presents an extensive stage disease (ES-SCLC) at diagnosis, the remaining 30%, a limited stage of disease (LS-SCLC). The prognosis of SCLC is poor, with a median overall survival (OS) of 10 months for patients with ES-SCLC and a survival up to 4 years for selected patients with LS-SCLC [2].

Platinum-based chemotherapy in combination with etoposide or irinotecan is the standard first-line treatment. Recently, immune-checkpoint inhibitors (ICIs) alone or in combination with chemotherapy have been approved for the treatment of SCLC [3].

Despite most patients initially responding to chemotherapy, alone or in combination with ICIs, with a high response rate, a rapid recurrence frequently occurs with an unfavorable prognosis [4]. The only approved second-line agent topotecan is associated with a low response rate and a short duration of survival [2]. Unlike non-small cell lung cancer (NSCLC) and other cancer types, in SCLC there are few therapeutic options and no targeted therapies are available for the management of patients in an advanced stage of disease.

Genomic profiling of SCLC revealed a high load of somatic mutations (about 8 mut/Mb) and molecular signatures associated with tobacco smoking, which plays a pivotal role in the pathogenesis of the disease [5,6]. Biallelic inactivation of TP53 and RB1 are nearly ubiquitary in SCLC [6]. Mutations in other genes, including CREBBP, EP300, NOTCH1, and amplification of MYC and SOX family genes, FGFR1 and IRS2 have been also observed [6,7]. Fusion genes, including a recurrent RLF1-MYCL1 fusion, have been also reported [7]. Recently, a molecular classification, based on gene expression profiling, of four distinct SCLC subtypes characterized by the differential expression of four transcription factors, achaete-scute homologue 1 (ASCL1), neurogenic differentiation factor 1 (NeuroD1), yes-associated protein 1 (YAP1) and POU class 2 homeobox 3 (POU2F3) has also been proposed [8]. Despite the genomic complexity of SCLC, few actionable mutations that offer potential for therapeutic intervention with targeted therapy have been identified in SCLC patients.

The high aggressiveness of this disease and the lack of active treatments underlie the need for the identification of biomarkers that can aid in the development of personalized medicine in SCLC. In this respect, SCLC patients rarely undergo surgery and tissue samples obtained for diagnosis are often inadequate for biomarker analyses. Non-invasive biomarkers in peripheral blood, including circulating tumor cells (CTCs) or cell free DNA (cfDNA), can offer the opportunity to achieve prognostic and/or predictive information, to study mechanisms of resistance and to discover novel targets for therapeutic approaches. Although cfDNA testing is the most advanced approach in clinical routine, a great number of the studies are focused on CTCs in SCLC [9].

CTCs are rare cells released from primary tumors and/or metastatic sites into peripheral blood (one CTC per 10^6–10^7 white blood cells) with a short half-life [10]. Patients with SCLC have a relatively higher CTC number as compared to NSCLC patients [11] and patients with ES-SCLC have more CTCs compared to patients with limited disease [12–15].

In the last few years, technical advancements in isolation methods along with the possibility to recover and molecularly characterize single CTCs, have helped to assess the potential role of CTCs as biomarker for monitoring disease progression in order to study tumor heterogeneity and understanding of the mechanisms of resistance to therapies. In addition, the employment of CTC-derived xenograft (CDX) models has allowed performing studies into SCLC biology in vivo.

In this review, we will discuss the different methodological approaches employed in CTC studies and their utility in improving the management of SCLC patients.

2. Methodological Approaches to CTC Studies in SCLC

Several technologies have been developed for CTC enrichment and detection (Table 1). The most widely used platform for CTC analysis is the CellSearch System, which allows CTC isolation and enumeration based on their expression of EpCAM, a cell surface marker overexpressed in many epithelial tumors [16]. Although SCLC often displays a neuroendocrine differentiation, the expression of EpCAM has been described in SCLC cells [17,18]. In this respect, our group was the first to demonstrate that the CellSearch System is able to isolate EpCAM-positive CTCs in SCLC patients [19]. Our original finding has been later confirmed by a number of studies [14,15,20,21]. However, other approaches have been developed to improve the capture of CTCs with low or without expression of epithelial markers, which might result in a higher efficiency in isolating CTCs from SCLC patients (Table 1).

Table 1. Overview of the main technologies used for enrichment and detection of CTCs in SCLC.

Technology [Refs]	CTC Enrichment	CTC Detection and Characterization	% of CTC Detection §	Comments
Protein marker-based devices				
CellSearch System [12,22]	EpCAM antibodies-coated ferromagnetic beads	IF for CK8, 18, 19, DAPI and CD45	≥85%	FDA-approved semi-automated system. Do not detect EpCAM-negative CTCs. Do not recover viable cells.
CellCollector [23]	Functionalized medical wire associated with EpCAM antibodies	IF for EpCAM, CK and DAPI	Not applicable	CE-approved as medical device for in vivo CTC isolation. Capacity to process large volumes of blood with a high CTC detection rate.
RosetteSep System [24,25]	Depletion of leukocytes and erythrocytes by specific antibodies followed by density gradient centrifugation	ICC	46.9%	Fast and easy-to-use. Collection of live cells with high purity for many applications (cell cultures, DNA/RNA extraction, implantation in mice).
Physical properties-based devices				
ISET [26,27]	Size-based filtration for isolation of CTCs	IF; FISH	95%	Isolation of clusters and viable cells of epithelial and non-epithelial origin. Low recovery and purity.
ClearCell FX [28,29]	Microfluidic technology for CTC enrichment based on drag and size-dependent lift forces	IF; FISH	85%	Capacity to capture viable and intact CTCs for in vivo and in vitro experiments and for NGS analysis. Small CTCs may escape detection.
CTC-iChip [30,31]	Microfluidic platform for size-based isolation in combination with EpCAM-based positive selection or CD45 negative depletion	IF; RT-PCR for tumor associated transcripts	>77%	Detection of both epithelial and non-epithelial CTCs. Capture and in vitro culture of viable CTCs for functional studies.
Parsortix [32]	Microfluidic platform for cell size and deformability-based separation	IF for CK, DAPI and CD45	78%	CE-marked for use as in vitro diagnostic device. Collection of viable CTCs for molecular and functional analysis.
VTX-1 Liquid Biopsy System [33,34]	Microfluidic separation of CTCs based on cell size and deformability	IF; FISH, RT-PCR; NGS for tumor-associated transcripts	69%-79.5%	High recovery and purity of intact CTCs. No red blood cell lysis required. Suitable for many applications (genomic and proteomic analyses, enumeration, IF staining).
DEPArray [35]	Requires a pre-enrichment step with other technologies (e.g., CellSearch or Parsortix)	IF for CK, CD45, DAPI or Hoechst staining	99.7%	Recovery of single viable cells.
Other Assays				
TelomeScan [36,37]	Detection of GFP-positive CTCs following incubation with a telomerase-specific conditionally replicating adenovirus expressing the GFP gene	IF	>70%	Isolation of live CTCs, including EpCAM negative cells and cells undergoing EMT. A modified assay has been developed to reduce false-positive results, based on targeting miR-142-3p to inhibit GFP-expressing blood cells.

§ calculated by spiking tumor cells into peripheral blood of healthy donors. Abbreviations: EpCAM: epithelial cell adhesion molecule; IF: immunofluorescence; CK: cytokeratins; DAPI: 4′,6-diamidino-2-phenylindole; ICC: immunocytochemistry; FDA: US Food and Drug Administration; CTCs: circulating tumor cells; NGS: next-generation sequencing; RT-PCR: reverse transcriptase polymerase chain reaction; FISH: fluorescence in situ hybridization; DEP: Dielectrophoresis; GFP: green fluorescent protein.

These methods have been described in several review articles [16,22,38]. Some approaches, based on the expression of cell surface markers, allow the positive or negative enrichment of CTCs in SCLC samples, including the possibility to recover viable CTCs [23,24] (Table 1).

Methods based on physical properties, such as size and deformability, have the advantage of enriching CTCs with epithelial and mesenchymal features [26,28,32,33].

Other technologies, such as the CTC-iChip, combine physical and biological properties for the enrichment of both epithelial and non-epithelial CTCs [30]. Some platforms, such as the DEPArray, can isolate single CTCs after enrichment with other methods [35]. Among alternative approaches to isolate CTCs from SCLC, the TelomeScan assay employs a green fluorescent protein (GFP) gene-expressing adenovirus in which telomerase regulates viral replication. As telomerase activity is higher in cancer cells rather than in normal cells, GFP-positive CTCs can be efficiently isolated [36,37] (Table 1).

After the enrichment step, CTCs can be detected and characterized using immunologic, molecular and functional assays.

Isolated CTCs offer different opportunities for studies in SCLC. In addition to CTC count that may provide prognostic and predictive information, molecular profiling of CTCs might allow the identification of biomarkers of sensitivity/resistance to therapy and deliver information on tumor heterogeneity. In addition, preclinical studies using CDXs and ex-vivo CTCs may offer the opportunity to acquire information on SCLC biology and facilitate the discovery of novel therapeutic approaches (Figure 1).

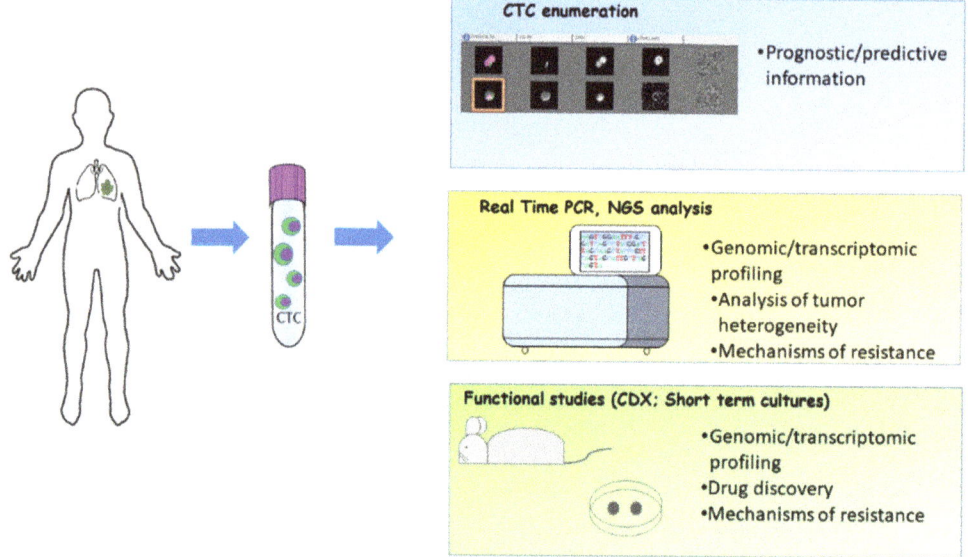

Figure 1. Methodological approaches to study CTCs in SCLC. CTCs enriched and isolated with various techniques offer the opportunity to perform different downstream assays such as CTC count, molecular analyses and in vivo functional studies.

2.1. CTC Count as Biomarker in SCLC

A number of studies have addressed the prognostic role of CTC count in patients with SCLC (Table 2). It is very difficult to summarize the main findings of these studies because of their high heterogeneity.

Although the CellSearch System has been the most used platform in studies assessing CTC count as a prognostic biomarker in SCLC, other technologies such as TelomeScan and methods based on negative immunomagnetic enrichment and immunocytochemistry have been also used [39,40] (Table 2). These approaches are based on different technologies and might detect different populations of CTCs, making their comparison difficult. Taking into account these considerations, we will focus our discussion only on studies that employed the CellSearch system, which still has several limits.

Table 2. Selected studies assessing the role of CTC number as prognostic or predictive biomarker in SCLC.

Study [Ref]	Disease Stage	Treatment	Blood Sample Collection	Number of Patients	CTC Detection Method	Optimal Cut-Off	Main Findings
Hou et al. [13]	LS- and ES-SCLC	Chemotherapy	Baseline, days 2 and 22 after the treatment	50	CellSearch	No cut-off	Patients with a high number of CTCs (> 300) had a shorter median OS than patients with a low number of CTCs (<2) (134 vs. 443 days). A persistently elevated CTC number at day 22 after treatment was considered an adverse prognostic factor at univariate analysis.
Hou et al. [34]	LS- and ES-SCLC	Chemotherapy	Baseline, post cycle 1	97	CellSearch	50 CTCs/ 7.5 mL blood	Patients with a CTC number > 50 had a shorter median PFS (4.6 versus 8.8 months) and OS compared to those with a CTC number < 50 (5.4 versus 11.5 months) at baseline. A number of CTC < 50 after one cycle of chemotherapy was associated with longer PFS and OS. At multivariate analysis, the CTC number at baseline was an independent prognostic factor for PFS (HR = 2.01) and OS (HR = 2.45).
Naito et al. [14]	LS- and ES-SCLC	Chemotherapy or chemoradio-therapy	Baseline, post treatment, at relapse	51	CellSearch	8 CTCs/7.5 mL blood	Patients with a CTC count < 8 at baseline had longer OS than patients with CTC ≥8. Patients with a CTC count ≥8 after treatment and at relapse had a worse OS as compared with those with <8 CTCs at the same time points.
Hiltermann et al. [15]	LS- and ES-SCLC	Chemotherapy	Baseline, post cycle 1 and 4	59	CellSearch	2 CTCs/7.5 mL blood	Patients with a CTC count < 2 had longer OS than patients with a CTC number > 215 (729 vs. 157 days). At multivariate analysis, CTC count was an independent prognostic factor for PFS and OS at all time points. No correlations were observed between the decrease in CTC number from baseline to after one cycle of chemotherapy, and/or the absolute number of CTCs after one cycle of chemotherapy and response to treatment.
Cheng et al. [22]	ES-SCLC	Chemotherapy	Baseline, post cycle 2 and at progression	91	CellSearch	10 CTCs/ 7.5 mL blood	Patients with a CTC count ≥ 10 at baseline had significantly shorter OS as compared with patients with a CTC count < 10 (8.2 vs. 16.6 months); no difference in PFS between the groups was observed.
Aggarwal et al. [21]	LS- and ES-SCLC	Chemotherapy or chemoradio-therapy	Baseline, during cycles 1, 2 (days 2, 3), 3,4 (day 1) and at relapse	50	CellSearch	5 CTCs/7.5 mL blood 50 CTCs/ 7.5 mL blood	Patients with a CTC count < 5 at baseline had better PFS than patients with CTCs ≥ 5 (11 vs. 6.7 months). Using a cut-off of 50 CTCs, for patients with <50 CTCs, PFS and OS were both significantly longer compared to patients with CTCs ≥ 50. At multivariate analysis, a higher CTC count at baseline was associated with a high hazard of death and progression. The decrease in CTCs during the course of therapy was not significantly associated with the response.

Table 2. *Cont.*

Study [Ref]	Disease Stage	Treatment	Blood Sample Collection	Number of Patients	CTC Detection Method	Optimal Cut-Off	Main Findings
Messaritakis et al. [20]	LS- and ES-SCLC	Chemotherapy	Baseline, after 1 cycle and at progression	83	CellSearch	5 CTCs/7.5 mL blood	Patients with a high number of CTCs had a significantly shorter median PFS and OS compared to patients with a low number of CTCs, irrespective of the time of CTC enumeration. At multivariate analysis, the detection of CTCs at baseline was considered as an independent factor associated with decreased PFS, whereas CTC count at progression was associated with a reduced OS. A significantly higher number of CTCs at baseline was observed in patients with PD compared to patients who experienced a CR/PR or SD.
Normanno et al. [43]	ES-SCLC	Chemotherapy	Baseline, post cycle 1	60	CellSearch	No cut-off	A CTC count reduction higher than 89% following chemotherapy was associated with a lower risk of death.
Huang et al. [44]	ES-SCLC	Chemotherapy	Baseline and within 4 weeks after chemotherapy	26	CellSearch	No cut-off	A trend toward significance was observed between baseline CTCs and the percentage of change from post-treatment to baseline and OS
Igawa et al. [39]	LS- and ES-SCLC	Chemotherapy or chemoradiotherapy	Baseline, at cycle 2 and 3, post cycle 4 and at progression	30	TelomeScan	2 CTCs/7.5 mL blood	Patients with a baseline CTC count < 2 had a significantly longer OS than patients with a CTC count ≥ 2.
Wang et al. [40]	LS- and ES-SCLC	Chemotherapy	Baseline, post cycle 1	42	Negative immunomagnetic enrichment	2 CTCs/7.5 mL blood	A CTC number ≥2 at baseline and after the first cycle of chemotherapy was significantly associated with worse PFS.
Tay et al. [45]	LS-SCLC	Chemoradiotherapy	Baseline	75	CellSearch	2 CTCs/7.5 mL blood 15 CTCs/ 7.5 mL blood 50 CTCs/ 7.5 mL blood	A number of 2 or 15 or 50 CTCs at baseline significantly correlated with PFS and OS. Patients with a CTC number < 15 had a better median PFS (19.0 months vs. 5.5 months) and OS (26.7 months vs. 5.9 months) than patients with a CTC number ≥15. At multivariate analysis only the 15 CTC cut-off emerged as an independent prognostic marker

Abbreviations: limited stage disease (LS-SCLC); extensive stage disease (ES-SCLC); progression-free survival (PFS); overall survival (OS).

While three studies with the CellSearch enrolled only ES- and one only LS-SCLC patients, the majority of the studies enrolled both ES- and LS-SCLC patients (Table 2). Patients with LS disease have a better prognosis as compared with patients with ES disease [2,46]. In addition, patients with ES disease have a number of CTCs, significantly higher than patients with LS-SCLC, thus making extremely heterogeneous the population of patients in studies that included both ES- and LS-SCLC [13–15,21]. The importance of the heterogeneity of the population of patients is confirmed by some studies that reported a prognostic value of CTC count only in the subgroup of patients with ES disease [14,21]. Only one study found that the CTC number at baseline is an independent prognostic factor for PFS and OS in LS patients treated with chemoradiotherapy [45].

The number of patients enrolled is limited in most studies, ranging between 14 and 120 (Table 2). The time points of CTC assessment are also different among the studies. In particular, in addition to the CTC count performed before the treatment, CTCs were collected at various days after treatment, after a various number of treatment cycles, and/or at progression. Finally, patients enrolled in the studies were subjected to different therapeutic regimens, i.e., chemotherapy or chemoradiotherapy.

Most studies employed one or more cut-off values to discriminate between patients with a high versus low CTC count. However, such cut-off values varied significantly. The identification of the optimal cut-off was influenced by the statistical methods employed for calculation, the size of samples, the diverse treatment regimens and, most likely, the fraction of ES vs. LS patients enrolled. All these variables might indeed explain the different cut-off values used to discriminate patients with a poor versus a good prognosis [20,41].

Although the above-described heterogeneity significantly limits the possibility to compare the results of the different studies on the prognostic role of CTC count in SCLC, some general findings are common to most of the reports published up to now.

All studies demonstrated that CTCs are detectable in most SCLC patients at baseline (i.e., before treatment), and that the number of CTCs is usually higher in SCLC as compared with most solid tumors [12] (Table 2).

More importantly, the majority of the studies are concordant in identifying a high baseline CTC count as a relevant prognostic factor in SCLC patients. Indeed, the CTC number at baseline was confirmed to be an independent prognostic factor for PFS and OS at multivariate analysis [15,21,41,45]. This evidence was also supported in a meta-analysis of seven studies enrolling 440 SCLC patients, in which a strong association between the presence of CTCs at baseline and a poor clinical outcome was demonstrated [47].

Although the timing for CTC enumeration after the treatment varied among the studies, the majority of the trials also found that the CTC count after one or more cycles of treatment predicts the outcome of SCLC patients. In the study of Hou and collaborators, a number of CTCs < 50 after one cycle of chemotherapy was associated with longer PFS and OS [41]. In a different study, patients with a CTC count ≥8 after treatment and at relapse had a worse OS as compared with those having <8 CTCs at the same time points [14]. Furthermore, the analysis of CTCs in 59 patients before, after one cycle and at the end of chemotherapy revealed that a number of CTCs < 2, after the first or the fourth cycle of chemotherapy, was a strong predictor for PFS and OS, although at multivariate analysis only the absolute number after the first cycle remained the most significant marker for OS [15]. Other studies showed that the CTC number after the second cycle of treatment is also a strong predictor of the outcome [21,42]. In the study of Messaritakis and collaborators, only the detection of CTCs at progression was considered an independent prognostic factor for OS at multivariate analysis [20].

Importantly, the change in the CTC number after chemotherapy was found to be a strong predictor of survival in different studies [14,41,43]. In particular, a study from our group in 60 ES SCLC patients suggested that the accuracy of the prognostic model was only marginally increased by the addition of CTC count to clinical information, whereas a reduction of CTCs greater than 89% following the first cycle of therapy had the strongest correlation with a lower risk of death (HR 0.24) with a significant increase of the prognostic accuracy [43]. These findings strongly suggest that CTC reduction might reflect the chemosensitivity of SCLC.

Although a correlation between CTC number and outcome was clearly demonstrated, a relationship between CTC count and response to treatment in SCLC patients was not found. In the study by Hiltermann, the decrease in CTC number from baseline to after one cycle of chemotherapy did not correlate with tumor response [15]. Similarly, Naito and colleagues did not find a significant correlation between response to treatment and the CTC number before and after chemotherapy [14]. These results are in agreement with the study of Aggarwal and colleagues who did not found a significant correlation between decrease in CTCs and a response to chemotherapy [21].

Clinical studies evaluating novel therapeutic agents for SCLC patients have planned CTC analysis as prognostic/predictive biomarker (Table 3). These studies employed the CellSearch system for CTC isolation and enumeration.

Table 3. Clinical studies incorporating exploratory CTC analysis in SCLC patients.

Investigational Drug	Phase	Number of Patients	Blood Sample Collection	CTC Detection Method	Optimal Cut-Off	Ref
Pazopanib	Phase II	56	Baseline, after the 1st cycle and at progression	CellSearch	5 CTCs	[48]
LY2510924 plus CE	Phase II	78	Baseline, cycle 1 (day 7), cycle 2 (day 1), and at 30-day follow-up after the last dose	CellSearch	6 CTCs/7.5 mL blood	[49]
Vismodegib or cixutumumab plus CE	Phase II	120	Baseline	CellSearch	100 CTCs/7.5 mL blood	[50]
Sonidegib plus CE	Phase I	14	Baseline, after cycles 1,2,4,6, every 3 cycles during maintenance therapy and at disease progression	CellSearch	No cut-off	[51]

Abbreviation: carboplatin-etoposide (CE).

In particular, in a clinical trial of the multi-kinase inhibitor pazopanib in patients with recurrent/refractory SCLC, a number of CTCs ≥ 5 was detected in 28/56 (50.0%) of patients [48]. Treatment with pazopanib for one cycle significantly decreased the number of patients with a high CTC number. Patients with PD as the best response had a significantly higher number of CTCs at baseline as compared with patients experiencing PR or SD. At multivariate analysis, an increased number of CTCs after one cycle was associated with poor OS [48].

An exploratory analysis of the predictive role of CTCs was performed in a phase II clinical trial enrolling 78 ES-SCLC patients who received chemotherapy plus the CXCR4 antagonist LY2510924 [49]. A CTC number ≥6 and a percentage of CXCR4-positive CTCs ≥ 7% were considered optimal cut-off values, based on receiver operating characteristic (ROC) analysis. A CTC number ≥6 at baseline and at cycle 2 predicted shorter PFS and OS. A frequency of CXCR4-positive CTCs > 7% at baseline was also a prognostic factor for shorter PFS [49].

The predictive role of CTCs was also explored in a randomized phase II study evaluating the efficacy of the Hedgehog inhibitor vismodegib or the insulin-like growth factor 1 receptor antibody cixutumumab in combination with standard chemotherapy in previously untreated patients with ES-SCLC [50]. Patients with a CTC number >100 at baseline (39/120, 32.5%) had a worse OS as compared with patients with a lower CTC count [50].

Finally, in a phase I clinical trial investigating the combination of the Hedgehog inhibitor sonidegib with standard chemotherapy in untreated ES-SCLC patients, CTCs were isolated and enumerated with the CellSearch System before, during and at disease progression [51]. Elevated CTC count at baseline (>200) was associated with worse OS at univariate analysis. A persistently high CTC number at cycle 2 also correlated with worse OS. An increase in CTCs from the nadir to progression was observed in 5/13 patients [51].

2.2. Molecular Characterization of CTCs in SCLC

Real time (RT)-PCR techniques were used for the detection of specific markers in CTCs isolated from SCLC patients. In this regard, the presence of transcripts of epithelial (*EpCAM* and *CK19*) and neuroendocrine (*CHGA, SYP, NCAM1* and enolase 2, *ENO2*) markers in CTCs enriched with a microfluidic system was investigated in a study enrolling 48 SCLC patients [52]. The expression of the neuroendocrine markers *SYP* and/or *CHGA* at diagnosis and at disease progression correlated with worse OS [52]. However, these results should be confirmed in additional studies. Interestingly, RT-PCR also revealed in 7.8% SCLC patients the presence of the delta-like 3 ligand (*DLL3*) transcript belonging to the Notch pathway and associated with neuroendocrine tumorigenesis. DLL3-positive patients had a significantly shorter OS than DLL3-negative patients (median OS 2 vs. 7 months) [52].

The employment of Next-Generation Sequencing (NGS) approaches that can interrogate a large number of genes in a single analysis, along with the development of technologies that allow isolating single CTCs, such as the DEPArray system, offered the possibility to perform a comprehensive genomic/transcriptomic profile of CTCs isolated from SCLC patients. Whole genome sequencing (WGS) of single CTCs enriched with the CellSearch System and individually isolated under a fluorescence microscope revealed that copy number variation (CNVs) profiles are specific for each cancer type [53]. In particular, the CNV profile of CTCs reflects the genetic landscape of metastasis and is highly reproducible from cell to cell and from patient to patient, in contrast with whole exome sequencing (WES) analysis of single nucleotide variations (SNV) and insertions/deletions (indels) that are highly heterogeneous from cell to cell [53].

The molecular profile of single CTCs from 13 SCLC patients, enriched with the CellSearch system and isolated using the DEPArray technology, was analyzed by WGS to generate 16 copy number alteration (CNA) profiles that stratified patients in chemosensitive or chemorefractory [54]. The CNA classifier was subsequently validated in an additional 18 patients. The CTC CNA classifier correctly assigned 83.3% of the cases as chemorefractory or chemosensitive. A homogeneous CNA classification was observed in the majority of patients (19/31). However, in 12/31 cases, intra-patient heterogeneity among single isolated CTCs was observed. When the CTC CNA classifier was applied before treatment, a statistically significant difference in PFS of chemosensitive compared to chemorefractory patients (median PFS, 2.8 months for chemorefractory; 5.8 months for chemosensitive; p value = 0.0166) was observed, suggesting a potential clinical utility of the CNA classifier. However, no changes were observed in CNA profiles in CTCs isolated at baseline from patients initially chemosensitive and CTCs isolated upon progressive disease, suggesting that other mechanisms may regulate the acquired resistance to chemotherapy [54].

In another study, single CTCs from 48 SCLC patients captured with the CellSearch were subjected to WES analysis to identify SNVs and indels and to WGS for CNA profile detection [55]. Ten CNA regions were selected for the establishment of a CNA score from CTCs obtained before treatment, as classifier for predicting the outcome of SCLC patients. Patients with a low CNA score (<0) after the first-line chemotherapy had a longer PFS and OS as compared with patients with a higher score ($\geq$0). Multivariate analysis showed that a high CNA score was an independent predictor of poor PFS and OS. Interestingly, the authors found an increase in genomic heterogeneity during disease progression, due to the allelic loss of CNAs in CTCs [55].

2.3. Functional Studies of CTCs in Preclinical Models

Functional analyses using preclinical models may offer complementary information to both genomic analyses and CTC count about the biology of SCLC and the discovery of therapeutic targets. The main requirement for these experiments is the isolation of viable CTCs. Functional studies of CTCs in mouse models are mainly performed using two approaches: the direct injection of CTCs into mice to generate CDX models or the establishment of cultures of CTCs ex-vivo.

Hodgkinson and colleagues was the first to demonstrate that CTCs isolated from SCLC patients are tumorigenic when injected in immunocompromised mice [56]. NGS analysis of CDXs confirmed a genomic profile characteristic of SCLC and showed a patient specific pattern of CNA gains and losses, with the loss of *RB1*, *TP53* and *PTEN*, commonly observed in SCLC. Moreover, the response of CDXs to cisplatin and etoposide was closely correlated with the outcome of the corresponding patients. The comparison of the genomic profiles of single CTCs with the corresponding CDX indicated a high correlation between CDXs and CTCs, despite in one patient heterogeneous CNA profiles between single CTCs being observed [56].

An automated microfluidic apparatus for viable CTC isolation was employed to generate CDXs with an efficiency of tumor growth in nude mice of 38% and a median latency of 112 days [57]. CTC-derived models retained a stable genome and the same alterations during serial passages, demonstrating to recapitulate the donors' tumors. Etoposide sensitivity in these models correlated with the clinical behavior of SCLC patients. Transcriptomic analysis revealed a *MYC* signature that was strongly correlated with etoposide resistance [57].

CDX models from SCLC patients with different sensitivity to chemotherapy have been used to analyze the mechanisms of resistance [58]. RNA-Seq analysis of CDX-derived single cells revealed the presence of neuroendocrine markers (*ASCL1*, *NEUROD1*), of *MYC* family genes and elevated epithelial-to-mesenchymal transition (EMT) scores. A high intratumor heterogeneity was described in chemotherapy-resistant CDXs at baseline, with upregulation of multiple signaling pathways associated with platinum resistance (including MYC, WNT and EMT pathways) within the same tumor. CTCs and CDXs collected at relapse were demonstrated to be more heterogeneous than at the time of diagnosis, suggesting that intratumor heterogeneity might be involved in the resistance to therapy [58].

CDXs from CTCs have the advantages of generating a large number of xenografts from patients for which tissue samples are not available and are able monitor the course of disease in a non-invasive manner. However, this approach has some limitations, such as the long time occurring to generate mouse models, the high cost of the in vivo pharmacology experiments and ethical implications. Ex vivo cultures of CTCs allow the generation of models in a shorter period with reduced costs. Ex vivo cell lines have been established from CTCs isolated in different cancer types, including breast, colon cancer and SCLC [59–61]. CTCs isolated from patients with extended SCLC allowed generation of ex-vivo cultures characterized by the presence of spheroidal morphology and stem cell markers that form tumorospheres with a mesenchymal-epithelial transition (MET) phenotype under culture [62]. Ex vivo cell lines resulted in being more sensitive to epirubicin and showed elevated cytotoxicity in response to the combination of epirubicin and topotecan as compared to SCLC continuous cell lines [63]. When CTC-derived cell lines spontaneously developed tumorospheres, the sensitivity to epirubicin and topotecan was reduced [64].

Finally, a recent study used CDX-derived cells to develop ex vivo short-term cultures [65]. CDX-derived cell lines maintained the same phenotypic and molecular characteristics of the corresponding CDXs. The response of ex vivo cell lines to chemotherapy correlated with the response observed in in vivo experiments. In addition, the authors demonstrated that short-term cultures generated from CDXs are a suitable approach for testing novel targeted agents [65].

3. Open Questions and Future Perspectives

SCLC is a highly aggressive subtype of lung cancer and its management is challenging, due to the rapid course of the disease and to the limited therapeutic options. The lack of tissue samples for preclinical and clinical studies has represented one of the major obstacles for studies about SCLC biology and drug development. Although the potential clinical utility of CTCs as surrogate of tumor tissue for prognostic and predictive information, for monitoring the course of the disease, and studying mechanisms of resistance has been demonstrated in different studies, CTC analysis is not currently employed in the clinical management of SCLC.

Several studies have demonstrated a prognostic role of the number of CTCs and/or the reduction of the absolute number of CTCs from baseline to first or subsequent cycles of chemotherapy [14,15,21,41,43,45]. However, the different technologies used for CTC enumeration, the heterogeneous patient populations included in the studies, a lack of a validated unique cut-off and the variability observed in the reduction of CTCs during the course of treatment, limited the utility of this biomarker in clinical practice. In this regard, the identification of a unique cut-off is a key issue for the development of CTC number as biomarker in SCLC. Indeed, not only have different techniques been employed for CTC analysis but also in the studies using the same technology (i.e., the CellSearch System) different cut-off values have been identified. Several factors may have influenced the identification of the threshold: (i) the low number of patients included in the majority of studies; (ii) the heterogeneity of the series analyzed with particular regard to the stage of the enrolled patients, given that patients with ES-SCLC generally have higher CTC levels than those of LS-SCLC patients; (iii) the different statistical approach used to identify the cut-off, often not justified by a priori hypotheses; (iv) the timing of the sampling which, with the exception of the baseline, was often performed at different times after the therapy. In addition, the majority of the studies in SCLC employed the CellSearch for CTC enrichment and isolation. However, the CellSearch technology is based on EpCAM for enrichment of CTCs and it might miss cells that have undergone an EMT phenotype. The employment of EpCAM-independent technologies might increase the detection rate of CTCs in SCLC. Nevertheless, the CTC count has been included in exploratory analyses in clinical studies evaluating novel targeted agents in SCLC [48–51], confirming the importance of the evaluation of the CTC number as a prognostic biomarker in this disease.

Molecular profiling of single CTCs confirmed the molecular complexity of SCLC characterized by the high tumor mutational burden, the ubiquitary presence of mutations in the *TP53* and *RB1* genes and a high number of CNAs [53–55,66]. Although it has been demonstrated that the CNA profiles of individual CTCs in each patient is homogeneous, some studies evidenced a heterogeneity at a single cell level both before and during the treatment, which might be associated with chemotherapy resistance [54,55]. However, to assess the involvement of intratumor heterogeneity in the evolution of the disease and the response to treatments, the genomic profile of a high number of single CTCs from multiple regions of the tumor or from different tumor sites at different time points should be analyzed. In this regard, the generation of CDXs and ex vivo cultures from CTCs might be of relevant importance in recapitulate tumor heterogeneity [67]. Interestingly, a study suggested that CDXs are more successfully generated from patients with a higher disease burden and a more aggressive disease [68]. Recently, transcriptomic analysis of a biobank of 38 CDXs was performed to analyze the mechanisms involved in tumor heterogeneity, confirming the presence of different molecular subtypes of SCLC [69].

The possibility to perform a molecular characterization of CTCs in combination with CTC count might provide information useful for patient selection in clinical studies. In this regard, patients with a high CTC number or a marginal reduction in the CTC number after the treatment and with a high level of intratumor heterogeneity could be enrolled in clinical trials with experimental agents, whereas patients with a low number of CTCs and with a homogeneous CTC population might be subjected to standard treatment (Figure 2).

A great potential of CTCs is the development of preclinical models for testing novel compounds. Unlike NSCLC, no targeted therapies have been developed in SCLC, due to the lack of actionable alterations in driver genes responsible of tumor development and progression. Different putative therapeutic targets are currently under investigation in SCLC, including DLL3, insulin-like growth factor 1 receptor (IGF1R), poly(ADP-ribose) polymerase (PARP), the DNA damage response (DDR) kinases ATM (ataxia-telangiectasia mutated), ATR (ATM- and Rad3-Related) and the cell cycle checkpoint kinases CHK1, WEE1 and aurora kinase A (AURKA) [70]. A number of compounds directed against these targets are in clinical development. Although preliminary data from clinical trials with agents targeting DLL3 showed modest clinical activity in heavily pre-treated SCLC patients [71], studies with novel agents and in the earlier phase of the disease will clear the relevance of DLL3 as a therapeutic target.

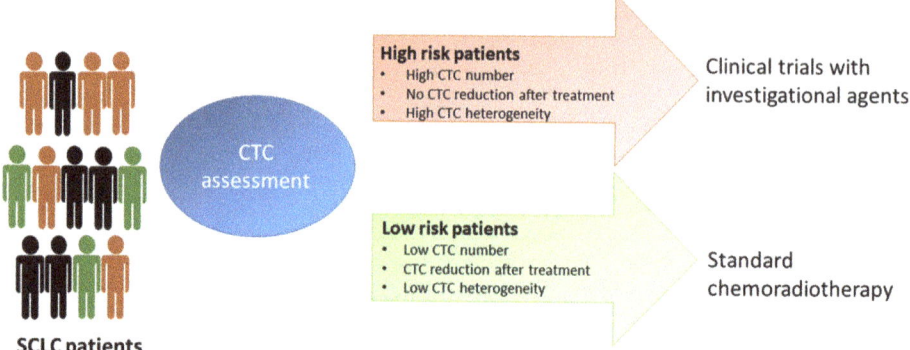

Figure 2. Possible SCLC patients' stratification based on CTC analysis. High risk patients, based on their CTC status, could be enrolled in clinical studies with investigational drugs, whereas low risk patients could receive standard treatments.

An association between the subtypes defined by the differential expression of ASCL1, NeuroD1, YAP1 and POU2F3 and specific targets have been identified [8], suggesting that specific subgroups of patients might benefit from these compounds. Interestingly, a recent study described in a CTC-derived mouse model a subtype switching that may be responsible for acquired resistance to chemotherapy [72].

4. Conclusions

A growing interest has recently emerged in the field of CTC research in SCLC for the potential utility of this biomarker in the clinic. CTC count coupled with genomic profiling might help to stratify patients for the optimal treatment. In addition, the analysis of the molecular profile of CTCs and the generation of CDXs are encouraging deeper knowledge of SCLC biology, with the major finding that SCLC is a very heterogeneous disease. The identification of different molecular subtypes and their vulnerability to unique pharmacological agents might aid in stratifying patients in clinical studies with investigational agents, with the aim to tailor a personalized treatment for each patient.

Author Contributions: Conceptualization, A.D.L. and N.N.; Writing—Original Draft Preparation, A.D.L. and N.N.; Writing—Review & Editing, M.G.; C.E.; A.M.; Supervision, N.N. All authors have read and agreed to the published version of the manuscript.

Funding: This work was in part sustained by funds from the Italian Department of Health to Ricerca Corrente Istituto Nazionale Tumori—IRCCS—Fondazione G. Pascale (Project M2/1) and by the POR Campania FESR 2014/2020.

Conflicts of Interest: N.N. declares the following speakers' bureau: Roche, Boehringer Ingelheim, AstraZeneca, MSD Oncology, BMS, Merck, Qiagen, Thermofisher, Illumina. The other authors declare no conflict of interest. The funders had no role in the writing of the manuscript, or in the decision to publish the results.

References

1. Siegel, R.L.; Miller, K.D.; Jemal, A. Cancer statistics, 2020. *CA Cancer J. Clin.* **2020**, *70*, 7–30. [CrossRef]
2. van Meerbeeck, J.P.; Fennell, D.A.; De Ruysscher, D.K. Small-cell lung cancer. *Lancet* **2011**, *378*, 1741–1755. [CrossRef]
3. Iams, W.T.; Porter, J.; Horn, L. Immunotherapeutic approaches for small-cell lung cancer. *Nat. Rev. Clin. Oncol.* **2020**, *17*, 300–312. [CrossRef] [PubMed]

8. Esposito, G.; Palumbo, G.; Carillio, G.; Manzo, A.; Montanino, A.; Sforza, V.; Costanzo, R.; Sandomenico, C.; La Manna, C.; Martucci, N.; et al. Immunotherapy in Small Cell Lung Cancer. *Cancers* **2020**, *12*, 2522. [CrossRef]
9. Alexandrov, L.B.; Nik-Zainal, S.; Wedge, D.C.; Aparicio, S.A.; Behjati, S.; Biankin, A.V.; Bignell, G.R.; Bolli, N.; Borg, A.; Borresen-Dale, A.L.; et al. Signatures of mutational processes in human cancer. *Nature* **2013**, *500*, 415–421. [CrossRef] [PubMed]
10. George, J.; Lim, J.S.; Jang, S.J.; Cun, Y.; Ozretic, L.; Kong, G.; Leenders, F.; Lu, X.; Fernandez-Cuesta, L.; Bosco, G.; et al. Comprehensive genomic profiles of small cell lung cancer. *Nature* **2015**, *524*, 47–53. [CrossRef]
11. Rudin, C.M.; Durinck, S.; Stawiski, E.W.; Poirier, J.T.; Modrusan, Z.; Shames, D.S.; Bergbower, E.A.; Guan, Y.; Shin, J.; Guillory, J.; et al. Comprehensive genomic analysis identifies SOX2 as a frequently amplified gene in small-cell lung cancer. *Nat. Genet.* **2012**, *44*, 1111–1116. [CrossRef] [PubMed]
12. Rudin, C.M.; Poirier, J.T.; Byers, L.A.; Dive, C.; Dowlati, A.; George, J.; Heymach, J.V.; Johnson, J.E.; Lehman, J.M.; MacPherson, D.; et al. Molecular subtypes of small cell lung cancer: A synthesis of human and mouse model data. *Nat. Rev. Cancer* **2019**, *19*, 289–297. [CrossRef]
13. Normanno, N.; De Luca, A.; Gallo, M.; Chicchinelli, N.; Rossi, A. The prognostic role of circulating tumor cells in lung cancer. *Expert Rev. Anticancer Ther.* **2016**, *16*, 859–867. [CrossRef]
14. Alix-Panabieres, C.; Pantel, K. Clinical Applications of Circulating Tumor Cells and Circulating Tumor DNA as Liquid Biopsy. *Cancer Discov.* **2016**, *6*, 479–491. [CrossRef]
15. Tanaka, F.; Yoneda, K.; Kondo, N.; Hashimoto, M.; Takuwa, T.; Matsumoto, S.; Okumura, Y.; Rahman, S.; Tsubota, N.; Tsujimura, T.; et al. Circulating tumor cell as a diagnostic marker in primary lung cancer. *Clin. Cancer Res* **2009**, *15*, 6980–6986. [CrossRef]
16. Allard, W.J.; Matera, J.; Miller, M.C.; Repollet, M.; Connelly, M.C.; Rao, C.; Tibbe, A.G.; Uhr, J.W.; Terstappen, L.W. Tumor cells circulate in the peripheral blood of all major carcinomas but not in healthy subjects or patients with nonmalignant diseases. *Clin Cancer Res.* **2004**, *10*, 6897–6904. [CrossRef] [PubMed]
17. Hou, J.M.; Greystoke, A.; Lancashire, L.; Cummings, J.; Ward, T.; Board, R.; Amir, E.; Hughes, S.; Krebs, M.; Hughes, A.; et al. Evaluation of circulating tumor cells and serological cell death biomarkers in small cell lung cancer patients undergoing chemotherapy. *Am. J. Pathol.* **2009**, *175*, 808–816. [CrossRef]
18. Naito, T.; Tanaka, F.; Ono, A.; Yoneda, K.; Takahashi, T.; Murakami, H.; Nakamura, Y.; Tsuya, A.; Kenmotsu, H.; Shukuya, T.; et al. Prognostic impact of circulating tumor cells in patients with small cell lung cancer. *J. Thorac. Oncol.* **2012**, *7*, 512–519. [CrossRef] [PubMed]
19. Hiltermann, T.J.N.; Pore, M.M.; van den Berg, A.; Timens, W.; Boezen, H.M.; Liesker, J.J.W.; Schouwink, J.H.; Wijnands, W.J.A.; Kerner, G.; Kruyt, F.A.E.; et al. Circulating tumor cells in small-cell lung cancer: A predictive and prognostic factor. *Ann. Oncol.* **2012**, *23*, 2937–2942. [CrossRef]
20. Gallo, M.; De Luca, A.; Frezzetti, D.; Passaro, V.; Maiello, M.R.; Normanno, N. The potential of monitoring treatment response in non-small cell lung cancer using circulating tumour cells. *Expert Rev. Mol. Diagn.* **2019**, *19*, 683–694. [CrossRef]
21. Brezicka, T. Expression of epithelial-cell adhesion molecule (Ep-CAM) in small cell lung cancer as defined by monoclonal antibodies 17-1A and BerEP4. *Acta Oncol.* **2005**, *44*, 723–727. [CrossRef] [PubMed]
22. Kularatne, B.Y.; Lorigan, P.; Browne, S.; Suvarna, S.K.; Smith, M.O.; Lawry, J. Monitoring tumour cells in the peripheral blood of small cell lung cancer patients. *Cytometry* **2002**, *50*, 160–167. [CrossRef]
23. Bevilacqua, S.; Gallo, M.; Franco, R.; Rossi, A.; De Luca, A.; Rocco, G.; Botti, G.; Gridelli, C.; Normanno, N. A "live" biopsy in a small-cell lung cancer patient by detection of circulating tumor cells. *Lung Cancer* **2009**, *65*, 123–125. [CrossRef]
24. Messaritakis, I.; Politaki, E.; Kotsakis, A.; Dermitzaki, E.K.; Koinis, F.; Lagoudaki, E.; Koutsopoulos, A.; Kallergi, G.; Souglakos, J.; Georgoulias, V. Phenotypic characterization of circulating tumor cells in the peripheral blood of patients with small cell lung cancer. *PLoS ONE* **2017**, *12*, e0181211. [CrossRef] [PubMed]
25. Aggarwal, C.; Wang, X.; Ranganathan, A.; Torigian, D.; Troxel, A.; Evans, T.; Cohen, R.B.; Vaidya, B.; Rao, C.; Connelly, M.; et al. Circulating tumor cells as a predictive biomarker in patients with small cell lung cancer undergoing chemotherapy. *Lung Cancer* **2017**, *112*, 118–125. [CrossRef] [PubMed]
26. Alix-Panabieres, C.; Pantel, K. Challenges in circulating tumour cell research. *Nat Rev Cancer* **2014**, *14*, 623–631. [CrossRef]
27. Gorges, T.M.; Penkalla, N.; Schalk, T.; Joosse, S.A.; Riethdorf, S.; Tucholski, J.; Lucke, K.; Wikman, H.; Jackson, S.; Brychta, N.; et al. Enumeration and Molecular Characterization of Tumor Cells in Lung Cancer Patients Using a Novel in Vivo Device for Capturing Circulating Tumor Cells. *Clin. Cancer Res.* **2016**, *22*, 2197–2206. [CrossRef]
28. Drucker, A.; Teh, E.M.; Kostyleva, R.; Rayson, D.; Douglas, S.; Pinto, D.M. Comparative performance of different methods for circulating tumor cell enrichment in metastatic breast cancer patients. *PLoS ONE* **2020**, *15*, e0237308. [CrossRef]
29. Xu, Y.; Liu, B.; Ding, F.; Zhou, X.; Tu, P.; Yu, B.; He, Y.; Huang, P. Circulating tumor cell detection: A direct comparison between negative and unbiased enrichment in lung cancer. *Oncol. Lett.* **2017**, *13*, 4882–4886. [CrossRef]
30. Vona, G.; Sabile, A.; Louha, M.; Sitruk, V.; Romana, S.; Schutze, K.; Capron, F.; Franco, D.; Pazzagli, M.; Vekemans, M.; et al. Isolation by size of epithelial tumor cells: A new method for the immunomorphological and molecular characterization of circulating tumor cells. *Am. J. Pathol.* **2000**, *156*, 57–63. [CrossRef]
31. Kallergi, G.; Politaki, E.; Alkahtani, S.; Stournaras, C.; Georgoulias, V. Evaluation of Isolation Methods for Circulating Tumor Cells (CTCs). *Cell Physiol. Biochem.* **2016**, *40*, 411–419. [CrossRef] [PubMed]
32. Lee, Y.; Guan, G.; Bhagat, A.A. ClearCell(R) FX, a label-free microfluidics technology for enrichment of viable circulating tumor cells. *Cytom. A* **2018**, *93*, 1251–1254. [CrossRef] [PubMed]

29. Hou, H.W.; Warkiani, M.E.; Khoo, B.L.; Li, Z.R.; Soo, R.A.; Tan, D.S.; Lim, W.T.; Han, J.; Bhagat, A.A.; Lim, C.T. Isolation and retrieval of circulating tumor cells using centrifugal forces. *Sci. Rep.* **2013**, *3*, 1259. [CrossRef] [PubMed]
30. Karabacak, N.M.; Spuhler, P.S.; Fachin, F.; Lim, E.J.; Pai, V.; Ozkumur, E.; Martel, J.M.; Kojic, N.; Smith, K.; Chen, P.I.; et al. Microfluidic, marker-free isolation of circulating tumor cells from blood samples. *Nat. Protoc.* **2014**, *9*, 694–710. [CrossRef]
31. Ozkumur, E.; Shah, A.M.; Ciciliano, J.C.; Emmink, B.L.; Miyamoto, D.T.; Brachtel, E.; Yu, M.; Chen, P.I.; Morgan, B.; Trautwein, J.; et al. Inertial focusing for tumor antigen-dependent and -independent sorting of rare circulating tumor cells. *Sci. Transl. Med.* **2013**, *5*, 179ra147. [CrossRef]
32. Chudziak, J.; Burt, D.J.; Mohan, S.; Rothwell, D.G.; Mesquita, B.; Antonello, J.; Dalby, S.; Ayub, M.; Priest, L.; Carter, L.; et al. Clinical evaluation of a novel microfluidic device for epitope-independent enrichment of circulating tumour cells in patients with small cell lung cancer. *Analyst* **2016**, *141*, 669–678. [CrossRef]
33. Sollier-Christen, E.; Renier, C.; Kaplan, T.; Kfir, E.; Crouse, S.C. VTX-1 Liquid Biopsy System for Fully-Automated and Label-Free Isolation of Circulating Tumor Cells with Automated Enumeration by BioView Platform. *Cytom. A* **2018**, *93*, 1240–1245. [CrossRef]
34. Lemaire, C.A.; Liu, S.Z.; Wilkerson, C.L.; Ramani, V.C.; Barzanian, N.A.; Huang, K.W.; Che, J.; Chiu, M.W.; Vuppalapaty, M.; Dimmick, A.M.; et al. Fast and Label-Free Isolation of Circulating Tumor Cells from Blood: From a Research Microfluidic Platform to an Automated Fluidic Instrument, VTX-1 Liquid Biopsy System. *SLAS Technol.* **2018**, *23*, 16–29. [CrossRef]
35. Di Trapani, M.; Manaresi, N.; Medoro, G. DEPArray system: An automatic image-based sorter for isolation of pure circulating tumor cells. *Cytom. A* **2018**, *93*, 1260–1266. [CrossRef] [PubMed]
36. Kojima, T.; Hashimoto, Y.; Watanabe, Y.; Kagawa, S.; Uno, F.; Kuroda, S.; Tazawa, H.; Kyo, S.; Mizuguchi, H.; Urata, Y.; et al. A simple biological imaging system for detecting viable human circulating tumor cells. *J. Clin. Investig.* **2009**, *119*, 3172–3181. [CrossRef] [PubMed]
37. Sakurai, F.; Narii, N.; Tomita, K.; Togo, S.; Takahashi, K.; Machitani, M.; Tachibana, M.; Ouchi, M.; Katagiri, N.; Urata, Y.; et al. Efficient detection of human circulating tumor cells without significant production of false-positive cells by a novel conditionally replicating adenovirus. *Mol. Ther. Methods Clin. Dev.* **2016**, *3*, 16001. [CrossRef] [PubMed]
38. Foy, V.; Fernandez-Gutierrez, F.; Faivre-Finn, C.; Dive, C.; Blackhall, F. The clinical utility of circulating tumour cells in patients with small cell lung cancer. *Transl. Lung Cancer Res.* **2017**, *6*, 409–417. [CrossRef]
39. Igawa, S.; Gohda, K.; Fukui, T.; Ryuge, S.; Otani, S.; Masago, A.; Sato, J.; Murakami, K.; Maki, S.; Katono, K.; et al. Circulating tumor cells as a prognostic factor in patients with small cell lung cancer. *Oncol. Lett.* **2014**, *7*, 1469–1473. [CrossRef]
40. Wang, Y.L.; Liu, C.H.; Li, J.; Ma, X.P.; Gong, P. Clinical significance of circulating tumor cells in patients with small-cell lung cancer. *Tumori* **2017**, *103*, 242–248. [CrossRef]
41. Hou, J.M.; Krebs, M.G.; Lancashire, L.; Sloane, R.; Backen, A.; Swain, R.K.; Priest, L.J.; Greystoke, A.; Zhou, C.; Morris, K.; et al. Clinical significance and molecular characteristics of circulating tumor cells and circulating tumor microemboli in patients with small-cell lung cancer. *J. Clin. Oncol.* **2012**, *30*, 525–532. [CrossRef] [PubMed]
42. Cheng, Y.; Liu, X.Q.; Fan, Y.; Liu, Y.P.; Liu, Y.; Liu, Y.; Ma, L.X.; Liu, X.H.; Li, H.; Bao, H.Z.; et al. Circulating tumor cell counts/change for outcome prediction in patients with extensive-stage small-cell lung cancer. *Future Oncol.* **2016**, *12*, 789–799. [CrossRef] [PubMed]
43. Normanno, N.; Rossi, A.; Morabito, A.; Signoriello, S.; Bevilacqua, S.; Di Maio, M.; Costanzo, R.; De Luca, A.; Montanino, A.; Gridelli, C.; et al. Prognostic value of circulating tumor cells' reduction in patients with extensive small-cell lung cancer. *Lung Cancer* **2014**, *85*, 314–319. [CrossRef]
44. Huang, C.H.; Wick, J.A.; Sittampalam, G.S.; Nirmalanandhan, V.S.; Ganti, A.K.; Neupane, P.C.; Williamson, S.K.; Godwin, A.K.; Schmitt, S.; Smart, N.J.; et al. A multicenter pilot study examining the role of circulating tumor cells as a blood-based tumor marker in patients with extensive small-cell lung cancer. *Front. Oncol.* **2014**, *4*, 271. [CrossRef] [PubMed]
45. Tay, R.Y.; Fernandez-Gutierrez, F.; Foy, V.; Burns, K.; Pierce, J.; Morris, K.; Priest, L.; Tugwood, J.; Ashcroft, L.; Lindsay, C.R.; et al. Prognostic value of circulating tumour cells in limited-stage small-cell lung cancer: Analysis of the concurrent once-daily versus twice-daily radiotherapy (CONVERT) randomised controlled trial. *Ann. Oncol.* **2019**, *30*, 1114–1120. [CrossRef]
46. Sabari, J.K.; Lok, B.H.; Laird, J.H.; Poirier, J.T.; Rudin, C.M. Unravelling the biology of SCLC: Implications for therapy. *Nat. Rev. Clin. Oncol.* **2017**, *14*, 549–561. [CrossRef]
47. Zhang, J.; Wang, H.T.; Li, B.G. Prognostic significance of circulating tumor cells in small-cell lung cancer patients: A meta-analysis. *Asian Pac. J. Cancer Prev.* **2014**, *15*, 8429–8433. [CrossRef]
48. Messaritakis, I.; Politaki, E.; Plataki, M.; Karavassilis, V.; Kentepozidis, N.; Koinis, F.; Samantas, E.; Georgoulias, V.; Kotsakis, A. Heterogeneity of circulating tumor cells (CTCs) in patients with recurrent small cell lung cancer (SCLC) treated with pazopanib. *Lung Cancer* **2017**, *104*, 16–23. [CrossRef]
49. Salgia, R.; Weaver, R.W.; McCleod, M.; Stille, J.R.; Yan, S.B.; Roberson, S.; Polzer, J.; Flynt, A.; Raddad, E.; Peek, V.L.; et al. Prognostic and predictive value of circulating tumor cells and CXCR4 expression as biomarkers for a CXCR4 peptide antagonist in combination with carboplatin-etoposide in small cell lung cancer: Exploratory analysis of a phase II study. *Investig. New Drugs* **2017**, *35*, 334–344. [CrossRef]
50. Belani, C.P.; Dahlberg, S.E.; Rudin, C.M.; Fleisher, M.; Chen, H.X.; Takebe, N.; Velasco, M.R., Jr.; Tester, W.J.; Sturtz, K.; Hann, C.L.; et al. Vismodegib or cixutumumab in combination with standard chemotherapy for patients with extensive-stage small cell lung cancer: A trial of the ECOG-ACRIN Cancer Research Group (E1508). *Cancer* **2016**, *122*, 2371–2378. [CrossRef]

1. Pietanza, M.C.; Litvak, A.M.; Varghese, A.M.; Krug, L.M.; Fleisher, M.; Teitcher, J.B.; Holodny, A.I.; Sima, C.S.; Woo, K.M.; Ng, K.K.; et al. A phase I trial of the Hedgehog inhibitor, sonidegib (LDE225), in combination with etoposide and cisplatin for the initial treatment of extensive stage small cell lung cancer. *Lung Cancer* **2016**, *99*, 23–30. [CrossRef]
2. Obermayr, E.; Agreiter, C.; Schuster, E.; Fabikan, H.; Weinlinger, C.; Baluchova, K.; Hamilton, G.; Hochmair, M.; Zeillinger, R. Molecular Characterization of Circulating Tumor Cells Enriched by A Microfluidic Platform in Patients with Small-Cell Lung Cancer. *Cells* **2019**, *8*, 880. [CrossRef] [PubMed]
3. Ni, X.; Zhuo, M.; Su, Z.; Duan, J.; Gao, Y.; Wang, Z.; Zong, C.; Bai, H.; Chapman, A.R.; Zhao, J.; et al. Reproducible copy number variation patterns among single circulating tumor cells of lung cancer patients. *Proc. Natl. Acad. Sci. USA* **2013**, *110*, 21083–21088. [CrossRef] [PubMed]
4. Carter, L.; Rothwell, D.G.; Mesquita, B.; Smowton, C.; Leong, H.S.; Fernandez-Gutierrez, F.; Li, Y.; Burt, D.J.; Antonello, J.; Morrow, C.J.; et al. Molecular analysis of circulating tumor cells identifies distinct copy-number profiles in patients with chemosensitive and chemorefractory small-cell lung cancer. *Nat. Med.* **2017**, *23*, 114–119. [CrossRef]
5. Su, Z.; Wang, Z.; Ni, X.; Duan, J.; Gao, Y.; Zhuo, M.; Li, R.; Zhao, J.; Ma, Q.; Bai, H.; et al. Inferring the Evolution and Progression of Small-Cell Lung Cancer by Single-Cell Sequencing of Circulating Tumor Cells. *Clin. Cancer Res.* **2019**, *25*, 5049–5060. [CrossRef] [PubMed]
6. Hodgkinson, C.L.; Morrow, C.J.; Li, Y.; Metcalf, R.L.; Rothwell, D.G.; Trapani, F.; Polanski, R.; Burt, D.J.; Simpson, K.L.; Morris, K.; et al. Tumorigenicity and genetic profiling of circulating tumor cells in small-cell lung cancer. *Nat. Med.* **2014**, *20*, 897–903. [CrossRef]
7. Drapkin, B.J.; George, J.; Christensen, C.L.; Mino-Kenudson, M.; Dries, R.; Sundaresan, T.; Phat, S.; Myers, D.T.; Zhong, J.; Igo, P.; et al. Genomic and Functional Fidelity of Small Cell Lung Cancer Patient-Derived Xenografts. *Cancer Discov.* **2018**, *8*, 600–615. [CrossRef]
8. Stewart, C.A.; Gay, C.M.; Xi, Y.; Sivajothi, S.; Sivakamasundari, V.; Fujimoto, J.; Bolisetty, M.; Hartsfield, P.M.; Balasubramaniyan, V.; Chalishazar, M.D.; et al. Single-cell analyses reveal increased intratumoral heterogeneity after the onset of therapy resistance in small-cell lung cancer. *Nat. Cancer* **2020**, *1*, 423–436. [CrossRef]
9. Yu, M.; Bardia, A.; Aceto, N.; Bersani, F.; Madden, M.W.; Donaldson, M.C.; Desai, R.; Zhu, H.; Comaills, V.; Zheng, Z.; et al. Cancer therapy. Ex vivo culture of circulating breast tumor cells for individualized testing of drug susceptibility. *Science* **2014**, *345*, 216–220. [CrossRef]
10. Cayrefourcq, L.; Mazard, T.; Joosse, S.; Solassol, J.; Ramos, J.; Assenat, E.; Schumacher, U.; Costes, V.; Maudelonde, T.; Pantel, K.; et al. Establishment and characterization of a cell line from human circulating colon cancer cells. *Cancer Res.* **2015**, *75*, 892–901. [CrossRef] [PubMed]
11. Hamilton, G.; Burghuber, O.; Zeillinger, R. Circulating tumor cells in small cell lung cancer: Ex vivo expansion. *Lung* **2015**, *193*, 451–452. [CrossRef]
12. Hamilton, G.; Hochmair, M.; Rath, B.; Klameth, L.; Zeillinger, R. Small cell lung cancer: Circulating tumor cells of extended stage patients express a mesenchymal-epithelial transition phenotype. *Cell Adh. Migr.* **2016**, *10*, 360–367. [CrossRef]
13. Hamilton, G.; Rath, B.; Holzer, S.; Hochmair, M. Second-line therapy for small cell lung cancer: Exploring the potential role of circulating tumor cells. *Transl. Lung Cancer Res.* **2016**, *5*, 71–77. [CrossRef]
14. Klameth, L.; Rath, B.; Hochmaier, M.; Moser, D.; Redl, M.; Mungenast, F.; Gelles, K.; Ulsperger, E.; Zeillinger, R.; Hamilton, G. Small cell lung cancer: Model of circulating tumor cell tumorospheres in chemoresistance. *Sci. Rep.* **2017**, *7*, 5337. [CrossRef]
15. Lallo, A.; Gulati, S.; Schenk, M.W.; Khandelwal, G.; Berglund, U.W.; Pateras, I.S.; Chester, C.P.E.; Pham, T.M.; Kalderen, C.; Frese, K.K.; et al. Ex vivo culture of cells derived from circulating tumour cell xenograft to support small cell lung cancer research and experimental therapeutics. *Br. J. Pharmacol.* **2019**, *176*, 436–450. [CrossRef] [PubMed]
16. Williamson, S.C.; Metcalf, R.L.; Trapani, F.; Mohan, S.; Antonello, J.; Abbott, B.; Leong, H.S.; Chester, C.P.; Simms, N.; Polanski, R.; et al. Vasculogenic mimicry in small cell lung cancer. *Nat. Commun.* **2016**, *7*, 13322. [CrossRef]
17. Shue, Y.T.; Lim, J.S.; Sage, J. Tumor heterogeneity in small cell lung cancer defined and investigated in pre-clinical mouse models. *Transl. Lung Cancer Res.* **2018**, *7*, 21–31. [CrossRef] [PubMed]
18. Vickers, A.J.; Frese, K.; Galvin, M.; Carter, M.; Franklin, L.; Morris, K.; Pierce, J.; Descamps, T.; Blackhall, F.; Dive, C.; et al. Brief report on the clinical characteristics of patients whose samples generate small cell lung cancer circulating tumour cell derived explants. *Lung Cancer* **2020**, *150*, 216–220. [CrossRef] [PubMed]
19. Simpson, K.L.; Stoney, R.; Frese, K.K.; Simms, N.; Rowe, W.; Pearce, S.P.; Humphrey, S.; Booth, L.; Morgan, D.; Dynowski, M.; et al. A biobank of small cell lung cancer CDX models elucidates inter- and intratumoral phenotypic heterogeneity. *Nat. Cancer* **2020**, *1*, 437–451. [CrossRef]
20. Taniguchi, H.; Sen, T.; Rudin, C.M. Targeted Therapies and Biomarkers in Small Cell Lung Cancer. *Front. Oncol.* **2020**, *10*, 741. [CrossRef] [PubMed]

71. Morgensztern, D.; Besse, B.; Greillier, L.; Santana-Davila, R.; Ready, N.; Hann, C.L.; Glisson, B.S.; Farago, A.F.; Dowlati, A.; Rudin, C.M.; et al. Efficacy and Safety of Rovalpituzumab Tesirine in Third-Line and Beyond Patients with DLL3-Expressing, Relapsed/Refractory Small-Cell Lung Cancer: Results from the Phase II TRINITY Study. *Clin. Cancer Res.* **2019**, *25*, 6958–6966. [CrossRef] [PubMed]
72. Gay, C.M.; Stewart, C.A.; Park, E.M.; Diao, L.; Groves, S.M.; Heeke, S.; Nabet, B.Y.; Fujimoto, J.; Solis, L.M.; Lu, W.; et al. Patterns of transcription factor programs and immune pathway activation define four major subtypes of SCLC with distinct therapeutic vulnerabilities. *Cancer Cell* **2021**, *39*, 346–360. [CrossRef] [PubMed]

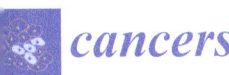

Review

Small Cell Lung Cancer: State of the Art of the Molecular and Genetic Landscape and Novel Perspective

Valeria Denninghoff [1], Alessandro Russo [2,3], Diego de Miguel-Pérez [2], Umberto Malapelle [4], Amin Benyounes [5], Allison Gittens [2], Andres Felipe Cardona [6,7,8] and Christian Rolfo [2,*]

1. National Council for Scientific and Technical Research (CONICET), University of Buenos Aires, Buenos Aires C1122AAH, Argentina; vdenninghoff@conicet.gov.ar
2. Marlene and Stewart Greenebaum Comprehensive Cancer Center, University of Maryland School of Medicine, Baltimore, MD 21201, USA; alessandro-russo@alice.it (A.R.); ddemiguelperez@som.umaryland.edu (D.d.M.-P.); agittens@umm.edu (A.G.)
3. Medical Oncology Unit, A.O. Papardo, 98158 Messina, Italy
4. Department of Public Health, University of Naples Federico II, 80138 Naples, Italy; umberto.malapelle@unina.it
5. Thoracic Oncology, Inova Schar Cancer Center, Fairfax, VA 22031, USA; Amin.Benyounes@inova.org
6. Clinical and Translational Oncology Group, Clínica del Country, Bogotá 110221, Colombia; andres.cardona@clinicadelcountry.com
7. Foundation for Clinical and Applied Cancer Research (FICMAC), Bogotá 110111, Colombia
8. Molecular Oncology and Biology Systems Research Group (Fox-G/ONCOLGroup), Universidad el Bosque, Bogotá 110121, Colombia
* Correspondence: c.rolfo@som.umaryland.edu; Tel.: +1-(410)-328-7224

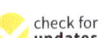

Simple Summary: Small cell lung cancer (SCLC) continues to carry a poor prognosis with a five-year survival rate of 3.5% and a 10-year survival rate of 1.8%. The pathogenesis remains unclear, and there are no known predictive or diagnostic biomarkers. The current SCLC classification as a single entity hinders effective targeted therapies against this heterogeneous neoplasm. Despite dedicated decades of research and clinical trials, there has been no change in the SCLC treatment paradigm. This review summarizes the body of literature available on SCLC's genomic landscape to describe SCLC's molecular/genetic aspects, regardless of therapeutic strategy.

Abstract: Small cell lung cancer (SCLC) is a highly proliferative lung cancer that is not amenable to surgery in most cases due to the high metastatic potential. Precision medicine has not yet improved patients' survival due to the lack of actionable mutations. Intra- and intertumoral heterogeneity allow the neoplasms to adapt to various microenvironments and treatments. Further studying this heterogeneous cancer might yield the discovery of actionable mutations. First-line SCLC treatment has added immunotherapy to its armamentarium. There has been renewed interest in SCLC, and numerous clinical trials are underway with novel therapeutic approaches. Understanding the molecular and genetic landscape of this heterogeneous and lethal disease will pave the way for novel drug development.

Keywords: small cell lung cancer; gene pathway; pathobiology; targeted therapy

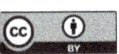

1. Small Cell Lung Cancer (SCLC) General Considerations

SCLC is a highly proliferative lung cancer that is not amenable to surgery in most cases due to the high metastatic potential. It is considered a high-grade neuroendocrine carcinoma with characterizing molecular alterations [1]. SCLC's estimated five-year survival rate is 3.5%, and the 10-year survival rate is 1.8% [2]. Smoking history is present in 95% of the cases, and therefore carcinogenesis is linked to tobacco and its substrates, possibly through a DNA damage mechanism; however, the exact mechanism is unknown.

The genes that affect oncogenes or tumor suppressor genes are usually acquired, not inherited. Tumor protein p53 (*TP53*) and retinoblastoma 1 (*RB1*) are the most common tumor suppressor genes (98% and 91%, respectively) [3]. These tumors are highly proliferative, as demonstrated by Ki67 immunohistochemistry [1,4–7]. SCLC is the deadliest lung cancer subtype and is uniformly fatal [8]. Lack of early detection and poor response to standard treatment are the main contributing factors to a poor outcome. SCLC usually responds to frontline therapy (60%–80% response rates); however, within 6–12 months, it becomes refractory to salvage treatments. Therefore, an understanding of resistance mechanisms is urgently needed. There has been renewed interest in SCLC, and numerous clinical trials are underway with novel therapeutic approaches. Understanding the molecular and genetic landscape of this heterogeneous and lethal disease will pave the way for novel drug development.

2. Molecular Pathways Involved in SCLC Development and Progression

Three pivotal comprehensive genomic analyses of SCLC shed light on SCLC development's principle molecular pathways [9–11]. The limitation of these analyses is the small number of samples, most likely due to the lack of clinical specimens, as this disease is not usually treated with surgery. Therefore, experimental models and/or cell lines are fundamental for genomic analysis and sensitivity to treatments. Although *TP53* and *RB1* are the most common mutations found in SCLC, these alterations cannot yet be targeted pharmacologically. Peifer et al. sequenced 29 SCLC exomes, two tumor genomes, and 15 tumor transcriptomes. They observed a high mutation rate of 7.4 ± 1 protein-changing mutations per million base pairs; loss of TP53 and RB1; mutations and amplifications of *MYCL1*, *MYCN*, and *MYC*; mutations in the histone-modifying genes CREBBP, EP300, and MLL; mutations in *PTEN*, *SLIT2*, and *EPHA7*; focal amplification in *FGFR1* tyrosine kinase gene [9]. George et al. conducted whole-genome sequencing of 110 first frozen tumor samples from patients with limited and extensive-stage small cell lung cancer and their matched normal DNA [11]. They observed an elevated mutation rate of 8.62 non-synonymous mutations per million base pairs (Mb). C: G->A: T transversions were seen in 28% of all mutations and were linked to heavy smoking. The signaling pathways affected in SCLC and frequently aberrant genes in SCLC are shown in Figure 1.

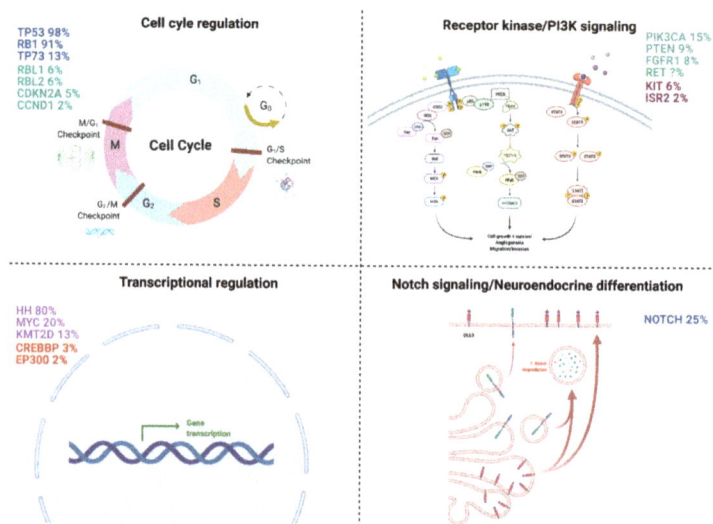

Figure 1. Signaling pathways recurrent affected in small cell lung cancer (SCLC) and frequently aberrant genes (created with BioRender.com, accessed on 28 March 2021).

SCLC neoplastic cells represent a broad molecular landscape. Thus, our current analysis techniques will detect the most frequent aberration within a given tumor sample. Intra- and intertumoral heterogeneity allow the neoplasms to adapt to various microenvironments and treatments. Further studying this heterogeneous cancer might yield the discovery of actionable mutations. Rubin et al. conducted a genetic study using RNA expression in mouse-derived SCLC cell lines and proposed a new classification. This classification identifies four main subdivisions based on the level of expression of *ASCL1* (achaete-scute homolog 1), classified as SCLC-A; *NEUROD1* (neurogenic differentiation factor one), classified as SCLC-N; *POU2F3* (pou class 2 homeobox 3), classified as SCLC-P; *YAP1* (yes-associated protein 1), classified as SCLC-Y. The expression of these four distinct genes has been established in both human ($n = 81$) and cell line tumor models ($n = 54$) [12]. The question is whether these molecular subtypes have different biologies and outcomes. Baine et al. studied protein expression by immunohistochemistry of these four molecular subtypes in a cohort of SCLC clinical specimens ($n = 174$). They also performed standard diagnostic stains, including neuroendocrine stains (SYP (synaptophysin), CgA (chromogranin A), CD56 (neural cell adhesion molecule 1), INSM1 (insulinoma-associated protein 1), TTF-1 (thyroid transcription factor 1), and DLL3 (delta-like ligand 3)) [13]. Based on the above results, the tumors were grouped into the following: ASCL1-dominant; NEUROD1-dominant; ASCL1/NEUROD1 double-negative with POU2F3 expression (POU2F3); ASCL1/NEUROD1 double-negative not otherwise specified (NOS) [13]. POU2F3 expression and the co-expression ASCL1/NEUROD1 were mutually exclusive. YAP1 was expressed in various subtypes and correlated with disease stage and survival. The authors suggested that YAP1 could be related to a transition phenotype between NSCLC and SCLC [13] and could induce multidrug resistance both in vivo and in vitro [14]. The SLCL-Y subtype seems to represent a well-differentiated tumor, with a marked inflamed microenvironment, rendering it perhaps more sensitive to immune checkpoint inhibitors [15]. DLL3 is absent in ASCL1/NEUROD1-negative tumors. This finding could be accounted for by the different techniques used across studies, protein vs. RNA analysis. These findings highlight the heterogeneity of SCLC. Identification of unique subtypes will allow the deployment of target treatments that will ultimately improve patient outcomes. Next, we review the genes and genomics/proteomic modifications related to the development, plasticity, and progression of SCLC, which could be identified as possible biomarkers for targeted therapy of this deadly disease.

2.1. Cell Cycle Regulation
2.1.1. TP53/RB1 (98%/91%)

Biallelic loss of *TP53* and *RB1* has been found in 100% and 93% of cases, respectively, in extensive genomic studies. Other simultaneously occurring molecular alterations have been seen, such as mutations, translocations, loss of heterozygosity. However, biallelic loss of *TP53* and *RB1* remains an essential hallmark of SCLC carcinogenesis [11]. *TP53* mutations are missense mutations that are involved the DNA-binding domain. RB1 is affected by translocations and results in mutations in the exon–intron junctions, which leads to splicing events and subsequently damages proteins, as confirmed by transcriptome sequencing. *TP53* is located in 17p13.1 and has 12 exons. *TP53* encodes a tumor suppressor protein and can bind DNA and activate transcription. It plays a vital role in cell cycle arrest, apoptosis, and DNA repair. It is subject to alternative promoters, which results in multiple transcription variations. Many human cancers carry this mutated gene (Gene ID: 5925, updated on 7 February 2021) [16]. The mutations of *TP53* are numerous, but the clinically relevant substitutions in SCLC include Y220C, R248W, R249M, M237I, and R273L. *RB1* acts as a transcriptional corepressor, is located in 13q14.2, has 28 exons, negatively regulates the cell cycle, and stabilizes the chromatin structure. When activated, it binds to the transcription factor E2F1 (Gene ID: 5925, updated on 7 February 2021) [16,17]. Inactivation of RB1 can occur through different mechanisms: Point mutations, deletion, exon inversions, splice site mutations, and loss of mRNA expression [18]. Although neuroendocrine differentiation is a hallmark of SCLC, specific subtypes lack neuroendocrine differentiation. This might be relevant, as this subtype could be susceptible to CDK4/6 inhibitors and resistant to DLL3-targeted agents [18]. Neither *TP53* nor *RB1* are therapeutically targetable.

2.1.2. TP73 (13%)

TP73 (tumor protein p73) is located in 1p36.32 and has 16 exons. This gene encodes a member of the p53 family of transcription factors involved in cellular responses to stress and development. Many transcript variants resulting from alternative splicing and/or use of alternate promoters have been found for this gene. Still, the biological validity and the full-length nature of some variants have not been determined (Gene ID: 7161, updated on 22 March 2021) [16]. *TP73* is frequently altered in the SCLC genome (13%) [3,11,19]. The *TP73* alterations include gene rearrangements that result in NH-terminal truncation (p73Δex2 and p73Δex2/3) or COOH-terminal deletion (p73Δex10).

2.2. Receptor Kinase/PI3K Signaling

2.2.1. PI3K3CA (15%)

The PI3K/AKT/mTOR pathway regulates cell cycle, proliferation, and survival. When activated, PIK3CA protein phosphorylates AKT, which leads to mTOR activation downstream and other factors such as CREB and PtdIns3P. In several solid tumors, the upregulation of the PI3K/AKT/mTOR pathway promotes carcinogenesis. Shibata et al. performed an extensive mutation screening of the *PIK3CA* gene and only found 3/13 (23%) mutations in SCLC cell lines and 2/15 (13%) mutations in samples of primary SCLC [20]. *PIK3CA* (phosphatidylinositol-4,5-bisphosphate 3-kinase catalytic subunit alpha) is located in 3q26.32 and has 23 exons. Phosphatidylinositol 3-kinase is composed of an 85 kDa regulatory subunit and a 110 kDa catalytic subunit. This gene has been found to be oncogenic and a pseudogene of this gene has been defined on chromosome 22 (Gene ID: 5291, updated on 22 March 2021) [16]. Missense mutations of *PIK3CA* mostly gain function and are located in the helical domain at G542, E545, and Q546 and the kinase domain H1047 in 80% of the cases. The most common mutation in *PIK3CA* is H1047R, which results in enzymatic over-activation. To evaluate the H1048 cell line (H1047R mutant) contribution of PI3K/AKT/mTOR signaling to SCLC cell proliferation, Umemura et al. used RNA interference to down-regulate the expression of *PIK3CA*, and a significant decrease in proliferation was observed [21]. PI3K inhibitors have been extensively used in clinical trials, but only a few have gained Food and Drug Administration (FDA) approval, mainly due to dose-limiting toxicities. Feng et al. recently published the effect of a Chinese medicinal formula, Baizhu Additive Powder (SLBZ-AP), on the pain control and survival of mice with metastatic lung cancer to the bone. It is postulated that SLBZ-AP partially exerts its effects through the PI3K/AKT/mTOR pathway [22].

2.2.2. PTEN (9%)

PTEN (phosphatase and tensin homolog) is located in 10q23.31 and has 10 exons. It serves as a tumor suppressor gene and regulates the AKT/PKB pathway. Multiple translation initiation codons allow transcription by alternative splicing of numerous variants that encode different isoforms (Gene ID: 5728, updated on 7 February 2021) [16]. *PTEN* mutations are ubiquitous across a broad range of cancers and in 4%–9% of SCLC [3,23]. The function of *PTEN* in SCLC is not known. A revealing study was conducted by inactivating *PTEN* on an *RB1/TP53*-deleted mouse model that simulated human SCLC in a metastatic pattern and neuroendocrine features [24]. On the one hand, when a single *PTEN* allele was inactivated, SCLC progression occurred rapidly, indicating *PTEN*'s tumor-suppressing function in SCLC. On the other hand, homozygous *PTEN* inactivation synergized with *RB1*, and *TP53* loss promoted transformation from adenocarcinoma to neuroendocrine carcinoma [25].

2.2.3. FGFR1 (8%)

The fibroblast growth factor receptor (FGFR) binds to the fibroblast growth factor (FGF) family. *FGFR1* (fibroblast growth factor receptor 1) is located in 8p11.23. It has 24 exons that encode an FGFR family member, where the amino acid sequence is highly conserved between members. Throughout evolution, they differ from one another in their ligand affinities and tissue distribution. *FGFR* has an extracellular ligand domain, a transmembrane domain, and an intracellular domain. The extracellular domain is composed of three immunoglobulin-like domains. The intracellular domain contains tyrosine kinase activity, setting in motion a cascade of downstream signals, ultimately influencing mitogenesis and differentiation [13]. Alternatively, spliced variants have been described; however, not all variants have been fully characterized (Gene ID: 2260, updated on 22 March 2021) [16]. It had been reported that a high copy number of the FGFR1 gene might be a possible therapeutic target [5,26]. Paracrine FGF signaling is described in SCLC and has a negative prognostic impact. Paracrine production of FGFs results in neo-angiogenesis in cancer cells through FGFR1 and FGFR2 [27]. However, aberrant FGFR signaling might only occur in the earlier stages of the disease. Biomarkers that assess FGFR inhibition response are missing and candidates are FGFR1 gene amplification, overexpression, or mRNA quantification [5]. To date, very few reports have been published on FGFR inhibitors in SCLC harboring FGFR signaling pathway aberrations [28].

2.2.4. RET

RET (rearranged during transfection) is a proto-oncogene located in 10q11.21, has 20 exons, and encodes transmembrane tyrosine kinase protein receptor. When activated, it leads to the downstream activation of numerous pathways: RAS-MAPK, PI3K-AKT, and STAT3. The activation of this proto-oncogene can occur through both activating point mutations and cytogenetic rearrangement [29]. Chromosomal rearrangements involving *RET* have several fusion partner genes, for example: *KIF5B, CCDC6, CUX1* (Gene ID: 5979, updated on 7 February 2021) [16]. The prevalence of RET alterations in SCLC is unknown. The low prevalence of lack of surgical SCLC specimens renders the tasks of studying *RET* in SCLC difficult. Neither Peifer et al. nor Rudin et al. identified RET in SCLC as a statistically significantly mutated gene [9,10]. Dabir and colleagues performed Sanger sequencing on an SCLC metastasis and found an M918T mutation [30]. A skin biopsy from the same patient did not contain this mutation, establishing its somatic nature. The specimen also stained for RET by immunohistochemistry. Currently, basket trials for cancers with *RET* mutations are not enrolling SCLC patients.

2.3. Transcriptional Regulation

2.3.1. Hedgehog Signaling Pathway (80%)

The Hedgehog (HH) pathway plays conserved roles in regulating a diverse spectrum of developmental processes: Cellular proliferation and differentiation [31,32]. The pathway is composed of three proteins: Sonic Hedgehog (SHH), Indian Hedgehog (IHH), and Desert Hedgehog (DHH). The pathway is associated with carcinogenesis; however, it has not been studied in depth in SCLC. HH appears to regulate stem cells that maintain and regenerate within adult tissues. Park et al. used a TP53/RB1 knockout mouse model and observed HH to be upregulated in SCLC independently of the pulmonary microenvironment. Activated Smoothened (sMO), a transmembrane protein part of HH, triggered clonality in human SCLC cell lines and appeared to initiate carcinogenesis in an SCLC mouse model. Deletion of *sMO* had the opposite effect [33]. HH signaling is important for the in vivo growth of SCLC, but the establishment of cell lines from SCLC tumors may lead to the loss of key HH pathway members' expression [34]. This pathway is related to carcinogenesis, and therefore the discovery and synthesis of HH-specific signaling antagonists warrant further investigation [31]. On this basis, HH inhibition is a promising therapeutic target.

2.3.2. MYC (20%)

MYC is a family of regulator genes and proto-oncogenes that encode for transcription factors, with three related human genes: c-myc (MYC), l-myc (MYCL), and n-myc (MYCN). MYC was the first gene to be discovered in this family. MYC (MYC proto-oncogene) is located in 8q24.21 and has three exons that encode a nuclear phosphoprotein. MYC is critical to cell cycle progression and apoptosis. MYC amplification is present in various human tumors, with 20% of SCLC (Gene ID: 4609, updated on 7 February 2021) [16]. MYCL (MYCL proto-oncogene) is located in 1p34.2 and has two exons (Gene ID: 4610, updated on 2 March 2021) [16]. MYCN (MYCN proto-oncogene) is located in 2p24.3 and has three exons that encode a protein with a basic helix–loop–helix (bHLH) domain. Multiple alternatively spliced transcript variants encoding different isoforms have been found for this gene (Gene ID: 4613, updated on 2 March 2021) [16]. SCLC is treated as a homogeneous disease without further molecular sub-classification. These tumors often acquire an MYC amplification (in one of the subtypes: MYCL1 [9%], MYC [6%], or MYCN [4%]), dramatically accelerating tumorigenesis and metastatic potential [9,11]. MYC-amplified SCLC responds to frontline chemotherapy to only develop refractoriness and disease progression to subsequent lines of therapy. MYC's effect on this subtype of SCLC's natural history has not been confirmed in vivo yet [35]. Mollaoglu et al. studied an SCLC model with loss of TP53/RB1 and elevated MYC expression [36]. This model was similar to the human one, as evidenced by elevated NEUROD1 and low neuroendocrine markers such as ASCL1. Animal models of SCLC with high levels of MYC are sensitive to aurora kinase inhibitors. Chalishazar et al. described that tumors with MYC overexpression are vulnerable to arginine deletion. Arginine deiminase (ADE-PEG 20) has been shown to have antineoplastic effects in mice with MYC-associated cancers [37]. Based on Rudin et al.'s molecular classification of SCLC, Ireland et al. used single-cell transcriptome analyses in both mouse and human models and observed that MYC plays a critical role in evolving the different SCLC molecular subtypes [12,38]. On the one hand, MYC triggers the transition of ASCL1+ to NEUROD1+ to YAP1+ subtype in neuroendocrine cells. On the other hand, MYC promotes POU2F3+ tumors from different cell types. Given SCLC's intratumoral heterogeneity, it is assumed that this evolution happens in vivo as well. It is worth noting that MYC requires activation of the NOTCH pathway to induce carcinogenesis. Patel et al. recently reported that MYC and MYCL1 regulate the plasticity between these histological subtypes and molecular subtypes, then the role of the MYC family in SCLC tumorigenesis could be redefined to develop effective therapies [39].

2.3.3. KMT2D (13%)

KMT2D (lysine methyltransferase 2D) is located in 12q13.12, has 56 exons, and is also known as MLL2 or MLL4. The protein methylates the Lys-4 position of histone H3. The encoded protein is part of a large protein complex called ASCOM, a transcriptional regulator of the beta-globin and estrogen receptor genes (Gene ID: 8085, updated on 16 March 2021) [16,23]. Most striking is the high frequency of truncating KMT2D mutations, which have been found in 17% of SCLC cell lines and 8% of SCLC tumors. Although truncating KMT2D mutations are occasionally homozygous, most are hemizygous, suggesting that decreased gene dosage may contribute to SCLC [40]. It is not clear whether KMT2D-mutant SCLC will benefit from therapeutic inhibition of the H3K4 demethylase lysine demethylase 1A (LSD1). Future work will need to determine which SCLC subsets are likely to benefit from current approaches to target chromatin dynamic states [41].

2.4. Notch Signaling/Neuroendocrine Differentiation
NOTCH (25%)

NOTCH receptor protein is a heterodimer transmembrane receptor that is proteolytically cleaved from a precursor protein (NOTCH1, NOTCH2, NOTCH3, or NOTCH4), and their fragment migrates to the nucleus. The ligand can be from within the same cell (cis-interaction) or from a different cell (trans-interaction) [42]. This fragmented protein in the nucleus is converted into a transcription regulatory protein inducing critical genes' expression [43]. NOTCH mutation in SCLC is more commonly seen in the primary tumor rather than in the metastatic site. NOTCH1 (NOTCH receptor 1) is located in 9q34.3 and has 34 exons that encode a member of this type I transmembrane protein family. This receptor is critical for developing various cells and tissues (Gene ID: 4851, updated on 7 February 2021) [16]. In SCLC, NOTCH1 signaling is suppressed and plays a tumor-suppressive role, is most widely mutated (25%), and the most mutations are missense mutations (82%). Mutations are associated with significantly improved survival [44]. Overexpression in NOTCH1 inhibits SCLC growth and neuroendocrine features [45]. NOTCH negatively regulates the transcription factor ASCL1. On the one hand, ASCL1 promotes neuroendocrine transcription programs and is necessary for SCLC cells' viability. On the other hand, when ASCL1 is deleted in vivo, marked tumorigenesis inhibition is observed [46]. In general, the ASCL1 transcription factor is not targetable. However, LSD1, a lysine-specific histone demethylase 1, activates the NOCTH family upstream by suppressing ASCL1 expression. SCLC highly expresses LSD1, which is attached to the NOTCH1 gene [47]. Delta-like protein 3 (DLL3) is over-expressed in 80% of SCLC membrane cells and is specific to SCLC compared to normal lung cells. It is expressed both in the cytoplasm and in the membrane of SCLC cells [48]. Hence, DLL3 is a potential therapeutic target; clinical trials using a DLL3-targeted antibody–drug conjugate failed to benefit from toxicity concerns leading to discontinuation of the product. Other possible mechanisms to target DLL3 are illustrated in Figure 2 and include BiTE molecules® (AMG757) and chimeric antigen receptor T cells (AMG119). AMG757 is a half-life extended bispecific T cell engager antibody construct that binds to DLL3 on cancer cells with one scFv domain and connects DLL3-positive cells to CD3-positive T cells, which causes tumor lysis and proliferation of autologous T cells (Phase 1 study NCT03319940) [49]. AMG119 is an autologous T cell that has been genetically engineered ex vivo to express a chimeric antigen T cell receptor directed toward DLL3 and results in tumor lysis and autologous proliferation T cells (Phase 1 study NCT03392064) [49].

Although NOTCH3 expression in SCLC is lower than normal lung tissue [50], NOTCH3 remains understudied, and further research is needed to determine its effect on SCLC biology.

2.5. Epigenetic and Proteomic Changes

How genetic and transcriptomic alterations affect the functional proteome in lung neoplasms is not fully understood. Epigenetics refers to ways to alter a phenotype's expression that do not change the DNA sequence. It often occurs via methylation and histone modification [51]. SLFN11 (Schlafen 11) epigenetic silencing, a putative DNA/RNA helicase, by the EZH1/2 (Enhancer of the Zeste Homolog 1 or 2), has allowed us to gain an understanding of the role of epigenetics in SCLC. SLFN11 seems to be a predictor of response to DNA-interfering agents such as topoisomerase I and II inhibitors, platinum, and PARP inhibitors [52]. For example, the clinical trial NCT03879798 was designed to evaluate whether EZH1/2 inhibitors could overcome chemotherapy resistance by reversing epigenetic silencing and restoring SLFN11 expression [7]. Other clinical trials have used the bromodomain and extra-terminal motif protein (BET) inhibitor. These can modify the expression of several genes involved in carcinogenesis, such as MYC, BCL2, CDK4, and CDK6. The single-agent activity is limited but seems more promising in combination with other agents (NCT02391480) [7]. Stewart and colleagues studied 108 SCLC patients by mass spectrometry-based proteomics integrated with parallel analyses of DNA and mRNA to define molecular subtypes and identify drivers. With genomic, transcriptomic, and proteomic datasets, they identified three SCLC subtypes at the proteomic level. However, 87% of SCLC patients were associated with either immune infiltration (Inflamed) or oxidation-reduction (Re-dox) subtype [53].

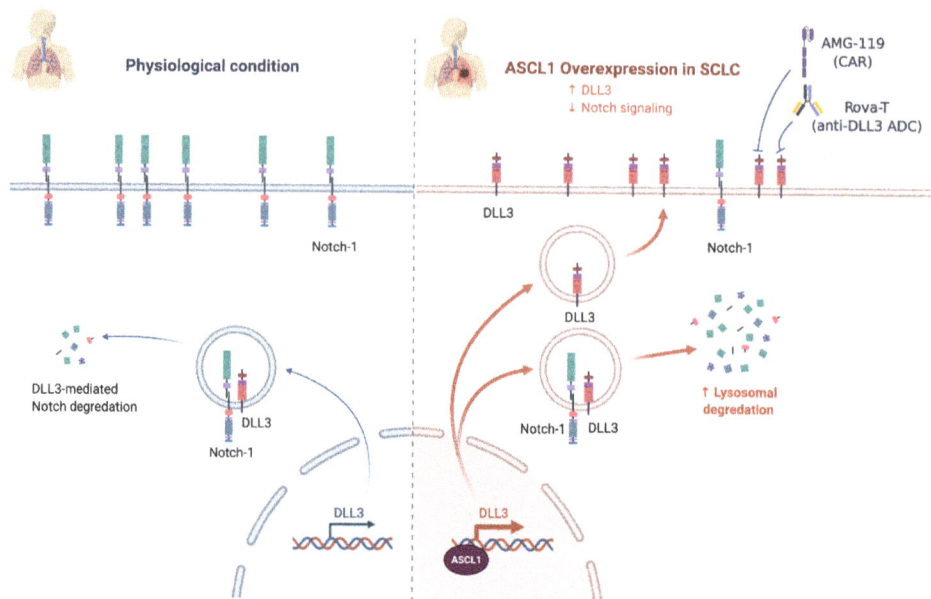

Figure 2. ASCL1 overexpression in SCLC and exploitation of DLL3 as therapeutic target (created with BioRender.com, accessed on 24 February 2021).

2.6. Transcriptional Addictions

SCLC cells can manipulate and regulate gene expression to favor their growth and survival. Pharmacologically modulating gene expression could be a promising therapeutic approach. For example, on the one hand, THZ1 is a selective and potent covalent CDK7 inhibitor that suppresses SCLC growth. Christensen et al. demonstrated the efficacy of THZ1 treatment on the expression of proto-oncogenes such as *MYC* and neuroendocrine factors [54]. Meanwhile, on the other hand, lurbinectedin inhibits oncogenic genes' active transcription, mainly in the GC-rich regulatory domains, and received the Food and Drug Administration's (FDA) granted accelerated approval for extensive-stage SCLC after platinum-based therapy [55]. At the time of this manuscript's submission, there is one ongoing clinical trial combining lurbinectedin with doxorubicin versus cyclophosphamide doxorubicin and vincristine for second-line SCLC after platinum based-therapy (NCT: 02566993).

3. Future Perspectives

SCLC has benefited little from the progress that the oncology field has seen in the last few decades. Diagnostically, a PET-radiotracer using 89Zr-SC16 is being developed. This radiotracer is directed toward DLL3; SCLC tracer uptake is correlated with DLL3 expression [7].

Bioinformatics strategy and extensive human sample collection will allow the study and discovery of potentially relevant molecular landscape and signaling pathways from a genomic perspective. Other potential areas of interest are epigenetic alterations in other genes (*CREBBP, KMT2D/MLL2,* and *MLL3*) and PIK3/mTOR pathway genes.

Although *PARP1* is overexpressed in SCLC, PARP inhibitors show little efficacy in SCLC with PIK3/mTOR pathway alterations. The same applies to *BCL2*. Although overexpressed as well in SCLC, BCL2 inhibitors show little benefit and significant hematological toxicity. Other DNA damage response proteins are also overexpressed in SCLC, such as *ATR* (ATR Serine/Threonine Kinase) [7].

Liquid biopsy is also a promising diagnostic tool that allows minimally invasive tumor genotyping and real-time monitoring [56]. Nong et al. performed deep-sequencing on 430 pretreatment SCLC biopsies and plasma samples from 22 SCLC patients at various treatment stages. They noted that average variant allele frequency is more predictive of survival than individual gene mutations, suggesting that clonal dynamics might be a vital determinant in SCLC biology [57]. Almodovar et al. developed a circulating free DNA (cfDNA) panel that detects 14 genes commonly mutated in SCLC [58]. They noted that most patients (85%) had genetic changes with mutant allele frequency between $\leq 0.1\%$ and 84%, and *TP53* and *RB1* were most commonly mutated (70% and 52%, respectively). Interestingly, cfDNA allowed for relapse detection before this became evident radiographically. Liquid biopsy, therefore, has the potential of non-invasively tracking the disease status and response to treatment and provide valuable information before this becomes clinically evident. Carter et al. demonstrated that the circulating tumor cells were reliable in evaluating chemotherapy response and impacted progression-free survival [59].

4. Conclusions

Small cell lung cancer (SCLC) continues to carry a poor prognosis with a five-year survival rate of 3.5% and a 10-year survival rate of 1.8% [2]. The pathogenesis remains unclear, and there are no known predictive or diagnostic biomarkers. In this manuscript, we provided an overview of published studies on SCLC's genomic landscape. Since there have been several comprehensive review articles published recently, this review summarizes the body of literature available on SCLC's genomic landscape to describe SCLC's molecular/genetic aspects, regardless of therapeutic strategy [3,4,10,60,61]. Further studies are needed to identify better genes and signaling pathways essential to SCLC cell survival and proliferation. Integration of preclinical and clinical data will be critical to understanding this lethal disease better. Bioinformatics is an integral part of this effort as it allows the analysis of SCLC "big data" in addition to next-generation sequencing, tumor genotyping, liquid biopsy, and transcriptomics. Once all of these techniques and efforts are assembled, it will be possible to develop novel therapeutic approaches to improve patient's survival with SCLC.

Author Contributions: Conceptualization, V.D. and C.R.; writing—original draft preparation, V.D. and A.R.; visualization, A.R.; writing—review and editing. D.d.M.-P., U.M., A.B., A.G., A.F.C., and C.R. All authors have read and agreed to the published version of the manuscript.

Funding: This research received no external funding.

Institutional Review Board Statement: Not applicable.

Informed Consent Statement: Not applicable.

Data Availability Statement: No new data were created or analyzed in this study. Data sharing is not applicable to this article.

Conflicts of Interest: V.D. received personal fees (as consultant and/or speaker bureau) from Bristol, Amgen, Novartis, MSD, and Roche, and their research is sponsored by BMS, Novartis, Amgen, AstraZeneca, and Roche, unrelated to the current work. A.F.C. discloses financial research support from Merck Sharp & Dohme, Boehringer Ingelheim, Roche, Bristol-Myers Squibb, and the Foundation for Clinical and Applied Cancer Research (FICMAC); additionally, he was linked and received honoraria as an advisor, participated in speakers' bureau, and gave expert testimony to Merck Sharp & Dohme, Boehringer Ingelheim, Roche, Bristol-Myers Squibb, Pfizer, Novartis, Celldex Therapeutics, Foundation Medicine, Eli Lilly, and the Foundation for Clinical and Applied Cancer Research (FICMAC). C.R. is a speaker for Merck Sharp and Dohme, AstraZeneca; has research collaborations with Guardant Health; advisory board activity: Archer, Inivata and MD Serono, Novartis, and BMS; non-financial support from Guardant Health; research grant from LCRF-Pfizer. A.R. reports an advisory role for AstraZeneca and MSD. U.M. received personal fees (as a consultant and/or speaker bureau) from Boehringer Ingelheim, Roche, MSD, Amgen, Thermo Fisher Scientifics, Diaceutics, GSK, Merck, and AstraZeneca, unrelated to the current work. The other authors declare no conflicts of interest.

References

1. Bunn, P.A.; Minna, J.D.; Augustyn, A.; Gazdar, A.F.; Ouadah, Y.; Krasnow, M.A.; Berns, A.; Brambilla, E.; Rekhtman, N.; Massion P.P.; et al. Small Cell Lung Cancer: Can Recent Advances in Biology and Molecular Biology Be Translated into Improved Outcomes? *J. Thorac. Oncol.* **2016**, *11*, 453–474. [CrossRef]
2. Lassen, U.; Osterlind, K.; Hansen, M.; Dombernowsky, P.; Bergman, B.; Hansen, H.H. Long-Term Survival in Small-Cell Lung Cancer: Posttreatment Characteristics in Patients Surviving 5 to 18+ Year—An Analysis of 1714 Consecutive Patients. *J. Clin. Oncol.* **1995**, *13*, 1215–1220. [CrossRef] [PubMed]
3. Wang, S.; Zimmermann, S.; Parikh, K.; Mansfield, A.S.; Adjei, A.A. Current Diagnosis and Management of Small-Cell Lung Cancer. *Mayo Clin. Proc.* **2019**, *94*, 1599–1622. [CrossRef] [PubMed]
4. Gazdar, A.F.; Bunn, P.A.; Minna, J.D. Small-Cell Lung Cancer: What We Know, What We Need to Know and the Path Forward. *Nat. Rev. Cancer* **2017**, *17*, 725–737. [CrossRef] [PubMed]
5. Dowlati, A.; Lipka, M.B.; McColl, K.; Dabir, S.; Behtaj, M.; Kresak, A.; Miron, A.; Yang, M.; Sharma, N.; Fu, P.; et al. Clinical Correlation of Extensive-Stage Small-Cell Lung Cancer Genomics. *Ann. Oncol.* **2016**, *27*, 642–647. [CrossRef] [PubMed]
6. Karachaliou, N.; Sosa, A.E.; Rosell, R. Unraveling the Genomic Complexity of Small Cell Lung Cancer. *Transl. Lung Cancer Res.* **2016**, *5*, 363–366. [CrossRef] [PubMed]
7. Poirier, J.T.; George, J.; Owonikoko, T.K.; Berns, A.; Brambilla, E.; Byers, L.A.; Carbone, D.; Chen, H.J.; Christensen, C.L.; Dive C.; et al. New Approaches to SCLC Therapy: From the Laboratory to the Clinic. *J. Thorac. Oncol.* **2020**, *15*, 520–540. [CrossRef] [PubMed]
8. Byers, L.A.; Rudin, C.M. Small Cell Lung Cancer: Where Do We Go from Here? SCLC: Where Do We Go From Here? *Cancer* **2015**, *121*, 664–672. [CrossRef] [PubMed]
9. Peifer, M.; Fernández-Cuesta, L.; Sos, M.L.; George, J.; Seidel, D.; Kasper, L.H.; Plenker, D.; Leenders, F.; Sun, R.; Zander, T.; et al. Integrative Genome Analyses Identify Key Somatic Driver Mutations of Small-Cell Lung Cancer. *Nat. Genet.* **2012**, *44*, 1104–1110 [CrossRef]
10. Rudin, C.M.; Durinck, S.; Stawiski, E.W.; Poirier, J.T.; Modrusan, Z.; Shames, D.S.; Bergbower, E.A.; Guan, Y.; Shin, J.; Guillory, J.; et al. Comprehensive Genomic Analysis Identifies SOX2 as a Frequently Amplified Gene in Small-Cell Lung Cancer. *Nat. Genet.* **2012**, *44*, 1111–1116. [CrossRef]
11. George, J.; Lim, J.S.; Jang, S.J.; Cun, Y.; Ozretić, L.; Kong, G.; Leenders, F.; Lu, X.; Fernández-Cuesta, L.; Bosco, G.; et al. Comprehensive Genomic Profiles of Small Cell Lung Cancer. *Nature* **2015**, *524*, 47–53. [CrossRef] [PubMed]
12. Rudin, C.M.; Poirier, J.T.; Byers, L.A.; Dive, C.; Dowlati, A.; George, J.; Heymach, J.V.; Johnson, J.E.; Lehman, J.M.; MacPherson, D.; et al. Molecular Subtypes of Small Cell Lung Cancer: A Synthesis of Human and Mouse Model Data. *Nat. Rev. Cancer* **2019**, *19*, 289–297. [CrossRef] [PubMed]
13. Baine, M.K.; Hsieh, M.-S.; Lai, W.V.; Egger, J.V.; Jungbluth, A.A.; Daneshbod, Y.; Beras, A.; Spencer, R.; Lopardo, J.; Bodd, F.; et al. SCLC Subtypes Defined by ASCL1, NEUROD1, POU2F3, and YAP1: A Comprehensive Immunohistochemical and Histopathologic Characterization. *J. Thorac. Oncol.* **2020**, *15*, 1823–1835. [CrossRef] [PubMed]
14. Song, Y.; Sun, Y.; Lei, Y.; Yang, K.; Tang, R. YAP1 Promotes Multidrug Resistance of Small Cell Lung Cancer by CD74-related Signaling Pathways. *Cancer Med.* **2020**, *9*, 259–268. [CrossRef] [PubMed]
15. Owonikoko, T.K.; Niu, H.; Nackaerts, K.; Csoszi, T.; Ostoros, G.; Mark, Z.; Baik, C.; Joy, A.A.; Chouaid, C.; Jaime, J.C.; et al. Randomized Phase II Study of Paclitaxel plus Alisertib versus Paclitaxel plus Placebo as Second-Line Therapy for SCLC: Primary and Correlative Biomarker Analyses. *J. Thorac. Oncol.* **2020**, *15*, 274–287. [CrossRef]
16. National Center for Biotechnology Information (NCBI). Bethesda (MD): National Library of Medicine (US), National Center for Biotechnology Information. 1988. Available online: https://www.Ncbi.Nlm.Nih.Gov/ (accessed on 14 February 2021).
17. Yokouchi, H.; Nishihara, H.; Harada, T.; Yamazaki, S.; Kikuchi, H.; Oizumi, S.; Uramoto, H.; Tanaka, F.; Harada, M.; Akie, K.; et al. Detection of Somatic TP53 Mutation in Surgically Resected Small-Cell Lung Cancer by Targeted Exome Sequencing: Association with Longer Relapse-Free Survival. *Heliyon* **2020**, *6*, e04439. [CrossRef] [PubMed]
18. Sonkin, D.; Vural, S.; Thomas, A.; Teicher, B.A. Neuroendocrine Negative SCLC Is Mostly RB1 WT and May Be Sensitive to CDK4/6 Inhibition. *BioRxiv* **2019**, 516351. [CrossRef]
19. Kim, K.-B.; Dunn, C.T.; Park, K.-S. Recent Progress in Mapping the Emerging Landscape of the Small-Cell Lung Cancer Genome. *Exp. Mol. Med.* **2019**, *51*, 1–13. [CrossRef] [PubMed]
20. Shibata, T.; Kokubu, A.; Tsuta, K.; Hirohashi, S. Oncogenic Mutation of PIK3CA in Small Cell Lung Carcinoma: A Potential Therapeutic Target Pathway for Chemotherapy-Resistant Lung Cancer. *Cancer Lett.* **2009**, *283*, 203–211. [CrossRef]
21. Umemura, S.; Mimaki, S.; Makinoshima, H.; Tada, S.; Ishii, G.; Ohmatsu, H.; Niho, S.; Yoh, K.; Matsumoto, S.; Takahashi, A.; et al. Therapeutic Priority of the PI3K/AKT/MTOR Pathway in Small Cell Lung Cancers as Revealed by a Comprehensive Genomic Analysis. *J. Thorac. Oncol.* **2014**, *9*, 1324–1331. [CrossRef] [PubMed]
22. Feng, Z.; Feng, Z.; Han, J.; Cheng, W.; Su, B.; Mo, J.; Feng, X.; Feng, S.; Chen, G.; Huang, P.; et al. Antinociceptive Effects of Shenling Baizhu through PI3K-Akt-MTOR Signaling Pathway in a Mouse Model of Bone Metastasis with Small-Cell Lung Cancer. *Evid. Based Complement. Altern. Med.* **2020**, *2020*, 1–12. [CrossRef]
23. Rudin, C.M.; Brambilla, E.; Faivre-Finn, C.; Sage, J. Small-Cell Lung Cancer. *Nat. Rev. Dis. Primer* **2021**, *7*, 3. [CrossRef]
24. Meuwissen, R.; Linn, S.C.; Linnoila, R.I.; Zevenhoven, J.; Mooi, W.J.; Berns, A. Induction of Small Cell Lung Cancer by Somatic Inactivation of Both Trp53 and Rb1 in a Conditional Mouse Model. *Cancer Cell* **2003**, *4*, 181–189. [CrossRef]

25. Cui, M.; Augert, A.; Rongione, M.; Conkrite, K.; Parazzoli, S.; Nikitin, A.Y.; Ingolia, N.; MacPherson, D. PTEN Is a Potent Suppressor of Small Cell Lung Cancer. *Mol. Cancer Res.* **2014**, *12*, 654–659. [CrossRef] [PubMed]
26. Ferone, G.; Song, J.-Y.; Krijgsman, O.; van der Vliet, J.; Cozijnsen, M.; Semenova, E.A.; Adams, D.J.; Peeper, D.; Berns, A. FGFR1 Oncogenic Activation Reveals an Alternative Cell of Origin of SCLC in Rb1/P53 Mice. *Cell Rep.* **2020**, *30*, 3837–3850.e3. [CrossRef] [PubMed]
27. Desai, A.; Adjei, A.A. FGFR Signaling as a Target for Lung Cancer Therapy. *J. Thorac. Oncol.* **2016**, *11*, 9–20. [CrossRef] [PubMed]
28. Russo, A.; McCusker, M.G.; Scilla, K.A.; Arensmeyer, K.E.; Mehra, R.; Adamo, V.; Rolfo, C. Immunotherapy in Lung Cancer: From a Minor God to the Olympus. In *Immunotherapy*; Naing, A., Hajjar, J., Eds.; Advances in Experimental Medicine and Biology; Springer International Publishing: Cham, Switzerland, 2020; Volume 1244, pp. 69–92. [CrossRef]
29. Li, A.Y.; McCusker, M.G.; Russo, A.; Scilla, K.A.; Gittens, A.; Arensmeyer, K.; Mehra, R.; Adamo, V.; Rolfo, C. RET Fusions in Solid Tumors. *Cancer Treat. Rev.* **2019**, *81*, 101911. [CrossRef]
30. Dabir, S.; Babakoohi, S.; Kluge, A.; Morrow, J.J.; Kresak, A.; Yang, M.; MacPherson, D.; Wildey, G.; Dowlati, A. RET Mutation and Expression in Small-Cell Lung Cancer. *J. Thorac. Oncol.* **2014**, *9*, 1316–1323. [CrossRef]
31. Lim, S.; Lim, S.M.; Kim, M.-J.; Park, S.Y.; Kim, J.-H. Sonic Hedgehog Pathway as the Prognostic Marker in Patients with Extensive Stage Small Cell Lung Cancer. *Yonsei Med. J.* **2019**, *60*, 898. [CrossRef]
32. Falkenstein, K.N.; Vokes, S.A. Transcriptional Regulation of Graded Hedgehog Signaling. *Semin. Cell Dev. Biol.* **2014**, *33*, 73–80. [CrossRef] [PubMed]
33. Park, K.-S.; Martelotto, L.G.; Peifer, M.; Sos, M.L.; Karnezis, A.N.; Mahjoub, M.R.; Bernard, K.; Conklin, J.F.; Szczepny, A.; Yuan, J.; et al. A Crucial Requirement for Hedgehog Signaling in Small Cell Lung Cancer. *Nat. Med.* **2011**, *17*, 1504–1508. [CrossRef]
34. Vestergaard, J.; Pedersen, M.W.; Pedersen, N.; Ensinger, C.; Tümer, Z.; Tommerup, N.; Poulsen, H.S.; Larsen, L.A. Hedgehog Signaling in Small-Cell Lung Cancer: Frequent in Vivo but a Rare Event in Vitro. *Lung Cancer* **2006**, *52*, 281–290. [CrossRef]
35. Sos, M.L.; Dietlein, F.; Peifer, M.; Schottle, J.; Balke-Want, H.; Muller, C.; Koker, M.; Richters, A.; Heynck, S.; Malchers, F.; et al. A Framework for Identification of Actionable Cancer Genome Dependencies in Small Cell Lung Cancer. *Proc. Natl. Acad. Sci. USA* **2012**, *109*, 17034–17039. [CrossRef]
36. Mollaoglu, G.; Guthrie, M.R.; Böhm, S.; Brägelmann, J.; Can, I.; Ballieu, P.M.; Marx, A.; George, J.; Heinen, C.; Chalishazar, M.D.; et al. MYC Drives Progression of Small Cell Lung Cancer to a Variant Neuroendocrine Subtype with Vulnerability to Aurora Kinase Inhibition. *Cancer Cell* **2017**, *31*, 270–285. [CrossRef] [PubMed]
37. Chalishazar, M.D.; Wait, S.J.; Huang, F.; Ireland, A.S.; Mukhopadhyay, A.; Lee, Y.; Schuman, S.S.; Guthrie, M.R.; Berrett, K.C.; Vahrenkamp, J.M.; et al. MYC-Driven Small-Cell Lung Cancer Is Metabolically Distinct and Vulnerable to Arginine Depletion. *Clin. Cancer Res.* **2019**, *25*, 5107–5121. [CrossRef]
38. Ireland, A.S.; Micinski, A.M.; Kastner, D.W.; Guo, B.; Wait, S.J.; Spainhower, K.B.; Conley, C.C.; Chen, O.S.; Guthrie, M.R.; Soltero, D.; et al. MYC Drives Temporal Evolution of Small Cell Lung Cancer Subtypes by Reprogramming Neuroendocrine Fate. *Cancer Cell* **2020**, *38*, 60–78.e12. [CrossRef] [PubMed]
39. Patel, A.S.; Yoo, S.; Kong, R.; Sato, T.; Sinha, A.; Karam, S.; Bao, L.; Fridrikh, M.; Emoto, K.; Nudelman, G.; et al. Prototypical Oncogene Family Myc Defines Unappreciated Distinct Lineage States of Small Cell Lung Cancer. *Sci. Adv.* **2021**, *7*, eabc2578. [CrossRef] [PubMed]
40. Augert, A.; Zhang, Q.; Bates, B.; Cui, M.; Wang, X.; Wildey, G.; Dowlati, A.; MacPherson, D. Small Cell Lung Cancer Exhibits Frequent Inactivating Mutations in the Histone Methyltransferase KMT2D/MLL2: CALGB 151111 (Alliance). *J. Thorac. Oncol.* **2017**, *12*, 704–713. [CrossRef]
41. Gardner, E.E.; Poirier, J.T.; Rudin, C.M. Histone Code Aberrancies in Small Cell Lung Cancer. *J. Thorac. Oncol.* **2017**, *12*, 599–601. [CrossRef]
42. Leonetti, A.; Facchinetti, F.; Minari, R.; Cortellini, A.; Rolfo, C.D.; Giovannetti, E.; Tiseo, M. Notch Pathway in Small-Cell Lung Cancer: From Preclinical Evidence to Therapeutic Challenges. *Cell. Oncol.* **2019**, *42*, 261–273. [CrossRef]
43. Terragni, J.; Zhang, G.; Sun, Z.; Pradhan, S.; Song, L.; Crawford, G.E.; Lacey, M.; Ehrlich, M. Notch Signaling Genes: Myogenic DNA Hypomethylation and 5-Hydroxymethylcytosine. *Epigenetics* **2014**, *9*, 842–850. [CrossRef]
44. Ardeshir-Larijani, F.; Wildey, G.; Fu, P.; Bhateja, P.; Dowlati, A. Frequency of NOTCH Pathway Mutation in Primary Tumor of SCLC Compared to Metastatic Biopsies and Association with Better Survival. *J. Clin. Oncol.* **2018**, *36* (Suppl. 15), e20574. [CrossRef]
45. Sriuranpong, V.; Borges, M.W.; Ravi, R.K.; Arnold, D.R.; Nelkin, B.D.; Baylin, S.B.; Ball, D.W. Notch Signaling Induces Cell Cycle Arrest in Small Cell Lung Cancer Cells. *Cancer Res.* **2001**, *61*, 3200–3205. [PubMed]
46. Mohammad, H.P.; Smitheman, K.N.; Kamat, C.D.; Soong, D.; Federowicz, K.E.; Van Aller, G.S.; Schneck, J.L.; Carson, J.D.; Liu, Y.; Butticello, M.; et al. A DNA Hypomethylation Signature Predicts Antitumor Activity of LSD1 Inhibitors in SCLC. *Cancer Cell* **2015**, *28*, 57–69. [CrossRef] [PubMed]
47. Augert, A.; Eastwood, E.; Ibrahim, A.H.; Wu, N.; Grunblatt, E.; Basom, R.; Liggitt, D.; Eaton, K.D.; Martins, R.; Poirier, J.T.; et al. Targeting NOTCH Activation in Small Cell Lung Cancer through LSD1 Inhibition. *Sci. Signal.* **2019**, *12*, eaau2922. [CrossRef] [PubMed]
48. Sharma, S.K.; Pourat, J.; Abdel-Atti, D.; Carlin, S.D.; Piersigilli, A.; Bankovich, A.J.; Gardner, E.E.; Hamdy, O.; Isse, K.; Bheddah, S.; et al. Noninvasive Interrogation of DLL3 Expression in Metastatic Small Cell Lung Cancer. *Cancer Res.* **2017**, *77*, 3931–3941. [CrossRef] [PubMed]

49. Owen, D.H.; Giffin, M.J.; Bailis, J.M.; Smit, M.-A.D.; Carbone, D.P.; He, K. DLL3: An Emerging Target in Small Cell Lung Cancer. *J. Hematol. Oncol.* **2019**, *12*, 61. [CrossRef]
50. Zhou, L.; Zhang, N.; Song, W.; You, N.; Li, Q.; Sun, W.; Zhang, Y.; Wang, D.; Dou, K. The Significance of Notch1 Compared with Notch3 in High Metastasis and Poor Overall Survival in Hepatocellular Carcinoma. *PLoS ONE* **2013**, *8*, e57382. [CrossRef]
51. Dupont, C.; Armant, D.; Brenner, C. Epigenetics: Definition, Mechanisms and Clinical Perspective. *Semin. Reprod. Med.* **2009**, *27*, 351–357. [CrossRef]
52. Krushkal, J.; Silvers, T.; Reinhold, W.C.; Sonkin, D.; Vural, S.; Connelly, J.; Varma, S.; Meltzer, P.S.; Kunkel, M.; Rapisarda, A.; et al. Epigenome-Wide DNA Methylation Analysis of Small Cell Lung Cancer Cell Lines Suggests Potential Chemotherapy Targets. *Clin. Epigenetics* **2020**, *12*, 93. [CrossRef]
53. Stewart, P.A.; Welsh, E.A.; Slebos, R.J.C.; Fang, B.; Izumi, V.; Chambers, M.; Zhang, G.; Cen, L.; Pettersson, F.; Zhang, Y.; et al. Proteogenomic Landscape of Squamous Cell Lung Cancer. *Nat. Commun.* **2019**, *10*, 3578. [CrossRef]
54. Christensen, C.L.; Kwiatkowski, N.; Abraham, B.J.; Carretero, J.; Al-Shahrour, F.; Zhang, T.; Chipumuro, E.; Herter-Sprie, G.S.; Akbay, E.A.; Altabef, A.; et al. Targeting Transcriptional Addictions in Small Cell Lung Cancer with a Covalent CDK7 Inhibitor. *Cancer Cell* **2014**, *26*, 909–922. [CrossRef]
55. Trigo, J.; Subbiah, V.; Besse, B.; Moreno, V.; López, R.; Sala, M.A.; Peters, S.; Ponce, S.; Fernández, C.; Alfaro, V.; et al. Lurbinectedin as Second-Line Treatment for Patients with Small-Cell Lung Cancer: A Single-Arm, Open-Label, Phase 2 Basket Trial. *Lancet Oncol.* **2020**, *21*, 645–654. [CrossRef]
56. Russo, A.; De Miguel Perez, D.; Gunasekaran, M.; Scilla, K.; Lapidus, R.; Cooper, B.; Mehra, R.; Adamo, V.; Malapelle, U.; Rolfo, C. Liquid Biopsy Tracking of Lung Tumor Evolutions over Time. *Expert Rev. Mol. Diagn.* **2019**, *19*, 1099–1108. [CrossRef]
57. Nong, J.; Gong, Y.; Guan, Y.; Yi, X.; Yi, Y.; Chang, L.; Yang, L.; Lv, J.; Guo, Z.; Jia, H.; et al. Circulating Tumor DNA Analysis Depicts Subclonal Architecture and Genomic Evolution of Small Cell Lung Cancer. *Nat. Commun.* **2018**, *9*, 3114. [CrossRef] [PubMed]
58. Almodovar, K.; Iams, W.T.; Meador, C.B.; Zhao, Z.; York, S.; Horn, L.; Yan, Y.; Hernandez, J.; Chen, H.; Shyr, Y.; et al. Longitudinal Cell-Free DNA Analysis in Patients with Small Cell Lung Cancer Reveals Dynamic Insights into Treatment Efficacy and Disease Relapse. *J. Thorac. Oncol.* **2018**, *13*, 112–123. [CrossRef] [PubMed]
59. Carter, L.; Rothwell, D.G.; Mesquita, B.; Smowton, C.; Leong, H.S.; Fernandez-Gutierrez, F.; Li, Y.; Burt, D.J.; Antonello, J.; Morrow, C.J.; et al. Molecular Analysis of Circulating Tumor Cells Identifies Distinct Copy-Number Profiles in Patients with Chemosensitive and Chemorefractory Small-Cell Lung Cancer. *Nat. Med.* **2017**, *23*, 114–119. [CrossRef]
60. Yang, S.; Zhang, Z.; Wang, Q. Emerging Therapies for Small Cell Lung Cancer. *J. Hematol. Oncol.* **2019**, *12*, 47. [CrossRef] [PubMed]
61. Saltos, A.; Shafique, M.; Chiappori, A. Update on the Biology, Management, and Treatment of Small Cell Lung Cancer (SCLC). *Front. Oncol.* **2020**, *10*, 1074. [CrossRef]

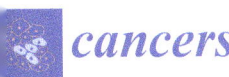

Review

Novel Cytotoxic Chemotherapies in Small Cell Lung Carcinoma

Diego Cortinovis [1,*], Paolo Bidoli [1,2], Stefania Canova [1], Francesca Colonese [1], Maria Gemelli [1], Maria Luisa Lavitrano [2], Giuseppe Luigi Banna [3], Stephen V. Liu [4] and Alessandro Morabito [5]

1. Department Medical Oncology—ASST-Monza Ospedale San Gerardo, via Pergolesi 33, 20090 Monza, Italy; paolo.bidoli@unimib.it (P.B.); s.canova@asst-monza.it (S.C.); f.colonese@asst-monza.it (F.C.); maria.gemelli@asst-monza.it (M.G.)
2. School of Medicine and Surgery, University of Milano-Bicocca, 20900 Monza, Italy; marialuisa.lavitrano@unimib.it
3. Department of Oncology, Portsmouth Hospitals University NHS Trust, Cosham, Portsmouth PO6 3LY, UK; giuseppe.banna@nhs.net
4. Lombardi Comprehensive Cancer Center, Georgetown University, 3800 Reservoir Road NW, Washington, DC 20007, USA; stephen.v.liu@gunet.georgetown.edu
5. SC Oncologia Medica Toraco-Polmonare, IRCCS Istituto Nazionale dei Tumori, Fondazione Pascale, 80100 Napoli, Italy; a.morabito@istitutotumori.na.it
* Correspondence: d.cortinovis@asst-monza.it; Tel.: +39-039-2336-040

Simple Summary: Small cell lung cancer is a subtype of lung cancer and one of the deadliest thoracic tumours. Historically, chemotherapy consisting of either platinum plus etoposide or anthracycline-based regimens have been associated with a high response rate and rapid development of acquired resistance, contributing to the poor overall prognosis. Only a fraction of patients with local or early disease can be cured, whilst the treatment is palliative in those with extensive disease. In recent decades, few novel drugs have been developed, which are herein described.

Abstract: Small cell lung cancer (SCLC) is one of the deadliest thoracic neoplasms, in part due to its fast doubling time and early metastatic spread. Historically, cytotoxic chemotherapy consisting of platinum–etoposide or anthracycline-based regimens has demonstrated a high response rate, but early chemoresistance leads to a poor prognosis in advanced SCLC. Only a fraction of patients with limited-disease can be cured by chemo-radiotherapy. Given the disappointing survival rates in advanced SCLC, new cytotoxic agents are eagerly awaited. Unfortunately, few novel chemotherapy drugs have been developed in the latest decades. This review describes the results and potential application in the clinical practice of novel chemotherapy agents for SCLC.

Keywords: small cell lung cancer; chemotherapy; immunotherapy; lurbinectedin

1. Introduction

Small cell lung cancer (SCLC) is an aggressive neuroendocrine tumour, accounting for 13–15% of new lung cancer diagnoses with a lower prevalence among lung cancer due to short survival. It is characterised by rapid cellular proliferation, deregulation of cell cycle control and apoptosis and high chemosensitivity followed by quick emergence of resistance to many therapies [1]. Cytotoxic chemotherapy currently represents the standard treatment to reduce tumour growth and limit metastatic spread [2], though its benefit is consistently transient. Chemotherapy given with radiotherapy can cure the limited-disease (LD) SCLC, but this is still only achieved by a fraction of patients, with a 5-year survival rate of 10–20% [3]. For patients with extensive-disease (ED) SCLC, chemotherapy has only a palliative intent, with anecdotal long-term survivors following this treatment but survival for most patients limited to 8–10 months.

Since 1985, the combination of platinum plus etoposide has been the standard treatment for both the LD- and ED-SCLC [4,5]. The superiority of regimens containing platinum-derivatives, as compared to non-platinum regimens, has been confirmed in several meta analyses [6–8]. Carboplatin and cisplatin have equivalent activity and efficacy in SCLC however, carboplatin has a more favourable toxicity profile than cisplatin, with the exception of more myelosuppression activity [9].

Beyond platinum and etoposide, other combinations have been tested with response rates ranging from 50 to 60%, median progression-free survival (PFS) and overall survival (OS) of 4–5 months and 8–12 months, respectively. Specifically, the combination of cisplatin and irinotecan showed a superior efficacy than cisplatin and etoposide in the Asiatic population [10], whereas combining cisplatin with topotecan or an anthracycline did not result as more effective as to etoposide [11,12].

Other attempts to exploit the chemosensitivity included dose intensification and the use of non-cross-resistant drugs with different mechanisms of action, which did not prove to be superior to the platinum and etoposide combination; the high-dose chemotherapy followed by bone marrow transplant was abandoned due to the lack of improved long-term survival despite the high incidence of serious adverse events [13–19]. Non-cross resistant chemotherapy agents are used to treat disease relapse in the second-line setting, with variable results depending on the treatment-free interval (i.e., > or ≤90 days from the end of the first-line therapy) [20].

For many decades, topotecan was the only FDA (Food and Drug Administration) and EMA (European Medicine Agency) approved drug for patients progressing to the first-line therapy based on an equivalent efficacy and better tolerability compared to the triplet of cyclophosphamide, doxorubicin and vincristine (i.e., the CAV regimen) [21]. In a randomised clinical trial, single-agent topotecan showed a median PFS of 2 months less than carboplatin and etoposide (2.7 vs. 4.7 months, respectively) in patients with a treatment-free interval >90 days; the mOS, however, was not different between the two arms [22]. In June 2020, lurbinectedin received accelerated FDA approval.

Since the end of the 1990s, the clinical recommendations on systemic chemotherapy had not changed. No drugs with novel mechanisms of action were available, other than alkylating agents or DNA intercalating drugs. Numerous clinical trials with conventional drugs failed to demonstrate any outcome improvement, and the efficacy of platinum plus etoposide was not surpassed, despite its modest results. This generated a basic nihilism that did not facilitate progress.

In recent years, some clinical trials paved the way for the development of new drugs with different mechanisms of action and new combinations for the SCLC.

More recently, the advent of immunotherapy has brought about new lifeblood in research applied to SCLC. In particular, in the first line, the increase in overall survival highlighted with the addition of anti-programmed-cell-death-1 (antiPD-1) and anti-PD-ligand-1 (antiPD-L1) led to a change in the standard of care. For this reason, the association of platinum and etoposide for 4–6 cycles can no longer be considered the gold standard. In fact, even in these more recent randomised studies, the standard chemotherapy arm resulted in OS between 9.7 and 10.5 months, comparable to what combination chemotherapy treatment has shown for about 40 years.

In further lines, on the contrary, chemotherapy treatment remains a standard of care, although the results in terms of clinical outcomes are unsatisfactory.

The purpose of this review is to discuss new chemotherapeutics and how old chemotherapeutics may have a new life through innovative approaches.

2. Older Chemotherapeutics as a Companion to Immune-Checkpoint Inhibitors (ICIs): New Insights to Exploit Synergy

In the last decade, immunotherapy significantly improved the clinical outcomes of patients with thoracic malignancies. The use of immunotherapy in ED-SCLC holds its rationale on the high mutational rate and chemotherapy tumour cell killing effect, potentially associated with the expression and release, respectively, of a high number of neoantigens. This could elicit and enhance the activity of ICIs, translating into a clinical benefit [23].

Three phase III studies investigated the combination of chemotherapy and ICIs in the ED-SCLC: the CASPIAN study, the IMpower 133 and the KEYNOTE-604 [24–26] (Table 1).

Table 1. Phase III trial results of chemotherapy + immune checkpoint inhibitors. Abbreviations: mOS = median Overall Survival; mPFS = median Progression Free Survival; HR = Hazard Ratio.

First Line-Chemo-Immunotherapy Trials	IMpower 133		CASPIAN			KEYNOTE 604	
	Atezolizumab	Placebo	Durvalumab	Durvalumab Tremelimumab	Placebo	Pembrolizumab	Placebo
mPFS, mos	5.2	4.3	5.1	4.9	5.4	4.5	4.3
HR (95%)	0.77 (0.63–0.95)		0.78 (0.65–0.94)	0.84 (0.7–1.01)		0.75 (0.61–0.91)	
mOS, mos	12.3	10.3	12.9	10.4	10.5	10.8	9.7
HR (95%)	0.70 (0.54–0.91)		0.75 (0.62–0.91)	0.82 (0.68–1)		0.8 (0.64–0.98)	
12-mos OS, %	51.9	39	52.8	43.8	40	45.1	39.6
24-mos OS, %	22	16.8	22.2	23.4	14.4	22.5	11.2

The CASPIAN study randomised patients with ED-SCLC in a 1:1:1 ratio to receive durvalumab plus platinum–etoposide, durvalumab plus tremelimumab plus platinum–etoposide, or platinum–etoposide alone. The updated analysis showed an improvement in the mOS in the durvalumab plus platinum–etoposide arm as compared to chemotherapy alone (12.9–95% confidence interval [CI] 11.3–14.7–versus 10.5 months–95% CI 9.3–11.2–respectively), with 22.2 versus 14.4% of patients, respectively, alive at 24 months. The addition of tremelimumab to durvalumab and platinum and etoposide did not improve survival compared to chemotherapy alone [24]. The IMpower133 study randomised in a 1:1 ratio of patients with ED-SCLC to atezolizumab plus carboplatin–etoposide or placebo plus carboplatin-etoposide. The addition of atezolizumab improved both the mOS (12.3 vs. 10.3 months, respectively, hazard ratio [HR] for death 0.70, 95% CI 0.54–0.91, $p = 0.007$) and median PFS (5.2 vs. 4.3 months, HR for progression 0.77, 95% CI 0.62–0.96, $p = 0.02$) [25]. The KEYNOTE-604 study randomised in a 1:1 ratio the addition of pembrolizumab to platinum–etoposide vs. placebo plus platinum–etoposide in patients with ED-SCLC. The addition of pembrolizumab statistically improved only the median PFS (4.5 vs. 4.3 months, HR 0.75, 95% CI 0.61–0.91, $p = 0.023$), whereas the median OS was not significantly prolonged according to the prespecified criteria for statistical significance [26].

These studies have similar design and survival primary endpoints, with key differences regarding the use of a programmed-cell-death-1 (PD-1) inhibitor (instead of a PD-ligand-1 (PD-L1)) in the KEYNOTE-604 study, the choice of the carboplatin as the only platinum compound in the IMpower 133 study, and the open-label design in CASPIAN study. Overall, a durable survival benefit emerged from the combination of ICIs with chemotherapy. Atezolizumab received FDA approval in March 2019 and EMA approval in July 2019, whereas durvalumab was approved by FDA in March 2020, both as first-line therapy for ED-SCLC [27]. Regarding safety, the immune-related adverse events (irAEs) from the chemo-immunotherapy in ES-SCLC had a mild impact on the overall toxicity, without any significant difference in grade 3–4 AEs as compared to the chemotherapy [28].

Despite the favourable outcomes of chemo-immunotherapy observed in clinical trials, their translation into the clinical practice has some limitations. For instance, patients with severe comorbidities, frailties and/or an Eastern Cooperative Oncology Group (ECOG) Performance Status (PS) ≥2 were excluded from clinical trials, although they represent up to 30 to 40% of patients with ED-SCLC [29]. Furthermore, only those patients with stable brain metastases were enrolled in clinical trials. Consequently, the proportion of patients with brain disease treated in clinical trials with chemo-immunotherapy (10.4% overall) was smaller than that observed in clinical practice (which is up to 24%) [28].

Finally, no predictive biomarker for chemo-immunotherapy is still available in ED-SCLC. As demonstrated in the CASPIAN and IMpower 133 studies, neither PD-L1 expression nor tumour mutational burden (TMB) using various thresholds was predictive for efficacy from the addition of immunotherapy to the chemotherapy [30,31].

It is also noteworthy the lack of an obvious effect from ICIs on the median duration of response (DOR) observed across the different above-mentioned studies and in contrast with evidence in other cancers. One possible explanation for this effect is that a high overall response rate (ORR) is already achieved with the chemotherapy in SCLC, as for the high chemosensitivity of this cancer. In addition, the short follow-up duration of the studies might have hidden the gain in the median DOR from the addition of the immunotherapy. Indeed, when a landmark endpoint such as the 12-month ORR was considered, the benefit from ICIs in terms of response duration was detectable [32].

These considerations raise another important point regarding the optimal chemotherapy backbone for immunotherapy. The chemotherapy and chemo-immunotherapy arms PFS and OS curves separated after 4–7 months in clinical trials, which might suggest the lack of a synergistic effect between platinum–etoposide and ICIs. In experimental models, this lack of synergy was explained by a mechanism involving calreticulin (CALR) in immunogenic cell death. CALR is a protein normally located in the endoplasmic reticulum; it translocates to the cell membrane in response to the endoplasmic reticulum (ER) stress and provides an "eat-me" signal to antigen-presenting cells. The anthracyclines, but not etoposide, are efficient immunogenic cell death inducers and strongly immunogenic in preclinical mouse models [23]. In the phase I CheckMate 012 study on patients with non-small-cell-lung cancer (NSCLC), nivolumab was evaluated in three different chemotherapy regimens, including gemcitabine–cisplatin (for the squamous histology) or pemetrexed–cisplatin (for the nonsquamous tumours) or paclitaxel–carboplatin (for all the histologies). Although it was for a limited number of patients, the combination of nivolumab 5 mg/kg with paclitaxel–carboplatin yielded a similar overall response rate and higher 24-month OS than pemetrexed–cisplatin [33]. Further studies are needed to confirm whether a different chemotherapy backbone and platinum-containing regimens than platinum–etoposide may produce more favourable outcomes in ED-SCLC by the addition of the immunotherapy. A combination of lurbinectedin and atezolizumab is currently ongoing in a phase I/II study, with atezolizumab at a fixed dose of 1200 mg followed by lurbinectedin at a starting dose of 3.2 mg/m^2 as a 1-hour infusion on day 1, every three weeks, in patients with SCLC progressing on first-line platinum-based chemotherapy (NCT04253145).

Furthermore, there is a renewed interest in developing new platinum compounds by exploiting the recent knowledge on the sensitivity and resistance mechanisms of cancer cells, their epigenetic modifications, which translate into a platinum drug-tolerant cancer phenotype, and the immunomodulatory effects of platinum compounds to limit immune cell exhaustion [34].

3. Oral Versus Intravenous (i.v.) Formulations of Chemotherapy

The severe acute respiratory syndrome coronavirus 2 (SARS-CoV-2) pandemic has been challenging the oncology services and how we currently administer systemic treatments to patients with cancers, particularly in the palliative setting [35]. Patients with lung cancer could represent a vulnerable population to this infection [36–38] with high related mortality in the range of 25–39% [36–42].

Oral alternatives to i.v. anticancer therapies have gained attention, given efforts to reduce visits to the hospitals and the associated risk of infective transmission [42,43]. There is also a benefit in terms of patient convenience and preference with PO (per os) anticancer drugs, provided that their efficacy is equivalent to their i.v. counterparts [44].

Oral formulations of either topotecan and etoposide, two of the most active and used drugs in SCLC, are available and have the following sufficient data to support their use.

3.1. Oral Topotecan

Oral topotecan (2.3 mg/m^2/d, from day 1 to day 5, every 21 days) has demonstrated an absolute benefit in OS (of 12 weeks), slower quality of life deterioration, and greater symptom control, as compared to best supportive care (BSC) by a phase III randomised clinical trial in 141 patients with relapsed SCLC, regardless of their treatment-free interval (< or ≥60 days) [45].

As a second-line treatment, a phase III randomised trial comparing oral topotecan (2.3 mg/m^2/d from day 1 to day 5) with i.v. topotecan (1.5 mg/m^2/d from day 1 to day 5, every 21 days) demonstrated similar activity and tolerability between the two formulations in 309 patients with SCLC sensitive to initial chemotherapy (i.e., with a treatment-free interval of > or = 90 days). The absolute difference in response rates between oral and i.v. topotecan was −3.6% (18.3 vs. 21.9% for oral and i.v., respectively), whilst no difference in OS was observed. The toxicity profile was different with more thrombocytopenia and diarrhea for oral topotecan, but less neutropenia and anemia, as compared to i.v. topotecan [46]. Another phase III randomised trial compared oral topotecan (2.3 mg/m^2 from day 1 to day 5) every 21 days for six cycles to carboplatin (area under the curve 5 mg/mL per min day 1) plus etoposide (100 mg/m^2 from day 1 to day 3), as a second-line treatment for 164 patients with sensitive relapsed (at least 90 days after completion of first-line treatment) SCLC [22]. The median PFS was significantly longer in the combination chemotherapy group than in the oral topotecan group with an absolute benefit of 2.0 months (HR 0.57, 90% CI 0.41–0.73; p = 0.0041), but no OS difference was observed (HR 1.03, 95% CI 0.87–1.19; p = 0.94). The toxicity was comparable between the two groups, although two treatment-related deaths occurred in the oral topotecan group (both were febrile neutropenia with sepsis) as compared to none in the combination group.

As first-line treatment, a phase III study randomised 784 patients with untreated ED-SCLC to either oral topotecan (1.7 mg/m^2/d from day 1 to day 5) with i.v. cisplatin (60 mg/m^2 on day 5) (TC) or i.v. etoposide (100 mg/m^2/d from day 1 to day 3) with i.v. cisplatin (80 mg/m^2 on day 1) (PE) every 21 days. No difference in OS was observed between the two groups with the absolute difference of −0.03 (95% CI, −6.53 to 6.47), meeting the predefined criteria for non-inferiority of TC relative to PE. The regimens were similarly tolerable, with more frequent grade 3/4 neutropenia with PE (84% vs. 59%), grade 3/4 anemia and thrombocytopenia with TC (38 vs. 21% and 38 vs. 23%, respectively) [11].

3.2. Oral Etoposide

As an alternative to the i.v. formulation, the use of oral etoposide is supported by randomised data and a registry real-world population-based study of 2066 chemotherapy naïve patients with LD- (n = 762) and ED-SCLC (n = 1264) [47]. These studies showed, both in the LD- and in the ED-SCLC, no significant difference in OS between i.v. versus oral etoposide, although the oral group did require more dose reductions as compared to the i.v. group [47]. The oral etoposide was given on days 2 and 3 at the doubled dose of 200 mg/m^2 than 100 mg/m^2 of the i.v.

3.3. Conclusions

Based on these data, oral topotecan and etoposide could be considered as convenient alternatives to other i.v. therapies either in first-line, as a substitute for i.v. etoposide in platinum-combinations, and, for the oral topotecan, in subsequent treatment lines, as compared to other i.v. options, particularly for the platinum-resistant disease. Furthermore, the reduced incidence and severity of neutropenia observed with oral topotecan in two of the three above-mentioned phase III studies, either when compared to the i.v. etoposide and to its i.v. formulation, may represent a further advantage during the SARS-CoV-2 pandemic and speculatively for novel chemo-immunotherapy combinations.

4. Lurbinectedin

Lurbinectedin is an oncogenic transcription inhibitor. The drug is an analogue of trabectedin which covalently binds guanine residues in the minor groove of DNA, creating adducts that are able to induce double-strand breaks. As a consequence, a cascade of events occurs affecting the activity of DNA binding proteins, involving transcription factors and DNA repair mechanisms, leading to double-strand breaks and finally to cell death [48]. According to its mechanism of action, lurbinectedin showed antiproliferative and cytotoxic functions in several tumour cell lines and increased activity in cell lines bearing defects in the DNA mismatch repair. Moreover, lurbinectedin causes ICD (immunogenic cell death) and elicits anticancer immunity [49]. A single preclinical study demonstrated a direct effect of lurbinectedin on the tumour microenvironment, as it decreases the tumour-associated macrophages and circulating monocytes, and the angiogenic factor VEGF (vascular endothelial growth factor), with consequent reduced blood vessel density [50]. Lurbinectedin received accelerated approval by the FDA in 2020 for adult patients with metastatic SCLC progressing on or after platinum-based chemotherapy after demonstrating favourable ORR and DOR in an open-label, single-arm phase II trial [51] (Table 2).

Table 2. Lurbinectedin trials on small cell lung cancer (SCLC). Median progression-free survival (mPFS) and median overall survival (mOS) expressed in months, overall response rate (ORR) as a percentage, with 95% CI in graphs. Abbreviations: N/A = not available; mOS = median Overall Survival; mPFS = median Progression Free Survival; ORR = Overall Response Rate; ITT = Intent To Treat population.

Ref	Phase	N	Intervention	ITT			Platinum Sensitive			Platinum Refractory		
				mOS	mPFS	ORR	mOS	mPFS	ORR	mOS	mPFS	ORR
[52]	II	105	Lurbinectedin 3.2 mg/m2 1q21	9.3 (6.3–11.8)	3.5 (2.6–4.3)	35.2% (26.2–45.2)	11.9 (9.7–16.2)	4.6 (2.8–6.5)	45.0% (32.1–58.4)	5.0 (4.1–6.3)	2.6 (1.3–3.9)	22.2% (11.2–37.1)
[53]	I	27	Doxorubicin 50 mg/m² Lurbinectedin 4.0 mg (dose escalation from 3.5 mg) 1q21	7.9 (5.0–12.0)	4.1 (1.4–5.8)	57.7% (36.9–76.6)	11.5 (13.5–8.5)	5.8 (3.6–10.9)	91.7% (61.5–9.8)	4.9 (7.3–2.8)	3.5 (1.1–8.0)	33.3% (7.5–70.1)
[54]	Ib/II	13	Irinotecan 75 mg/m² 1,8q21 lurbinectedin 2.0 mg day 1q21 (dose escalation from 1.0 mg)	N/A	5.4	61.5%	N/A	N/A	N/A	N/A	N/A	N/A
[55]	III	613	Lurbinectedin 2.0 + Doxorubicin 40.0 mg1q21 versus cyclophosphamide + doxorubicin + vincristine (CAV) versus topotecan	N/A	N/A	50%	N/A	N/A	N/A	N/A	N/A	N/A
[56]	Ib/II	7	Paclitaxel 80 mg/mq 1,8q21 + lurbinectedin 2.2 mg day 1q21 (dose escalation from 1.0 mg)	N/A	4.8	71%	N/A	N/A	N/A	N/A	N/A	N/A

5. Clinical Development

5.1. Phase I Trials

A phase I study indicated the dose of 4 mg/m² or a flat dose of 7 mg i.v. every 21 days as safe dosing for lurbinectedin [57]. Based on preclinical data of synergy, another phase I study investigated the combination of lurbinectedin at 4 mg flat dose with doxorubicin 50 mg/m² [53]. The study enrolled 27 relapsed SCLC patients. When administered as second-line, the combination showed relevant activity as 91.7% of patients with a platinum-sensitive disease (defined as with platinum-free interval ≥ 90 days) and 33.3% of those with a platinum-resistant disease (with platinum-free interval < 90 days) achieved a disease response, with a PFS of 5.8 and 3.5 months, respectively. As a third-line treatment, all patients had a platinum-resistant disease, and the median PFS was 1.2 months. The major toxicities were hematologic, with high rates of grade 3–4 neutropenia (95%), leukopenia (79%), anemia (47%) and thrombocytopenia (26%). Aiming at improving the safety of this combination, an expansion cohort with a reduced dose of both drugs (lurbinectedin 2 mg/m^2 and doxorubicin 40 mg/m^2) was implemented, with an observed ORR of 37% and 53% in patients with a resistant and sensitive disease, respectively. The median PFS was 3.4 months in all patients, 1.5 and 5.7 months in those with a resistant and sensitive disease, respectively. The median OS was 7.9 months in all patients, 4.9 and 11.5 months in those with a resistant and sensitive disease, respectively [58].

Another combination with lurbinectedin and irinotecan has been explored in a phase Ib/II trial for advanced solid tumours (NCT02611024). Patients with SCLC included in this study were 13. The study investigates an escalating dose of lurbinectedin starting from 1 mg/m^2 on day one with a fixed dose of irinotecan 75 mg/m^2 on days 1 and 8, every 21 days. The recommended dose of lurbinectedin was 2.0 mg/m^2, and the maximum tolerated dose was 2.4 mg/m^2 in combination with irinotecan 75 mg/m^2 and prophylactic granulocyte-colony stimulating factor (G-CSF). In the SCLC cohort, the ORR was 61.5% [54,56].

5.2. Phase II Trial

Recently, the results of a phase II, open-label, basket trial exploring the safety and efficacy of lurbinectedin as a single-agent in several tumour types were published, including 105 patients with progressive SCLC [52]. The eligibility criteria required previous platinum-based chemotherapy and the absence of central nervous system (CNS) involvement. Forty-five and 60 patients had chemotherapy-resistant and -sensitive disease, respectively, with a chemotherapy-free interval of ≥90 days. The median follow-up was 17.1 months. The ORR was 35.2% (95% CI, 26.2–45.2), the median DOR and mOS were 5.3 and 10.8 months, respectively, in all SCLC patients. Patients with platinum-sensitive disease showed better outcomes as compared to platinum-resistant disease, with a median DOR of 6.2 months (95% CI, 3.5–7.3) and 4.7 months (95% CI, 2.6–5.6), respectively. The most frequent grade 3–4 AEs were hematological. Furthermore, a preplanned subset analysis of patients with chemotherapy-free interval ≥ 180 days was conducted on 20 patients. The ORR was 60% (95% CI, 36.1–86.9) in these patients, with a median DOR of 5.5. months (95% CI, 2.9–11.2) and a disease control rate (DCR) of 95% (95% CI, 75.1–99.9). The median PFS was 4.6 months (95% CI, 2.6–7.3), and the median OS 16.2 months (95% CI, 9.6-not reached). The most common grade 3–4 adverse events were hematological and increased liver function tests [59].

5.3. Phase III Trial

The phase III ATLANTIS study (NCT02566993) compared the combination of lurbinectedin and doxorubicin to topotecan or CAV at the physician's choice. Sixty-hundred-thirteen patients with SCLC progressing to one prior platinum-based chemotherapy were randomised 1:1. Lurbinectedin was given at 2 mg/m^2, lower than that of 3.2 mg/m^2 approved by the FDA. Patients were stratified by their chemotherapy-free interval, ECOG PS of 0 or 1–2, CNS involvement, prior use of ICIs (anti-PD-1/PD-L1 agents), and investigator's preference of topotecan or CAV. The recent press release from Jazz Pharmaceuticals and PharmaMar announced that the experimental treatment with lurbinectedin and doxorubicin missed its prespecified OS endpoint [55]. The secondary outcome endpoints and subgroup analyses, however, favoured the investigational combination in the intent-to-treat patient population, including the analysis of OS differences between the subgroup of patients treated with lurbinectedin and doxorubicin versus CAV; the OS and PFS in patients with and without CNS metastases; the ORR and DOR as assessed by an independent review committee.

Patients with relapsed SCLC still represent an unmet medical need as they have limited treatment options, lack of druggable targets, and poor prognosis. Despite the innovative mechanism of action and promising phase I and II trial results, lurbinectedin in combination with doxorubicin did not meet its prespecified OS endpoint in the phase III trial. As above-mentioned, however, there is still rationale and room for exploring combinations of lurbinectedin with ICIs +/− other chemotherapy agents, based on its immunomodulatory effects. (Table 2).

6. Novel Formulations of Traditional Chemotherapy Agents and "Promising" Drug Derivatives

Few cytotoxic agents with modest benefit and poor tolerability are currently available for SCLC, especially in later treatment lines. Although potentially associated with prolonged survival, their toxicity profile often represents a barrier to their administration at the full recommended dose. In addition to new agents with a different mechanism of action, the development of newer formulations of traditional chemotherapy drugs might represent a promising strategy to improve either activity and safety (Table 3).

6.1. Nanoparticle Albumin Bound-Paclitaxel (Nab-Paclitaxel)

Paclitaxel, alone or in combination with carboplatin, has shown activity in the refractory relapsed SCLC; however, its use is limited by potentially severe infusion reactions and peripheral neurotoxicity [60–62]. A solvent-free formulation of paclitaxel, the nanoparticle albumin-bound (nab)-paclitaxel, has been developed to improve the tolerability of paclitaxel, confirming efficacy and a safer profile than paclitaxel in pancreatic, breast cancer and NSCLC [63]. The activity of single-agent weekly nab-paclitaxel was tested in phase II, single-arm, NABSTER trial on 68 patients with relapsed SCLC, divided into two cohorts based on platinum-sensitivity (with a cut-off of 60 days). The primary endpoint was investigator-assessed ORR; PFS and OS were secondary endpoints. The RR was 8% and 14% in the refractory and sensitive cohort, respectively. The median PFS was similar in both the cohorts (1.8 and 1.9 months), whilst the median OS was longer in the sensitive than in the refractory cohort (6.6 vs. 3.6 months, respectively). The treatment was well tolerated with grade 3–4 neutropenia in 10% of patients and anemia in 4%. The study did not meet the primary endpoint on ORR, and the authors concluded that further investigations and a head-to-head comparison with topotecan were not justified [64].

6.2. Liposomal Irinotecan (Nal-IRI)

Liposomal formulations of chemotherapy agents, such as irinotecan and topotecan, have been developed to improve their efficacy through a slow and controlled release of the drug expected to prolong the exposure of tumour cells to these agents [65,66]. Irinotecan is active in the first-line treatment of SCLC in combination with cisplatin and is commonly used in Japan. In the second-line setting, single-agent irinotecan showed similar outcomes to those from topotecan and is included in several guidelines as a possible treatment option [67–69].

The liposomal encapsulation of irinotecan has been designed to prolong its circulation levels, exploiting the tumour vascular permeability and accumulation in the tumour tissue, where the macrophages can activate the drug [65]. Compared to irinotecan, its liposomal formulation demonstrated a longer persistence of plasma levels of SN-38, the active metabolite (50 vs. 8 h in mice), resulting in sustained topoisomerase-1 inhibition, increased DNA damage and cell death [70].

In metastatic pancreatic cancer, liposomal irinotecan in combination with fluorouracil and folinic acid showed significant improvement in OS in phase III Napoli-1 trial and was approved by the FDA and EMA as second-line treatment after failure of gemcitabine-based chemotherapy [71].

Table 3. Novel formulations of traditional chemotherapy and drug derivatives clinical trials results. mPFS and mOS expressed in months, ORR as percentage, with 95% CI in graphs. Abbreviations: ITT = Intent To Treat population; N/A = not available; mOS = median Overall Survival; mPFS = median Progression Free Survival; ORR = Overall Response Rate.

Drug	Phase	Intervention	ITT mOS	ITT mPFS	ITT ORR	Toxicities (G3–4 AEs)
Nab-paclitaxel	II (NABSTER)	Nab-paclitaxel 100 mg/mq die 1–8-15q28	3.65 refractory 6.64 sensitive	1.84 refractory 1.88 sensitive	11.8%	Fatigue (54%) Anaemia (38%) Neutropenia (29%) Leukopenia (26%) Diarrhea (21%)
Liposomal Irinotecan (Nal-IRI)	Ib/II	Nal-IRI 70 mg/m² or 85 mg/m² every 2 weeks	N/A	N/A	33.3%	Diarrhea ($n = 5$) Neutropenia ($n = 4$) Anemia ($n = 2$) Thrombocytopenia ($n = 2$)
Belotecan	II	Belotecan 0.5 mg/m² 1–5q21	9.9	2.2	24%	Neutropenia (grade 3–4) (88%) Thrombocytopenia (40.0%)
Belotecan	II	Belotecan 0.5 mg/m² 1–5q21	6.5 sensitive 4.0 refractory	2.8 sensitive 1.5 refractory	20% sensitive 10% refractory	Neutropenia (54%) Thrombocytopenia (38%) Anemia (32%)
Belotecan	IIb	Belotecan 0.5 mg/m² 1–5q21 vs. Topotecan 1.5 mg/m² 1–5q21	13.2 vs. 8.2 $p = 0.018$	4.8 vs. 3.8 $p = 0.96$	33 vs. 21% $p = 0.09$	Hematological disorders ($\geq 10\%$) Neutropenia Thrombocytopenia Anaemia
Amrubicin	II	amrubicin (40 mg/m² on days 1 through 3) or topotecan (1.0 mg/m² on days 1 through 5) every 3 weeks	8.1 vs. 8.4	3.5 vs. 2.2	38% (95% CI, 20 to 56%) vs. 13% (95% CI, 1 to 25%)	Neutropenia (79%) Febrile Neutropenia (14%) Anemia (21%) Thrombocytopenia (28%)
Amrubicin	II	Amrubicin 40 mg/m² on days 1 to 3 every 3 weeks	11.2	2.6 refractory 4.2 sensitive	52%	Neutropenia (83%) Thrombocytopenia (20%) Anemia (33%) Febrile neutropenia (5%)
Amrubicin	II	Amrubicin (40 mg/m²/d for 3 every 21 days) (NB: refractory patients)	6.0 (95% CI, 4.8 to 7.1)	3.2 (95% CI, 2.4 to 4.0)	21.3% (95% CI, 12.7 to 32.3%)	Neutropenia (67%) Thrombocytopenia (41%) Anemia (30%) Febrile neutropenia (12%)
Amrubicin	II	amrubicin (40 mg/m² on days 1 through 3) or topotecan (1.0 mg/m² on days 1 through 5) every 3 weeks NB: platinum sensitive	9.2 vs. 7.6	4.5 vs. 3.3	44 vs. 15%; $p = 0.021$	Neutropenia (61%) Thrombocytopenia (39%) Leukopenia (39%) Anemia (25%) Febrile neutropenia (10%)
Amrubicin	III	amrubicin (40 mg/m² on days 1 through 3) or topotecan (1.0 mg/m² on days 1 through 5) every 3 weeks	7.5 vs. 7.8 (HR = 0.880; $p = 0.170$)	4.1 vs. 3.5 (HR, 0.802; $p = 0.018$)	31.1 vs. 16.9% (odd ratio 2.223; $p = 0.001$)	Neutropenia (41%) Thrombocytopenia (21%) Anemia (16%) Infections (16%) Febrile neutropenia (10%) Cardiac disorders (5%) Need of transfusion (32%)
Amrubicin	III	cisplatin (60 mg/m², day 1) amrubicin (40 mg/m², days 1–3) vs. cisplatin and etoposide (100 mg/m², days 1–3) once every 21 days.	11.8 vs. 10.3 ($p = 0.08$)	6.8 vs. 5.7 months ($p = 0.35$)	69.8 vs. 57.3%	Neutropenia (54.4%) Leukopenia (34.9%) Thrombocytopenia (16.1%)
Temozolomide (TMZ)	II	TMZ 75 mg/mq/die 1→21q28	NA	NA	22% sensitive 19% refractory	Thrombocytopenia and neutropenia (14%)
Temozolomide (TMZ)	II	TMZ 200 mg/mq/die 1→5 q28	1.8	5.8	12%	Anemia, thrombocytopenia and neutropenia (20%)

SCLC is highly vascularised and enriched by tumour-associated-macrophages (TAM). These two characteristics suggest a possible high penetration of liposomal irinotecan (nal-IRI) in the tumour tissue and activation by local phagocytic through high CES (carboxylesterase) levels, the enzyme that converts irinotecan in its active metabolite SN-38 resulting in effective cytotoxic activity [72–74]. In preclinical models, nal-IRI showed superior antitumour activity than topotecan and irinotecan, either in cell-line derived models and patients-derived xenograft models built after progression to carboplatin and etoposide [75]. These preclinical data supported the clinical development of nal-IRI in patients with SCLC.

The RESILIENT study is an ongoing two-part phase II/III trial assessing the potential use of nal-IRI in patients with SCLC who progressed on or after platinum-based regimens. Part one of the trial involved dose-finding and dose-escalation analyses, whilst in the second part, patients were randomised to liposomal irinotecan or topotecan to compare efficacy in terms of PFS and OS. In the dose-finding phase, patients were divided into two cohorts to receive liposomal irinotecan every 2 weeks at 70 mg/m^2 or 85 mg/m^2. The cohort treated with 85 mg/m^2 dose was closed early for dose-limiting toxicities. In the second cohort, 12 patients received the 70 mg/m^2 dose, which was deemed by the investigators as tolerable. Among these patients, preliminary exploratory efficacy endpoints were promising, with a RR of 33.3%, the median time to response of 6 weeks and an overall DCR of 58.3% [76]. This led to a dose-expansion phase with additional 13 patients, whose safety data were presented at the 2020 World Conference on Lung Cancer (WCLC). Among the 25 patients who received the 70 mg/m^2 dose, the grade $\geq$3 treatment-emergent AEs occurred in 40% (n = 10) of patients, mostly represented by diarrhea (n = 5), neutropenia (n = 4), anemia (n = 2) and thrombocytopenia (n = 2) [77]. The trial is still recruiting for the second part (www.ClinicalTrials.gov Identifier: NCT03088813; accessed on 20 January 2021).

6.3. Belotecan

Belotecan is a new camptothecin analogue and topoisomerase I inhibitor. Preclinical data on mice models suggested superior antitumour efficacy and wider therapeutic margins than topotecan [78]. In phase II clinical trials, belotecan monotherapy showed encouraging activity and good tolerability in patients with relapsed SCLC [79,80]. More recently, second-line belotecan has been compared to topotecan in a phase IIb trial on 164 SCLC patients progressing to platinum-based chemotherapy. Patients were randomised in a 1:1 ratio to receive five consecutive daily intravenous infusions of topotecan (1.5 mg/m^2) or belotecan (0.5 mg/m^2) every 3 weeks for six cycles. The study was powered to assess the non-inferiority of belotecan to topotecan in ORR. Belotecan significantly improved ORR (33 vs. 21%, respectively, p = 0.09) and DCR (85 vs. 70%, p = 0.030) as compared to topotecan. Furthermore, the median OS was significantly longer with belotecan than topotecan (13.2 vs. 8.2 months, HR = 0.69, 95% CI 0.48–0.99), with a favourable safety profile. On the basis of these promising results, belotecan might be another treatment option for second-line treatment in SCLC, pending phase III trials to confirm its efficacy in this setting [81].

6.4. Amrubicin

Amrubicin is a third-generation synthetic anthracycline with potent inhibiting activity on the topoisomerase II. Among drugs belonging to the same class, amrubicin has fewer chronic cardiological effects (e.g., cardiomyopathy) and no cumulative-dose heart damage in animal models [82]. Amrubicin is approved in Japan as a single-agent for SCLC after the failure of platinum-based chemotherapy, whilst it is under evaluation in other countries. In this setting, it has been investigated by several studies on Asian patients, showing ORR ranging from 36 to 52% and median OS of 7–12 months [83–87]. Two phase II studies demonstrated clinical efficacy in the Caucasian population also, with higher ORR as compared to topotecan (44 vs. 15%, respectively) [88,89]. A phase III study compared amrubicin with topotecan in patients with SCLC progressing to platinum–etoposide chemotherapy. A total of 637 patients were randomly assigned in a 2:1 ratio to receive amrubicin 40 mg/m^2 on days 1–3 every three weeks or topotecan 1.5 mg/m^2 on days 1–5 of 21 days cycles. Amrubicin did not improve the primary endpoint of OS as compared to topotecan (7.5 vs. 7.8 months, HR 0.88, p = 0.170), despite an improvement in the median PFS (4.1 vs. 3.5 months, HR, 0.80, p = 0.018) and ORR (31.1 vs. 16.9%, odds ratio [OR] 2.22, p < 0.001). A slight survival benefit of two weeks was observed in the subgroup of patients with refractory disease. The safety profile favoured amrubicin as far as hematologic events are concerned; however, higher rates of infections (16 vs. 10%, respectively) and febrile neutropenia (10 vs. 3%, respectively) were linked to amrubicin [90].

In the first-line setting of ED-SCLC, the combination of amrubicin plus cisplatin has been compared to cisplatin–etoposide in phase III non-inferiority study in Chinese patients. The amrubicin–cisplatin regimen was non-inferior to standard platinum–etoposide chemotherapy on OS (median OS of 11.8 vs. 10.3 months, p = 0.08), with a slight non-significant improvement of 1.5 months [91].

The potential interest of this drug derives from its possible synergy with other agents. Although the results of the lurbinectedin/doxorubicin combination showed by the ATLANTIS trial press release were disappointing [55], amrubicin still remains a plausible alternative to the doxorubicin as a potential companion drug for lurbinectedin in future clinical trials. Furthermore, based on its immunomodulatory effect, the association of amrubicin and pembrolizumab is under evaluation in a phase II trial in patients with refractory SCLC [92]. Therefore, despite the modest activity showed in non-Asian patients as single-agent, amrubicin may still have a role as a new companion for combination strategies in clinical trials.

6.5. Temozolomide

Temozolomide is an oral alkylating agent that induces cytotoxic damage and apoptosis through single-strand DNA breaks. The rationale for its application in SCLC is strong, as temozolomide has a good penetration through the blood–brain barrier, which can be useful for brain metastasis, and SCLC has aberrantly methylated O6-methylguanine-DNA methyltransferase MGMT, the enzyme involved in the repair mechanism of the DNA damage induced by temozolomide [93].

Two phase II single-arm studies investigated the role of the single agent temozolomide in SCLC patients who progressed to one or two lines of chemotherapy, stratified on the basis of platinum sensitiveness. In the first by Pietanza et al., 64 patients were enrolled and received temozolomide 75 mg/m^2/die for 21 days in a 28-day cycle. The primary endpoint was ORR in the platinum-sensitive and refractory cohort. The ORR was 22% (95% CI, 9–40%) and 19% (95% CI, 7–36%), respectively. One complete remission was observed in the platinum-sensitive cohort. The main limiting toxicities were grade 3 thrombocytopenia and neutropenia, which were observed in nine patients (14%) [94].

In the second study by Zauderer MG et al., a different schedule was used to improve tolerability on hematologic toxicities. Temozolomide was given 200 mg/m^2/die for 5 days in a 28-day cycle. Among 25 SCLC patients, five patients have grade 3–4 events (mostly anemia, thrombocytopenia and neutropenia). The ORR was 12% (95% CI 3–31%), with two responses also observed in refractory patients, median PFS was 1.8 months (95% CI 0.9–3.5 months) and median OS 5.8 months (95% CI: 3.3–9.8 months) [95].

Data on brain metastasis response were conflicting among the two studies. In the first study, at the standard dose, 38% had a CR (complete response) or PR (partial response) (95% CI, 14–68%) [94], whilst no response was seen in the eight patients with target brain lesions of the second study (four had stable disease and four progression) [95].

MGMT promoter methylation is a well-known predictive factor of response to temozolomide in glioma [96]. For this reason, it was evaluated in both the aforementioned studies. In the first one, ORR improved in patients with methylated MGMT promoter with respect to patients without methylation (38 vs. 7%; p = 0.08) [94]. In the second one, 50% of patients had methylation in MGMT promoter, but the number of patients was too small to derive statistical conclusions on response [95].

However, due to the scarce data on efficacy and hematologic toxicity, temozolamide single agent is not routinely used in clinical practice.

More recently, the association of temozolamide with PARP (poly ADP-ribose polymerase)-inhibitors, veliparib and olaparib, has been investigated [97,98]. Alterations in the PARP-dependent base excision repair pathway are an established resistance mechanism to temozolamide, and preclinical models validated the rationale for the clinical development of combinations with temozolamide and PARP-inhibitors [99]. The combination of temozolamide plus veliparib or olaparib improved ORR compared to temozolamide alone in phase II trials [97,98]. However, data on larger cohorts and phase III trials are ongoing to assess the possible application in clinical practice.

7. Conclusions

After many years of inactivity, the treatment of SCLC has been observing a renewed interest thanks to the introduction of immunotherapy in the first-line setting.

Cytotoxic agents remain so far the backbone treatment for immunotherapy in the first-line and the only current options in later therapeutic lines, although limited benefit and relevant toxicity, particularly in the platinum-resistant population.

Re-interpreting and exploiting the mechanisms of action of old cytotoxic agents, such as cisplatin and anthracyclines, with a view to their immunomodulatory effects, can unveil new therapeutic scenarios with combination strategies based on ICIs and different chemotherapeutic agents or their new formulations.

Despite the limitations highlighted by all the chemotherapy molecules currently investigated, the discovery of transcription factors and their overexpression will allow the segmentation of SCLC into different molecular subgroups, which could benefit from combinations of chemotherapy with other small molecules (such as PARP inhibitors, Aurora kinase inhibitors).

The chemotherapy chapter for SCLC is not yet closed, and new studies are needed to better understand its role in these future therapeutic scenarios.

Funding: This research received no external funding.

Acknowledgments: The authors thank Elisa Sala, Ph.D. medical writer, for her contribution in drafting and editing the text.

Conflicts of Interest: The authors declare no conflict of interest.

References

1. Gazdar, A.F.; Bunn, P.A.; Minna, J.D. Small-cell lung cancer: What we know, what we need to know and the path forward. *Nat. Rev. Cancer* **2017**, *17*, 725–737. [CrossRef]
2. Van Meerbeeck, J.P.; Fennell, D.A.; De Ruysscher, D.K. Small-cell lung cancer. *Lancet* **2011**, *378*, 1741–1755. [CrossRef]
3. Rami-Porta, R. *Staging Handbook in Thoracic Oncology*, 2nd ed.; IASLC: Denver, CO, USA, 2016.
4. Evans, W.K.; Shepherd, F.A.; Feld, R.; Osoba, D.; Dang, P.; Deboer, G. VP-16 and cisplatin as first-line therapy for small-cell lung cancer. *J. Clin. Oncol.* **1985**, *3*, 1471–1477. [CrossRef]
5. Roth, B.J.; Johnson, D.H.; Einhorn, L.H.; Schacter, L.P.; Cherng, N.C.; Cohen, H.J.; Crawford, J.; Randolph, J.A.; Goodlow, J.L.; Broun, G.O. Randomized study of cyclophosphamide, doxorubicin, and vincristine versus etoposide and cisplatin versus alternation of these two regimens in extensive small-cell lung cancer: A phase 3 trial of the Southeastern Cancer Study Group. *J. Clin. Oncol.* **1992**, *10*, 282–291. [CrossRef]
6. Pujol, J.L.; Carestia, L.; Daures, J.P. Is there a case for cisplatin in the treatment of small-cell lung cancer? A meta-analysis of randomized trials of a cisplatin-containing regimen versus a regimen without this alkylating agent. *Br. J. Cancer* **2000**, *83*, 8–15. [CrossRef] [PubMed]
7. Mascaux, C.; Paesmans, M.; Berghmans, T.; Branle, F.; Lafitte, J.J.; Lemaitre, F.; Meert, A.P.; Vermylen, P.; Sculier, J.P. European Lung Cancer Working Party (ELCWP). A systematic review of the role of etoposide and cisplatin in the chemotherapy of small cell lung cancer with methodology assessment and meta-analysis. *Lung Cancer* **2000**, *30*, 23–36. [CrossRef]
8. Amarasena, I.U.; Walters, J.A.; Wood-Baker, R.; Fong, K.M. Platinum versus non-platinum chemotherapy regimens for small cell lung cancer. *Cochr. Database Syst. Rev.* **2008**, *4*, CD006849.

9. Rossi, A.; Di Maio, M.; Chiodini, P.; Rudd, R.M.; Okamoto, H.; Skarlos, D.V.; Früh, M.; Qian, W.; Tamura, T.; Samantas, E.; et al. Carboplatin- or cisplatin-based chemotherapy in first-line treatment of small-cell lung cancer: The COCIS meta-analysis of individual patient data. *J. Clin. Oncol.* **2012**, *30*, 1692–1698. [CrossRef]
10. Liu, Z.L.; Wang, B.; Liu, J.Z.; Liu, W.W. Irinotecan plus cisplatin compared with etoposide plus cisplatin in patients with previously untreated extensive-stage small cell lung cancer: A meta-analysis. *J. Cancer Res. Ther.* **2018**, *14*, S1076–S1083.
11. Eckardt, J.R.; Von Pawel, J.; Papai, Z.; Tomova, A.; Tzekova, V.; Crofts, T.E.; Brannon, S.; Wissel, P.; Ross, G. Open-label, multicenter, randomized, phase 3 study comparing oral topotecan/cisplatin versus etoposide/cisplatin as treatment for chemo-therapy-naive patients with extensive-disease small-cell lung cancer. *J. Clin. Oncol.* **2006**, *24*, 2044–2051. [CrossRef] [PubMed]
12. O'Brien, M.E.; Konopa, K.; Lorigan, P.; Bosquee, L.; Marshall, E.; Bustin, F.; Margerit, S.; Fink, C.; Stigt, J.A.; Dingemans, A.M.; et al. Randomised phase ii study of amrubicin as single agent or in combination with cisplatin versus cisplatin etoposide as first-line treatment in patients with extensive stage small cell lung cancer—eortc 08062. *Eur. J. Cancer* **2011**, *47*, 2322–2330. [CrossRef] [PubMed]
13. Baka, S.; Agelaki, S.; Kotsakis, A.; Veslemes, M.; Papakotoulas, P.; Agelidou, M.; Agelidou, A.; Tsaroucha, E.; Pavlakou, G.; Gerogianni, A.; et al. Phase 3 study comparing sequential versus alternate administration of cisplatin–etoposide and topotecan as first-line treatment in small cell lung cancer. *Anticancer Res.* **2010**, *30*, 3031–3038.
14. Ignatiadis, M.; Mavroudis, D.; Veslemes, M.; Boukovinas, J.; Syrigos, K.; Agelidou, M.; Agelidou, A.; Gerogianni, A.; Pavlakou, G.; Tselepatiotis, E.; et al. Sequential versus alternating administration of cisplatin/etoposide and topotecan as first-line treatment in extensive-stage small-cell lung cancer: Preliminary results of a phase 3 trial of the Hellenic Oncology Research Group. *Clin. Lung Cancer* **2005**, *7*, 183–189. [CrossRef] [PubMed]
15. Masutani, M.; Ochi, Y.; Kadota, A.; Akusawa, H.; Kisohara, A.; Takahashi, N.; Koya, Y.; Horie, T. Dose-intensive weekly alternating chemotherapy for patients with small cell lung cancer: Randomized trial, can it improve survival of patients with good prognostic factors? *Oncol. Rep.* **2000**, *7*, 305–310. [CrossRef] [PubMed]
16. Sculier, J.P.; Paesmans, M.; Lecomte, J.; Van Cutsem, O.; Lafitte, J.J.; Berghmans, T.; Koumakis, G.; Florin, M.C.; Thiriaux, J.; Michel, J.; et al. A three-arm phase 3 randomised trial assessing, in patients with extensive- disease small-cell lung cancer, accelerated chemotherapy with support of haematological growth factor or oral anti- biotics. *Br. J. Cancer* **2001**, *85*, 1444–1451. [CrossRef]
17. Ueoka, H.; Kiura, K.; Tabata, M.; Kamei, H.; Gemba, K.; Sakae, K.; Hiraki, Y.; Hiraki, S.; Segawa, Y.; Harada, M. A randomized trial of hybrid administration of cyclophosphamide, doxorubicin, and vincristine (cav)/cisplatin and etoposide (pvp) versus sequential administration of cav-pvp for the treatment of patients with small cell lung carcinoma: Results of long term follow-up. *Cancer* **1998**, *83*, 283–290.
18. Humblet, Y.; Symann, M.; Bosly, A.; Delaunois, L.; Francis, C.; Machiels, J.; Beauduin, M.; Doyen, C.; Weynants, P.; Longueville, J. Late intensification chemotherapy with autologous bone marrow transplantation in selected small-cell carcinoma of the lung: A randomized study. *J. Clin. Oncol.* **1987**, *5*, 1864–1873. [CrossRef]
19. Banna, G.L.; Simonelli, M.; Santoro, A. High-dose chemotherapy followed by autologous hematopoietic stem-cell transplantation for the treatment of solid tumors in adults: A critical review. *Stem Cell Res. Ther.* **2007**, *2*, 65–82.
20. Lara, P.N.; Moon, J.; Redman, M.W.; Semrad, T.J.; Kelly, K.; Allen, J.W.; Gitlitz, B.J.; Mack, P.C.; Gandara, D.R. Relevance of platinum sensitivity status in relapsed/refractory extensive stage small cell lung cancer (ES-SCLC) in the modern era: A patient level analysis of SWOG trials. *J. Thorac. Oncol.* **2016**, *10*, 110–115. [CrossRef]
21. Von Pawel, J.; Schiller, J.H.; Shepherd, F.A.; Fields, S.Z.; Kleisbauer, J.P.; Chrysson, N.G.; Stewart, D.J.; Clark, P.I.; Palmer, M.C.; Depierre, A.; et al. Topotecan versus cyclophosphamide, doxorubicin, and vincristine for the treatment of recurrent small-cell lung cancer. *J. Clin. Oncol.* **1999**, *17*, 658–667. [CrossRef] [PubMed]
22. Baize, N.; Monnet, I.; Greillier, L.; Geier, M.; Lena, H.; Janicot, H.; Vergnenegre, A.; Crequit, J.; Lamy, R.; Auliac, J.B.; et al. Carboplatin plus etoposide versus topotecan as second-line treatment for patients with sensitive relapsed small-cell lung cancer: An open-label, multicentre, randomised, phase 3 trial. *Lancet Oncol.* **2020**, *21*, 1224–1233. [CrossRef]
23. Mankor, J.M.; Zwiereng, F.; Dumoulin, D.W.; Neefjes, J.; Aerts, J. A brief report on combination chemotherapy and antiepro-grammed death (ligand) 1 treatment in small-cell lung cancer: Did we choose the optimal chemotherapy backbone? *Eur. J. Cancer* **2020**, *137*, 40–44. [CrossRef]
24. Goldman, J.W.; Dvorkin, M.; Chen, Y.; Reinmuth, N.; Hotta, K.; Trukhin, D.; Statsenko, G.; Hochmair, M.J.; Özgüroğlu, M.; Ji, J.H.; et al. Durvalumab, with or without tremelimumab, plus platinum-etoposide versus platinum-etoposide alone in first-line treatment of extensive-stage small-cell lung cancer (CASPIAN): Updated results from a randomised, controlled, open-label, phase 3 trial. *Lancet Oncol.* **2020**, *4*, S1470–S2045.
25. Horn, L.; Mansfield, A.S.; Szczęsna, A.; Havel, L.; Krzakowski, M.; Hochmair, M.J.; Huemer, F.; Losonczy, G.; Johnson, M.L.; Nishio, M.; et al. First-line atezolizumab plus chemotherapy in extensive-stage small-cell lung cancer. *N. Engl. J. Med.* **2018**, *379*, 2220–2229. [CrossRef] [PubMed]
26. Rudin, C.M.; Awad, M.M.; Navarro, A.; Gottfried, M.; Peters, S.; Csőszi, T.; Cheema, P.K.; Rodriguez-Abreu, D.; Wollner, M.; Yang, J.C.; et al. Pembrolizumab or placebo plus etoposide and platinum as first-line therapy for extensive-stage small-cell lung cancer: Randomized, double-blind, phase 3 KEYNOTE-604 study. *J. Clin. Oncol.* **2020**, *38*, 2369–2379. [CrossRef]
27. Melosky, B.; Cheema, P.K.; Brade, A.; McLeod, D.; Liu, G.; Price, P.W.; Jao, K.; Schellenberg, D.D.; Juergens, R.; Leighl, N.; et al. Prolonging survival: The role of immune checkpoint inhibitors in the treatment of extensive-stage small cell lung cancer. *Oncologist* **2020**, *25*, 981–992. [CrossRef]

28. Facchinetti, F.; Di Maio, M.; Tiseo, M. Adding PD-1/PD-L1 inhibitors to chemotherapy for the first-line treatment of extensive stage small cell lung cancer (SCLC): A meta-analysis of randomized trials. *Cancers* **2020**, *12*, 2645. [CrossRef] [PubMed]
29. Okamoto, H.; Watanabe, K.; Kunikane, H.; Yokoyama, A.; Kudoh, S.; Asakawa, T.; Shibata, T.; Kunitoh, H.; Tamura, T.; Saijo, N. Randomised phase 3 trial of carboplatin plus etoposide vs split doses of cisplatin plus etoposide in elderly or poor-risk patients with extensive disease small-cell lung cancer: JCOG 9702. *Br. J. Cancer* **2007**, *97*, 162–169. [CrossRef] [PubMed]
30. Liu, S.V.; Horn, L.; Mok, T.; Mansfield, A.; De Boer, R.; Losonczy, G.; Sugawara, S.; Dziadziuszko, R.; Krzakowski, M.; Smolin, A. 1781MO IMpower133: Characterisation of long-term survivors treated first-line with chemotherapy ± atezolizumab in extensive-stage small cell lung cancer. *Ann. Oncol.* **2020**, *31*, S1032–S1033. [CrossRef]
31. Paz-Ares, L.G.; Dvorkin, M.; Chen, Y.; Reinmuth, N.; Hotta, K.; Trukhin, D.; Statsenko, G.; Hochmair, M.; Özgüroglu, M.; Ji, J.H. Durvalumab±tremelimumab+ platinum-etoposideinfirst-lineextensive-stage SCLC (ES-SCLC): Updated results from the phase 3 CASPIAN study. *J. Clin. Oncol.* **2020**, *38*, 9002. [CrossRef]
32. Landre, T.; Chouahnia, K.; Des Guetz, G.; Duchemann, B.; Assié, J.B.; Chouaïd, C. First-line immune-checkpoint inhibitor plus chemotherapy versus chemotherapy alone for extensive-stage small-cell lung cancer: A meta-analysis. *Ther. Adv. Med. Oncol* **2020**, *12*. [CrossRef] [PubMed]
33. Rizvi, N.A.; Hellmann, M.D.; Brahmer, J.R.; Juergens, R.A.; Borghaei, H.; Gettinger, S.; Chow, L.Q.; Gerber, D.E.; Laurie, S.A.; Goldman, J.W.; et al. Nivolumab in combination with platinum-based doublet chemotherapy for first-line treatment of advanced non-small-cell lung cancer. *J. Clin. Oncol.* **2016**, *34*, 2969–2979. [CrossRef] [PubMed]
34. Rottenberg, S.; Disler, C.; Perego, P. The rediscovery of platinum-based cancer therapy. *Nat. Rev. Cancer* **2021**, *21*, 37–50. [CrossRef] [PubMed]
35. Curigliano, G.; Banerjee, S.; Cervantes, A.; Garassino, M.C.; Garrido, P.; Girard, N.; Haanen, J.; Jordan, K.; Lordick, F.; Machiels, J.P.; et al. Managing cancer patients during the COVID-19 pandemic: An ESMO multidisciplinary expert consensus. *Ann. Oncol.* **2020**, *31*, 1320–1335. [CrossRef] [PubMed]
36. Liang, W.; Guan, W.; Chen, R.; Wang, W.; Li, J.; Xu, K.; Li, C.; Ai, Q.; Lu, W.; Liang, H.; et al. Cancer patients in SARS-CoV-2 infection: A nationwide analysis in China. *Lancet Oncol.* **2020**, *21*, 335–337. [CrossRef]
37. Zhang, L.; Zhu, F.; Xie, L.; Wang, C.; Wang, J.; Chen, R.; Jia, P.; Guan, H.Q.; Peng, L.; Chen, Y.; et al. Clinical characteristics of COVID-19-infected cancer patients: A retrospective case study in three hospitals within Wuhan, China. *Ann. Oncol.* **2020**, *31*, 894–901. [CrossRef]
38. Yu, J.; Ouyang, W.; Chua, M.L.K.; Xie, C. SARS-CoV-2 transmission in patients with cancer at a tertiary care hospital in Wuhan, China. *JAMA Oncol.* **2020**, *6*, 1108–1110. [CrossRef]
39. Garassino, M.C.; Whisenant, J.G.; Huang, L.C.; Trama, A.; Torri, V.; Agustoni, F.; Baena, J.; Banna, G.; Berardi, R.; Bettini, A.C.; et al. COVID-19 in patients with thoracic malignancies (TERAVOLT): First results of an international, registry-based, cohort study. *Lancet Oncol.* **2020**, *21*, 914–922. [CrossRef]
40. Guan, W.; Ni, Z.; Hu, Y.; Liang, W.; Ou, C.; He, J.; Liu, L.; Shan, H.; Lei, C.; Hui, D.S.C.; et al. Clinical characteristics of Coronavirus disease 2019 in China. *N. Eng. J. Med.* **2020**, *382*, 1708–1720. [CrossRef]
41. Grasselli, G.; Zangrillo, A.; Zanella, A.; Antonelli, M.; Cabrini, L.; Castelli, A.; Cereda, D.; Coluccello, A.; Foti, G.; Fumagalli, R.; et al. Baseline characteristics and outcomes of 1591 patients infected with SARS-CoV-2 admitted to ICUs of the Lombardy region, Italy. *JAMA* **2020**, *323*, 1574–1581. [CrossRef] [PubMed]
42. Burki, T.K. Cancer guidelines during the COVID-19 pandemic. *Lancet Oncol.* **2020**, *21*, 629–630. [CrossRef]
43. Banna, G.; Curioni-Fontecedro, A.; Friedlaender, A.; Addeo, A. How we treat patients with lung cancer during the SARS-CoV-2 pandemic: Primum non nocere. *ESMO Open* **2020**, *5*. [CrossRef]
44. Banna, G.L.; Collova, E.; Gebbia, V.; Lipari, H.; Giuffrida, P.; Cavallaro, S.; Condorelli, R.; Buscarino, C.; Tralongo, P.; Ferrau, F. Anticancer oral therapy: Emerging related issues. *Cancer Treat. Rev.* **2010**, *36*, 595–605. [CrossRef]
45. O'Brien, M.E.; Ciuleanu, T.E.; Tsekov, H.; Shparyk, Y.; Cucevia, B.; Juhasz, G.; Thatcher, N.; Ross, G.A.; Dan, G.C.; Crofts, T. Phase 3 trial comparing supportive care alone with supportive care with oral topotecan in patients with relapsed small-cell lung cancer. *J. Clin. Oncol.* **2006**, *24*, 5441–5447. [CrossRef]
46. Eckardt, J.R.; von Pawel, J.; Pujol, J.L.; Papai, Z.; Quoix, E.; Ardizzoni, A.; Poulin, R.; Preston, A.J.; Dane, G.; Ross, G. Phase 3 study of oral compared with intravenous topotecan as second-line therapy in small-cell lung cancer. *J. Clin. Oncol.* **2007**, *25*, 2086–2092. [CrossRef] [PubMed]
47. Karachiwala, H.; Tilley, D.; Abdel-Rahman, O.; Morris, D. Comparison of oral versus intravenous etoposide in the management of small-cell lung cancer: A real-world, population-based study. *Clin. Resp. J.* **2020**. [CrossRef]
48. Leal, J.F.; Martínez-Díez, M.; García-Hernández, V.; Moneo, V.; Domingo, A.; Bueren-Calabuig, J.A.; Negri, A.; Gago, F.; Guillén-Navarro, M.J.; Avilés, P.; et al. PM01183, a new DNA minor groove covalent binder with potent in vitro and in vivo anti-tumour activity. *Br. J. Pharmacol.* **2010**, *161*, 1099–1110. [CrossRef]
49. Xie, W.; Forveille, S.; Iribarren, K.; Sauvat, A.; Senovilla, L.; Wang, Y.; Humeau, J.; Perez-Lanzon, M.; Zhou, H.; Martínez-Leal, J.F.; et al. Lurbinectedin synergizes with immune checkpoint blockade to generate anticancer immunity. *Oncoimmunology* **2019**, *8*, e1656502. [CrossRef]
50. Belgiovine, C.; Bello, E.; Liguori, M.; Craparotta, I.; Mannarino, L.; Paracchini, L.; Beltrame, L.; Marchini, S.; Galmarini, C.M.; Mantovani, A.; et al. Lurbinectedin reduces tumour-associated macrophages and the inflammatory tumour microenvironment in preclinical models. *Br. J. Cancer* **2017**, *117*, 628–638. [CrossRef] [PubMed]

1. FDA Grants Accelerated Approval to Lurbinectedin for Metastatic Small Cell Lung Cancer. 2020. Available online: https://bit.ly/3g8LliK (accessed on 3 December 2020).
2. Trigo, J.; Subbiah, V.; Besse, B.; Moreno, V.; López, R.; Sala, M.A.; Peters, S.; Ponce, S.; Fernández, C.; Alfaro, V.; et al. Lurbinectedin as second line treatment for patients with small-cell lung cancer: A single-arm, open-label, phase 2 basket trial. *Lancet Oncol.* **2020**, *21*, 645–654. [CrossRef]
3. Calvo, E.; Moreno, V.; Flynn, M.; Holgado, E.; Olmedo, M.E.; Lopez Criado, M.P.; Kahatt, C.; Lopez-Vilariño, J.A.; Siguero, M.; Fernandez-Teruel, C.; et al. Antitumor activity of lurbinectedin (PM01183) and doxorubicin in relapsed small-cell lung cancer: Results from a phase I study. *Ann. Oncol.* **2017**, *28*, 2559–2566. [CrossRef] [PubMed]
4. Ponce Aix, S.; Cote, G.M.; Gonzalez, A.F.; Falcon Gonzalez, A.; Sepulveda, J.M.; Aguilar, E.J.; Sanchez-Simon, I.; Flor, M.J.; Nuñez, R.; Gonzalez, E.M.; et al. Lurbinectedin (LUR) in combination with irinotecan (IRI) in patients (pts) with advanced solid tumors: Updated results from a phase Ib-II trial. *J. Clin. Oncol.* **2020**, *38*, 3514. [CrossRef]
5. Jazz Pharmaceuticals and PharmaMar Announce Results of ATLANTIS Phase 3 Study Evaluating Zepzelca™ in Combination with Doxorubicin for Patients with Small Cell Lung Cancer Following One Prior Platinum-Containing Line. 2020. Available online: https://bit.ly/3qupxmC (accessed on 3 December 2020).
6. Ponce Aix, S.; Flor, M.J.; Falcon, A.; Sanchez-Simon, I.; Aguilar, E.J.; Coté, G.; Nuñez, R.; Siguero, M.; Insa, M.; Cullell-Young, M.; et al. Lurbinectedin (LUR) in combination with irinotecan (IRI) in patients (pts) with advanced solid tumours. *Ann. Oncol.* **2019**, *30*, v178.
7. Elez, M.E.; Tabernero, J.; Geary, D.; Macarulla, T.; Kang, S.P.; Kahatt, C.; Soto-Matos Pita, A.; Teruel, C.F.; Siguero, M.; Cullell-Young, M.; et al. First-in-human phase I study of Lurbinectedin (PM01183) in patients with advanced solid tumors. *Clin. Cancer Res.* **2014**, *20*, 2205–2214. [CrossRef]
8. Forster, M.; Moreno, V.; Calvo, E.; Olmedo, M.E.; Lopez-Criado, M.P.; Lopez-Vilarino, J.; Nunez, R.; Kahatt, C.; Soto-Matos, A. Overall Survival with Lurbinectedin Plus Doxorubicin in Relapsed SCLC. Results from an Expansion Cohort of a Phase Ib Trial. *J. Thorac. Oncol.* **2018**, *13*, S581. [CrossRef]
9. Subbiah, V.; Paz-Ares, L.; Besse, B.; Moreno, V.; Peters, S.; Sala, M.A.; López-Vilariño, J.A.; Fernández, C.; Kahatt, C.; Alfaro, V.; et al. Antitumor activity of lurbinectedin in second-line small cell lung cancer patients who are candidates for re-challenge with the first-line treatment. *Lung Cancer* **2020**, *150*, 90–96. [CrossRef] [PubMed]
10. Smit, E.F.; Fokkema, E.; Biesma, B.; Groen, H.J.; Snoek, W.; Postmus, P.E. A phase II study of paclitaxel in heavily pretreated patients with small-cell lung cancer. *Br. J. Cancer* **1998**, *77*, 347–351. [CrossRef]
11. Groen, H.J.; Fokkema, E.; Biesma, B.; Kwa, B.; van Putten, J.W.; Postmus, P.E.; Smit, E. Paclitaxel and carboplatin in the treatment of small-cell lung cancer patients resistant to cyclophosphamide, doxorubicin, and etoposide: A non-cross-resistant schedule. *J. Clin. Oncol.* **1999**, *17*, 927–932. [CrossRef]
12. De Jong, W.K.; Groen, H.J.; Koolen, M.G.; Biesma, B.; Willems, L.N.; Kwa, H.B.; van Bochove, A.; van Tinteren, H.; Smit, E. Phase 3 study of cyclophosphamide, doxorubicin, and etoposide compared with carboplatin and paclitaxel in patients with extensive disease small-cell lung cancer. *Eur. J. Cancer* **2007**, *43*, 2345–2350. [CrossRef] [PubMed]
13. Ojima, I.; Lichtenthal, B.; Lee, S.; Wang, C.; Wang, X. Taxane anticancer agents: A patent perspective. *Expert Opin. Ther. Pat.* **2016**, *26*, 1–20. [CrossRef]
14. Gelsomino, F.; Tiseo, M.; Barbieri, F.; Riccardi, F.; Cavanna, L.; Frassoldati, A.; Delmonte, A.; Longo, L.; Dazzi, C.; Cinieri, S.; et al. Phase II study of NAB-paclitaxel in sensitive and refractory relapsed SCLC (NABSTER TRIAL). *Ann. Oncol.* **2018**, *29*, v3599. [CrossRef]
15. Drummond, D.C.; Noble, C.O.; Guo, Z.; Hayes, M.E.; Connolly-Ingram, C.; Gabriel, B.S.; Hann, B.; Liu, B.; Park, J.W.; Hong, K.; et al. Development of a highly stable and targetable nanoliposomal formulation of topotecan. *J. Control Release* **2010**, *141*, 13–21. [CrossRef] [PubMed]
16. Gerrits, C.J.; de Jonge, M.J.; Schellens, J.H.; Stoter, G.; Verweij, J. Topoisomerase I inhibitors: The relevance of prolonged exposure for present clinical development. *Br. J. Cancer* **1997**, *76*, 952–962. [CrossRef] [PubMed]
17. Jiang, J.; Liang, X.; Zhou, X.; Huang, L.; Huang, R.; Chu, Z.; Zhang, Q. A meta-analysis of randomized controlled trials comparing irinotecan/platinum with etoposide/platinum in patients with previously untreated extensive-stage small cell lung cancer. *J. Thorac. Oncol.* **2010**, *5*, 867–873. [CrossRef]
18. Sevinc, A.; Kalender, M.E.; Altinbas, M.; Ozkan, M.; Dikilitas, M.; Camci, C. Irinotecan as a second-line monotherapy for small cell lung cancer. *Asian Pac. J. Cancer Prev.* **2011**, *12*, 1055–1059.
19. National Comprehensive Cancer Network. NCCN Guidelines Small Cell Lung Cancer. Available online: https://www.nccn.org/professionals/physician_gls/pdf/sclc.pdf (accessed on 26 November 2020).
20. Kalra, A.V.; Kim, J.; Klinz, S.G.; Paz, N.; Cain, J.; Drummond, D.; Nielsen, U.B.; Fitzgerald, J.B. Preclinical activity of nanoliposomal irinotecan is governed by tumor deposition and intratumor prodrug conversion. *Cancer Res.* **2014**, *74*, 7003–7013. [CrossRef]
21. Wang-Gillam, A.; Li, C.P.; Bodoky, G.; Dean, A.; Shan, Y.S.; Jameson, G.; Macarulla, T.; Lee, K.; Cunningham, D.; Blanc, J.F.; et al. Nanoliposomal irinotecan with fluorouracil and folinic acid in metastatic pancreatic cancer after previous gemcitabine-based therapy (NAPOLI-1): A global, randomised, open-label, phase 3 trial. *Lancet* **2016**, *387*, 545–557. [CrossRef]
22. Dowell, J.E. Small cell lung cancer: Are we making progress? *Am. J. Med. Sci.* **2010**, *339*, 68–76. [CrossRef] [PubMed]
23. Van Ark-Otte, J.; Kedde, M.A.; van der Vijgh, W.J.; Dingemans, A.M.; Jansen, W.J.; Pinedo, H.M.; Boven, E.; Giaccone, G. Determinants of CPT-11 and SN-38 activities in human lung cancer cells. *Br. J. Cancer* **1998**, *77*, 2171–2176. [CrossRef]

74. Hedbrant, A.; Wijkander, J.; Seidal, T.; Delbro, D.; Erlandsson, A. Macrophages of M1 phenotype have properties that influence lung cancer cell progression. *Tumour Biol.* **2015**, *36*, 8715–8725. [CrossRef]
75. Leonard, S.C.; Lee, H.; Gadd, D.F.; Klinz, S.G.; Paz, N.; Kalra, A.V.; Drummond, D.C.; Chan, D.C.; Bunn, P.A.; Fitzgerald, J.; et al. Extended topoisomerase 1 inhibition through liposomal irinotecan results in improved efficacy over topotecan and irinotecan in models of small-cell lung cancer. *AntiCancer Drugs* **2017**, *28*, 1086–1096. [CrossRef]
76. Paz-Ares, L.G.; Spigel, D.R.; Zielinski, C.; Chen, Y.; Jove, M.; Vidal, O.; Chu, D.; Rich, P.; Hayes, T.M.; Gutierrez Calderon, M.V.; et al. RESILIENT: Study of irinotecan liposome injection (nal-IRI) in patients with small cell lung cancer—Preliminary findings from part 1 dose-defining phase. *J. Clin. Oncol.* **2019**, *37*, 8562. [CrossRef]
77. Paz-Ares, L.; Spigel, D.; Chen, Y.; Jove, M.; Juan, O.; Rich, P.; Hayes, T.; Guitierrez Calderon, V.; Bernabe, R.; Navarro, A.; et al. Initial efficacy and safety results of irinotecan liposome injection (NAL-IRI) in patients with small cell lung cancer. In Proceedings of the International Association for the Study of Lung Cancer 20th World Conference on Lung Cancer, Barcelona, Spain, 7–10 September 2019.
78. Lee, J.H.; Lee, J.M.; Kim, J.K.; Ahn, S.K.; Lee, S.J.; Kim, M.Y.; Jew, S.S.; Park, J.C.; Hong, C.I. Antitumor activity of 7-[2-(N-isopropylamino)ethyl]-(20S)-camptothecin, CKD602, as a potent DNA topoisomerase I inhibitor. *Arch. Pharm. Res.* **1998**, *21*, 581–590. [CrossRef]
79. Rhee, C.K.; Lee, S.H.; Kim, J.S.; Kim, S.J.; Kim, S.C.; Kim, Y.K.; Kang, H.H.; Yoon, H.K.; Song, L.S.; Moon, H.S.; et al. A multicenter phase II study of belotecan, a new camptothecin analogue, as a second-line therapy in patients with small cell lung cancer. *Lung Cancer* **2011**, *72*, 64–67. [CrossRef] [PubMed]
80. Kim, G.M.; Kim, Y.S.; Kang, A.; Jeong, J.; Kim, S.M.; Hong, Y.K.; Sung, J.H.; Lim, S.T.; Kim, J.H.; Kim, S.K.; et al. Efficacy and toxicity of belotecan for relapsed or refractory small cell lung cancer patients. *J. Thorac. Oncol.* **2012**, *7*, 731–736. [CrossRef] [PubMed]
81. Kang, J.; Lee, H.; Kim, D.; Kim, S.; Kim, H.R.; Kim, J.; Choi, J.; An, H.J.; Kim, J.; Jang, J.; et al. A randomised phase 2b study comparing the efficacy and safety of belotecan vs. topotecan as monotherapy for sensitive-relapsed small-cell lung cancer. *Br. J. Cancer* **2020**. [CrossRef]
82. Kohda, A.; Noda, T.; Horii, K.; Inoue, K.; Ozaki, M.; Kato, T. Single intravenous toxicity study of amrubicin hydrochloride (SM-5887) in dogs. *Jpn. Pharmacol. Ther.* **1999**, *27*, s37–s62.
83. Inoue, A.; Sugawara, S.; Yamazaki, K.; Maemondo, M.; Suzuki, T.; Gomi, K.; Takanashi, S.; Inoue, C.; Inage, M.; Yokouchi, H.; et al. Randomized phase II trial comparing amrubicin with topotecan in patients with previously treated small-cell lung cancer: North Japan Lung Cancer Study Group Trial 0402. *J. Clin. Oncol.* **2008**, *26*, 5401–5406. [CrossRef] [PubMed]
84. Kaira, K.; Sunaga, N.; Tomizawa, Y.; Yanagitani, N.; Shimizu, K.; Imai, H.; Utsugi, M.; Iwasaki, Y.; Iijima, H.; Tsurumaki, H.; et al. A phase II study of amrubicin, a synthetic 9-aminoanthracycline, in patients with previously treated lung cancer. *Lung Cancer* **2010**, *69*, 99–104. [CrossRef]
85. Onoda, S.; Masuda, N.; Seto, T.; Eguchi, K.; Takiguchi, Y.; Isobe, H.; Okamoto, H.; Ogura, T.; Yokoyama, A.; Seki, N.; et al. Phase II trial of amrubicin for treatment of refractory or relapsed small-cell lung cancer: Thoracic Oncology Research Group Study 0301. *J. Clin. Oncol.* **2006**, *24*, 5448–5453. [CrossRef]
86. Hasegawa, Y.; Takeda, K.; Kashii, T.; Katayama, H.; Sumitani, M.; Takifuji, N.; Condro Negoro, S.L. Clinical experience of amrubicin hydrochloride (Calsed) monotherapy in previously treated patients with small-cell lung cancer. *Jpn. J. Lung Cancer* **2005**, *45*, 811–815. [CrossRef]
87. Hirose, T.; Shirai, T.; Kusukoto, S.; Kusumoto, S.; Sugiyama, T.; Yamaoka, T.; Okuda, K.; Ohnishi, T.; Ohmori, T.; Adachi, M. Phase II study of amrubicin and carboplatin in patients with the refractory or relapsed small cell lung cancer (SCLC). *J. Clin. Oncol.* **2010**, *28*, 528s. [CrossRef]
88. Ettinger, D.S.; Jotte, R.; Lorigan, P.; Gupta, V.; Garbo, L.; Alemany, C.; Conkling, P.; Spigel, D.R.; Dudek, A.Z.; Shah, C.; et al. Phase II study of amrubicin as second-line therapy in patients with platinum-refractory small-cell lung cancer. *J. Clin. Oncol.* **2010**, *28*, 2598–2603. [CrossRef] [PubMed]
89. Jotte, R.; Conkling, P.; Reynolds, C.; Galsky, M.D.; Klein, L.; Fitzgibbons, J.F.; McNally, R.; Renschler, M.F.; Oliver, J.W. Randomized phase II trial of single-agent amrubicin or topotecan as second-line treatment in patients with small-cell lung cancer sensitive to first-line platinum based chemotherapy. *J. Clin. Oncol.* **2011**, *29*, 287–293. [CrossRef]
90. Von Pawel, J.; Jotte, R.; Spigel, D.R.; O'Brien, M.R.E.; Socinski, M.A.; Mezger, J.; Steins, M.; Bosquée, L.; Bubis, J.; Nackaerts, K.; et al. Randomized phase 3 trial of amrubicin versus topotecan as second-line treatment for patients with small-cell lung cancer. *J. Clin. Oncol.* **2014**, *32*, 4012–4019. [CrossRef] [PubMed]
91. Sun, Y.; Cheng, Y.; Hao, X.; Wang, J.; Hu, C.; Han, B.; Liu, X.; Zhang, L.; Wan, H.; Xia, Z.; et al. Randomized phase 3 trial of amrubicin/cisplatin versus etoposide/cisplatin as firstline treatment for extensive small-cell lung cancer. *BMC Cancer* **2016**, *16*, 265. [CrossRef]
92. Pembrolizumab Plus Amrubicin in Patients with Refractory Small-cell Lung Cancer, Wakayama Medical University (ClinicalTrials.gov Identifier: NCT03253068). Available online: https://clinicaltrials.gov/ct2/show/NCT03253068 (accessed on 6 March 2021).
93. Toyooka, S.; Toyooka, K.O.; Maruyama, R.; Virmani, A.K.; Girard, L.; Miyajima, K.; Harada, K.; Ariyoshi, Y.; Takahashi, T.; Sugio, K.; et al. DNA methylation profiles of lung tumors. *Mol. Cancer Ther.* **2001**, *1*, 61–67.

4. Pietanza, M.C.; Kadota, K.; Huberman, K.; Sima, C.S.; Fiore, J.J.; Sumner, D.K.; Travis, W.D.; Heguy, A.; Ginsberg, M.S.; Holodny, A.I.; et al. Phase II trial of temozolomide in patients with relapsed sensitive or refractory small cell lung cancer, with assessment of methylguanine-DNA methyltransferase as a potential biomarker. *Clin. Cancer Res.* **2012**, *18*, 1138–1145. [CrossRef]
5. Zauderer, M.G.; Drilon, A.; Kadota, K.; Huberman, K.; Sima, C.S.; Bergagnini, I.; Sumner, D.K.; Travis, W.D.; Heguy, A.; Ginsberg, M.S.; et al. Trial of a 5-day dosing regimen of temozolomide in patients with relapsed small cell lung cancers with assessment of methylguanine-DNA methyltransferase. *Lung Cancer* **2014**, *86*, 237–240. [CrossRef] [PubMed]
6. Hegi, M.E.; Diserens, A.C.; Gorlia, T.; Hamou, M.F.; de Tribolet, N.; Weller, M.; Kros, J.M.; Hainfellner, J.A.; Mason, W.; Mariani, L.; et al. MGMT gene silencing and benefit from temozolomide in glioblastoma. *N. Engl. J. Med.* **2005**, *352*, 997–1003. [CrossRef] [PubMed]
7. Pietanza, M.C.; Waqar, S.N.; Krug, L.M.; Dowlati, A.; Hann, C.L.; Chiappori, A.; Owonikoko, T.K.; Woo, K.M.; Cardnell, R.J.; Fujimoto, J.; et al. Randomized, double-blind, phase ii study of temozolomide in combination with either veliparib or placebo in patients with relapsed-sensitive or refractory small-cell lung cancer. *J. Clin. Oncol.* **2018**, *36*, 2386–2394. [CrossRef] [PubMed]
8. Farago, A.F.; Yeap, B.Y.; Stanzione, M.; Hung, Y.P.; Heist, R.S.; Marcoux, J.P.; Zhong, J.; Rangachari, D.; Barbie, D.A.; Phat, S.; et al. Combination olaparib and temozolomide in relapsed small-cell lung cancer. *Cancer Discov.* **2019**, *9*, 1372–1387. [CrossRef] [PubMed]
9. Tentori, L.; Graziani, G. Chemopotentiation by PARP inhibitors in cancer therapy. *Pharmacol. Res.* **2005**, *52*, 25–33. [CrossRef] [PubMed]

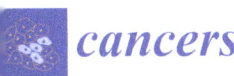

Review

History of Extensive Disease Small Cell Lung Cancer Treatment: Time to Raise the Bar? A Review of the Literature

Chiara Lazzari [1,†], Aurora Mirabile [1,†], Alessandra Bulotta [1], Maria Grazia Viganó [1], Francesca Rita Ogliari [1], Stefania Ippati [1], Italo Dell'Oca [2], Mariacarmela Santarpia [3], Vincenza Lorusso [1], Martin Reck [4] and Vanesa Gregorc [1,*]

1. Department of Oncology, IRCCS San Raffaele Hospital, via Olgettina 60, 20132 Milano, Italy; Lazzari.Chiara@hsr.it (C.L.); mirabile.aurora@hsr.it (A.M.); bulotta.alessandra@hsr.it (A.B.); vigano.mariagrazia@hsr.it (M.G.V.); ogliari.francesca@hsr.it (F.R.O.); ippati.stefania@hsr.it (S.I.); lorusso.vincenza@hsr.it (V.L.)
2. Department of Radiotherapy, IRCSS San Raffaele Hospital, via Olgettina 60, 20132 Milano, Italy; dell'oca.italo@hsr.it
3. Medical Oncology Unit, Department of Human Pathology of Adult and Evolutive Age "G. Barresi", University of Messina, 98121 Messina, Italy; msantarpia@unime.it
4. Airway Research Center North, German Center for Lung Research, Department of Thoracic Oncology, Lung Clinic, 22927 Grosshansdorf, Germany; m.reck@lungenclinic.de
* Correspondence: gregorc.vanesa@hsr.it
† Aurora Mirabile and Chiara Lazzari equally contributed for manuscript development.

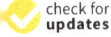

Citation: Lazzari, C.; Mirabile, A.; Bulotta, A.; Viganó, M.G.; Ogliari, F.R.; Ippati, S.; Dell'Oca, I.; Santarpia, M.; Lorusso, V.; Reck, M.; et al. History of Extensive Disease Small Cell Lung Cancer Treatment: Time to Raise the Bar? A Review of the Literature. *Cancers* **2021**, *13*, 998. https://doi.org/10.3390/cancers 13050998

Academic Editor: Jeffrey A. Borgia

Received: 26 January 2021
Accepted: 19 February 2021
Published: 27 February 2021

Publisher's Note: MDPI stays neutral with regard to jurisdictional claims in published maps and institutional affiliations.

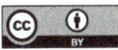

Copyright: © 2021 by the authors. Licensee MDPI, Basel, Switzerland. This article is an open access article distributed under the terms and conditions of the Creative Commons Attribution (CC BY) license (https:// creativecommons.org/licenses/by/ 4.0/).

Simple Summary: Small cell lung cancer (SCLC) remains the most aggressive form of neuroendocrine tumor of the lung, for which treatment options remain limited. The introduction of immune checkpoint inhibitors has modified for the first time the therapeutic strategies in patients with extensive disease after decades. New therapeutic approaches are required. Deeper knowledge of tumor biology is required to gain new insights into this complex disease.

Abstract: Several trials have tried for decades to improve the outcome of extensive disease small cell lung cancer (ED-SCLC) through attempts to modify the standard treatments. Nevertheless, platinum/etoposide combination and topotecan have remained respectively the first and the second line standard treatments for the last 40 years. With the advent of immunotherapy, this scenario has finally changed. Our review aims to provide an overview of the primary studies on the actual therapeutic strategies available for ED-SCLC patients, and to highlight emerging evidence supporting the use of immunotherapy in SCLC patients.

Keywords: small cell lung cancer; chemotherapy; Immunotherapy; extensive disease

1. Introduction

Small cell lung cancer (SCLC) is an aggressive tumor, with a high mitotic rate and early metastasis occurrence. It is observed in approximately 15% of new cases of lung cancer. Smoking represents the main risk factor for its development. For a long time, SCLC has been classified according to the Veteran's Administration Lung Cancer Study Group as limited stage (tumor located in the thorax and included in a single radiation field) or extensive stage (when not confined into a single radiation field, or in the presence of distant metastases). To better define patients' prognosis, in 2009, the International Association for the Study of Lung Cancer proposed the use of the tumor, node, and metastasis (TNM) staging system [1]. Following the introduction of the eighth TNM edition for the classification of non-small cell lung cancer (NSCLC), and the survival analysis of patients with SCLC, classified according to the seventh or the eighth TNM editions, the eighth TNM classification was adopted, and it is currently used [2]. Approximately 60–70% of patients are diagnosed with metastatic disease at the onset [3]. During the last four decades, platinum–etoposide has been the only recognized treatment in the first-line setting. Despite the response rate of 60–80%, responses are not durable, and patients develop resistance and unfortunately die within ten months. Less than 7% of patients are still alive at five years [4,5]. While aiming to improve patients' outcomes, several treatment strategies have been tested, but with poor results. At odds with NSCLC, where the deep understanding of tumor biology and the identification of actionable molecular alterations have been translated into efficient molecularly targeted therapies, no driver-targetable molecular alterations have been identified in SCLC, and its therapeutic portfolio has not been improved for several years. Recently, immune checkpoint inhibitors have significantly prolonged patient survival, thus resulting in a practice-changing strategy for the first time.

The current review provides an overview of the progress made in treating patients with extensive disease SCLC (ED-SCLC).

2. First Line Chemotherapy in ED-SCLC

Originally, cyclophosphamide, doxorubicin, and vincristine (CAV) represented the standard treatment used in untreated patients with ED-SCLC. For a long time, research has focused on identifying the most effective combinatorial chemotherapy regimen to prolong patients' survival with acceptable toxicity and good quality of life. Table 1 summarizes the main phase III trials conducted in naive patients with ED-SCLC.

Because of the high proliferative rate of SCLC, the high chemosensitivity, and the high percentage of relapses, in order to increase tumor-cell death, among the strategies evaluated, the use of alternating non-cross-resistant regimens was tested. A phase III study was designed to compare in 437 patients with ED-SCLC, stratified according to performance status (PS), cisplatin–etoposide (EP) with CAV for four cycles, or the alternation of CAV/EP for six cycles [6]. Overall survival (OS) was the primary end-point of the trial. No significant difference was observed in terms of objective response rate (ORR) or OS. The alternating regimen was associated with a significantly prolonged time to progression (TTP) in comparison to CAV, but with more hematologic toxicity. Moreover, CAV and EP resulted in comparable efficacies in terms of OS, TTP, and ORR.

Results from a meta-analysis, including data from 36 randomized phase II and III trials, demonstrated, for the first time, OS improvement with etoposide alone, or in combination with cisplatin [7], in patients with ED-SCLC. A further meta-analysis evaluated the differences between cisplatin and carboplatin [8] in terms of efficacy and toxicity. The results were comparable for OS and PFS, and were associated with a different spectrum of toxicity. The included a higher percentage of hematologically adverse events with carboplatin, and more non-hematological events with cisplatin, including nausea, vomiting, and renal failure. Based on these findings and the good efficacy/toxicity ratio of EP, this regimen has become the standard first-line treatment. The choice between cisplatin or carboplatin is secondary to the expected toxicity profile, the organ function, the PS, and the patients' co-morbidities [8].

Different phase III studies have explored the efficacy of adding one or two drugs to EP chemotherapy, the use of alternative compounds to etoposide, such as irinotecan, topotecan or amrubicine, or the use of a high dose of chemotherapy [9]. A phase III trial evaluated the benefit of ifosfamide combined with EP (VIP) in 171 patients with ED-SCLC [10]. Patients were stratified according to PS and randomized between EP or VIP. Patients with brain metastases were eligible and received concurrent whole-brain radiotherapy. The study was designed to demonstrate an OS increase of 50% in the VIP arm compared with the EP regimen. No significant difference was shown in terms of ORR, while prolonged median progression-free survival (PFS) and OS were observed in patients receiving VIP over EP. However, the benefit was less than expected, and VIP was associated with more hematologic and non-hematologic toxicity. Another phase III study tested the advantage of combining cyclophosphamide and epidoxorubicin with EP (PCDE) as a strategy to intensify and improve the therapeutic options in patients with ED-SCLC [11]. Two hundred twenty-six patients lacking previous treatment were randomized between EP or PCDE. Brain metastases represented an exclusion criterion to enter the study. The primary end-point was OS, and the trial was designed to demonstrate a 15% improvement at 1 year with PCDE over EP. At the end of chemotherapy, prophylactic cranial irradiation was recommended for patients with complete responses, while thoracic radiotherapy was suggested for those with partial responses in the case of a residual tumor. PDCE significantly increased ORR, and prolonged PFS and 1-year survival, over EP, with higher hematologic toxicity, and without affecting the quality of life. However, these results did not translate into a practice-changing strategy. In addition, the attempt to use a high dose of EP failed to demonstrate any significant advantage over standard EP in terms of ORR or OS, and was associated with increased toxicity [12]. Another strategy tested was the comparison of a combination therapy containing carboplatin, etoposide, and vincristine with paclitaxel, etoposide and carboplatin, in a phase III study enrolling 614 naive patients with SCLC of any stage [13]. The primary end-point was OS. The results showed a statistically significant increase in median and long-term survival, PFS, and a decrease in toxicities for patients with SCLC receiving a paclitaxel-containing regimen compared with standard chemotherapy.

The preliminary efficacy observed with the topoisomerase I inhibitor irinotecan [14], and the positive findings from a phase II study showing an ORR of 86%, with a median OS of 13.2 months in patients with ED-SCLC receiving cisplatin combined with irinotecan (IC) [15], led to the design of four phase III trials to compare the efficacy of IC to that of EP. All the studies included OS as the primary end-point. The Japanese JCOG 9511, designed to enroll 230 patients, was prematurely closed, following the inclusion of 154 patients [16]. The preliminary results, observed during the interim analysis and showing an OS difference in favor of IC combination, which was further confirmed at the second interim analysis, led to the early termination of patient accrual. The definitive results showed a significant improvement of ORR, PFS, and OS in the IC arm. Patients in the EP arm experienced higher grade 3–4 neutropenia and thrombocytopenia, but lower grade 3–4 diarrhea, than the IC group. However, these results were not confirmed by another phase III trial, designed to compare EP with IC in a larger number of patients from North America [17]. Three hundred thirty-one patients were enrolled. Conversely, from the Japanese trial, no significant difference in terms of ORR, PFS, or OS was observed between the two arms. Different reasons might explain the divergent findings of the two studies, including the differences in the characteristics of the patients enrolled (with a lower percentage of cases with more advanced disease in the JCOG study), the different dose and schedule of IC used, with an increased dose of irinotecan administered in the Japanese trial, and pharmacogenomic differences between the North American and Japanese populations. Similar findings were reported by the phase III SWOG S0124 study, enrolling 651 patients and designed using the same eligibility criteria and treatment regimens as the JCOG 9511 [18]. No difference was observed in ORR, PFS, or OS between the two arms, with less hematologic and greater gastrointestinal toxicity for IC over EP. The different results of the JCOG 9511 trial might be related to the smaller number of patients enrolled, and imbalances in the distribution of patients, including less patients with PS2, more women, and fewer cases with brain metastases in the Japanese study. Moreover, the differences in the ethnicities and the genetic backgrounds of the populations included might have influenced the final results. Conversely, when irinotecan in combination with carboplatin was compared with oral etoposide in combination with carboplatin in a phase III study, enrolling 220 patients with ED-SCLC, irinotecan prolonged OS without affecting the quality of life [19]. More recently, a meta-analysis, including data from six randomized trials [20] enrolling 1476 naive patients with ED-SCLC, compared the efficacy and toxicity of irinotecan/platinum with etoposide/platinum. Two trials were phase II studies, and in two trials carboplatin was used instead of cisplatin. Although the results showed that the combination of irinotecan/platinum improves ORR and prolongs OS over EP, the subgroup meta-analysis performed after excluding the two trials using carboplatin failed to confirm this advantage. The heterogeneity of the population, the different drugs, and the doses used has not allowed for a conclusion on the most efficient regimen, and EP has remained the reference standard treatment for western countries. Another topoisomerase I inhibitor, topotecan, has been explored in combination with cisplatin (TP) in untreated patients with ED-SCLC. Seven hundred and ninety-five patients were enrolled in a phase III trial, designed to assess OS superiority or at least the non-inferiority of TP over EP [21]. Despite a higher ORR, a prolonged PFS, and a comparable OS observed in the TP arm, the higher percentage of hematological toxicities, including anemia and thrombocytopenia requiring transfusions associated with a higher rate of treatment-related deaths, has not allowed the replacement of standard EP with TP. Similarly, the topoisomerase II inhibitor amrubicin, an anthracycline with the advantage of not determining cardiovascular toxicity, was tested in a phase III study designed to evaluate its non-inferiority in terms of OS, and eventually its superiority over EP when combined with cisplatin in 300 naive Chinese patients with ED-SCLC [22]. The results showed significantly higher ORR in the AP arm, with comparable PFS and OS, but this was associated with a higher percentage of hematopoietic toxicities in the amrubicine group.

Table 1. Phase III trials exploring chemotherapy in first-line setting of patients wing extensive disease small cell lung cancer (ED-SCLC).

Author (Ref)	Treatment	Primary End-Point	OS (m)	p	TTP/PFS (m)	p	ORR (%)
Ihde [12]	high EP	RR	10.7	0.68	7.0	0.96	86
	standard EP		11.4		6.9		83
Roth [6]	EP	OS	4.3	0.425	4.3	0.052	61
	CAV		4.0		4.0		51
	EP/CAV		5.2		5.2		60
Loehrer [10]	EP	OS	7.3	0.045	6.0	0.039	67
	VIP		9.1		6.8		73
Pujol [11]	EP	OS	9.3	0.0067	7.2	<0.00001	61
	PCDE		10.5		6.3		76
Reck [13]	TEC	OS	12.7	0.024	8.1	0.033	72.1
	CEV		11.7		7.5		69.4
Noda [16]	IC	OS	12.8	0.002	6.9	0.03	84.4
	EP		9.4		4.8		67.5
Hanna [17]	IC	OS	10.2	0.68	4.1	0.37	48.7
	EP		9.3		4.6		43.6
Lara [18]	IC	OS	9.1	0.071	5.8	0.07	60
	EP		9.9		5.2		57
Hermes [19]	CBDCA + E (*)	OS	8.5	0.02	-	-	-
	CBDCA + I		7.1				
Fink [21]	TP	OS	44.9 weeks	0.029	27.4 weeks	0.01	55.5
	EP		40.9 weeks		24.3 weeks		45.5
Sun [22]	AP	OS	11.8	0.008	6.8	0.035	69.8
	EP		10.3		5.7		57.3

EP: cisplatin–etoposide. CAV: cyclophosphamide, doxorubicin and vincristine. VIP: ifosfamide, cisplatin, etoposide. PDCE: cyclophosphamide, epidoxorubicin, cisplatin, etoposide. CEV: carboplatin, etoposide, and vincristine. TEC: paclitaxel, etoposide, and carboplatin. IC: irinotecan, cisplatin. CBDCA: carboplatin. E: etoposide. I: irinotecan. * oral. TP: topotecan, cisplatin. AP: amrubicin, cisplatin. OS: overall survival. PFS: progression-free survival. TTP: time to progression. m: months.

In conclusion, due to the toxicity and the lack of substantial efficacy, all the alternative regimens tested in patients with untreated ED-SCLC were unsuitable for becoming a new standard, and EP has remained the first therapeutic choice.

3. Immune Checkpoint Inhibitors in the Treatment of Patients with ED-SCLC

Recently, in patients with ED-SCLC, the treatment landscape has evolved because of the advent of immune checkpoint inhibitors. The genomic instability of SCLC [23] favors the accumulation of DNA damages, which in turn favor the development of immunogenic clones recognized by the antigen-presenting cells and the dendritic cells. As a consequence, CD8+ T cells are simulated. The activation of the immune system contributes to the killing of tumor cells.

Due to the correlation between SCLC and smoking, many somatic mutations occur. A higher T cells ratio was found in long-term survivors with SCLC compared to patients with recurrent disease [24], thus suggesting the potential efficacy of immune checkpoint inhibitors in SCLC. As such, immunotherapy has been tested in patients with ED-SCLC as a single agent, combined with chemotherapy or different immune checkpoint inhibitors, in the first-line setting, the maintenance, and the second line (Table 2).

Few data are available regarding the immune composition of SCLC tumors. Retrospective analyses indicate the expression of PD-L1 in a variable percentage of cases (0–71.6%). PD-L1 upregulation has been found in patients with high levels of CD3ε and CD68 mRNA, and in those with increased levels of CD8. CD8 T cells are detectable in 13% of patients [25]. However, a lower percentage of CD8 has been observed in SCLC compared with patients affected by NSCLC. These differences might partly explain the different outcomes obtained with immune checkpoint inhibitors in NSCLC in comparison with SCLC.

Recently, chemotherapeutic agents' immunologic effects on the tumor microenvironment's modulation have been established [26]. Preclinical evidence suggests that chemotherapy upregulates PD-L1 on tumor cells, increases the expression of nuclear factor kappa-light on B cells, favors the activation of antigen-presenting cells, and inhibits the infiltration of immunosuppressive cells in the tumor [27–30]. Based on these findings, clinical trials have been designed to evaluate platinum–etoposide's synergistic effect with immune checkpoint inhibitors in SCLC [31].

3.1. Immune Checkpoint Inhibitors in First Line Setting-CTLA4 Blockade

The anti-CTLA-4 monoclonal antibody ipilimumab was the first immune checkpoint inhibitor evaluated in combination with chemotherapy in untreated patients with ED-SCLC in a phase II study [32]. To define the best timing for chemotherapy and immunotherapy administration, two regimens were tested in 130 patients: ipilimumab concurrent with paclitaxel/carboplatin, or ipilimumab in combination with paclitaxel/carboplatin following two cycles of chemotherapy alone (phased regimen). The primary end-point of the study was immune-related progression-free survival (irPFS). Results showed improved irPFS in the group receiving the phased regimen over chemotherapy alone, while no difference was observed with the concurrent regimen, thus suggesting that induction chemotherapy might favor the release of tumor antigens, thus resulting in a more effective treatment strategy. Based on these promising findings, the phase III CA 184-156 study was designed to compare ipilimumab or placebo in combination with etoposide and platinum [33]. The phased regimen was selected. One thousand one hundred and thirty-two patients were enrolled to demonstrate an OS improvement in the experimental arm. Conversely, from what was expected, ipilimumab did not result in a statistically significantly improved OS over chemotherapy alone, and immunotherapy did not enter into the therapeutic armamentarium of patients with ED-SCLC.

3.2. Immune Checkpoint Inhibitors in First-Line Setting-PD-1/PD-L1 Blockade

Previous reports showed that PD-L1 is expressed in immune cells infiltrating the SCLC stroma, thus suggesting the potential of enhancing tumor-specific T-cell immunity by targeting the PD-1/PD-L1 pathway. Three phase III studies and one phase II study have been designed to evaluate the safety and efficacy of atezolizumab, durvalumab, pembrolizumab and nivolumab in combination with platinum–etoposide-based chemotherapy.

The efficacy of atezolizumab combined with carboplatin etoposide was evaluated in the phase III IMpower 133, designed to demonstrate the OS and PFS improvement of the combination over carboplatin–etoposide in 403 patients with naïve ED-SCLC. Patients were stratified according to sex, ECOG PS, and the presence of brain metastases [34]. In the presence of clinical benefit, patients were allowed to continue therapy beyond progression. Prophylactic cranial irradiation was allowed following the first four cycles, during the atezolizumab/placebo maintenance phase. The trial reached the primary end-points, showing a statistically significant reduction in the risk of death of 30%, and a progression of 23% in patients receiving atezolizumab. One-year OS rate was 13% higher in the atezolizumab group than in the placebo group (51.7 vs. 38.2%). The benefit was independent of the biomarkers analyzed, since neither PD-L1 expression nor blood tumor molecular burden were predictive of the outcome, and this was observed in all the subgroups analyzed except for those patients with treated brain metastases. However, this was an exploratory, and not a pre-planned, analysis performed on a limited number of cases, and no definitive conclusion can be drawn. Based on these results, the combination of carboplatin, etoposide and atezolizumab has become the new referral standard treatment for naive patients with ED-SCLC.

The CASPIAN trial was a randomized, phase III study, designed to compare the efficacy of the PD-L1 inhibitor durvalumab, with or without the CTLA-4 inhibitor tremelimumab, in combination with platinum–etoposide in 805 patients with untreated ED-SCLC [35]. In the case of progression, continuation of treatment was allowed in the presence of clinical benefits. The co-primary end-points were OS for durvalumab platinum–etoposide versus chemotherapy, and for durvalumab tremelimumab platinum–etoposide versus chemotherapy. The adding of durvalumab tremelimumab did not significantly prolong OS over chemotherapy. Conversely, as already observed in the IMpower 133 trial, the combination of durvalumab with platinum–etoposide significantly improved OS. No significant difference was evidenced in terms of PFS between the treatment arms. A survival benefit was also found with durvalumab in the group of patients with untreated brain metastases. These results confirm the lack of any additional benefit with the CTLA-4 blockade in unselected patients with ED-SCLC. Based on these findings, durvalumab in combination with cisplatin or carboplatin etoposide has been approved by the Food and Drug Administration (FDA) and the European Medicine Agency (EMA) for use in untreated patients with ED-SCLC.

The phase III KEYNOTE 604 trial was designed to investigate the efficacy of the PD-1 inhibitor pembrolizumab, combined with platinum–etoposide, over chemotherapy alone in 453 naive patients with ED-SCLC [36]. The co-primary end-points were OS and PFS. The trial reached one of its primary end-points, showing a significant PFS improvement in chemotherapy and immunotherapy, which did not translate into prolonged OS, despite the numerical benefit in OS being comparable to those achieved by IMpower 133 and CASPIAN. However, double the percentage of patients in the experimental arm were alive at two years compared with chemotherapy alone, thus suggesting that a subgroup of patients obtain a durable benefit from the combination. Compared to the IMpower 133 and the CASPIAN trials, more patients with brain metastases (with ECOG PS of 1) with large tumor dimensions, elevated LDH, and more metastatic sites were enrolled in the KEYNOTE 604 trial. These differences in the populations might have influenced the final results.

Finally, the PD-1 inhibitor nivolumab was tested in combination with platinum–etoposide in the phase II EA5161 trial, enrolling 160 naive patients with ED-SCLC [37]. The study reached its primary end-point, showing a significant PFS improvement in the experimental arm.

In conclusion, the durable benefit observed with the addition of PD-1 or PD-L1 inhibitors to platinum–etoposide has modified the therapeutic strategies recommended in patients with ED-SCLC after several decades. This is particularly remarkable in such an aggressive disease, where, historically, it has been challenging to overcome the long-term survival benefit obtained with platinum–etoposide.

3.3. Immune Checkpoint Inhibitors as a Maintenance Strategy

Aiming to prolong survival, immune checkpoint inhibitors have been tested in the maintenance setting in those patients with stable or responsive ED-SCLC following four to six cycles of platinum–etoposide, but with poor results.

Pembrolizumab was evaluated in a phase II study, designed to demonstrate in 45 patients a PFS improvement of 50%, compared with historical data [38]. Pembrolizumab was administered within eight weeks from the end of chemotherapy. Despite no significant PFS or OS improvement being observed among the patients enrolled, the 1-year PFS and OS rates were 13% and 37%, respectively, thus suggesting that a subgroup of patients might receive durable benefits from this strategy.

Similar results were found in the phase III CA 451 study, designed to compare nivolumab with the combination of ipilimumab + nivolumab or a placebo in 834 patients with ED-SCLC, who did not progress following four cycles of platinum-based chemotherapy [39]. The study failed to demonstrate OS improvement in nivolumab + ipilimumab patients over placebo patients, and of nivolumab over placebo.

These findings suggest that the timing of checkpoint inhibitors administration is important in improving the survival benefit in patients with ED-SCLC, and a maintenance strategy with immune checkpoint inhibitors is not suggested.

3.4. Immune Checkpoint Inhibitors in Recurrent Patients

Controversial results have been observed in the studies evaluating the efficacy of pembrolizumab, nivolumab, durvalumab and atezolizumab in patients progressing after platinum–etoposide-based chemotherapy.

The activity of pembrolizumab as a monotherapy in the second/third-line setting was assessed in two trials, the phase Ib KEYNOTE 028 trial and the phase II KEYNOTE 058 trial. The KEYNOTE 028 trial [40] was a multi-cohort phase Ib study, designed to define the preliminary effects of pembrolizumab in different cohorts of patients with solid tumors. The presence of PD-L1 expression in at least 1% of tumors and inflammatory cells represented one of the inclusion criteria to enter the study, the primary end-point of which was to determine the percentage of objective responses. One of the cohorts included 24 patients with ED-SCLC progressing to at least one previous line of chemotherapy. Among these, approximately half of them had received the second line with topotecan or irinotecan. An ORR of 33.3% was identified, with a median duration of response of 19.4 months, thus suggesting a promising clinical activity of pembrolizumab in this setting. In order to confirm these findings in a larger population, the phase II KEYNOTE 058 trial enrolled patients progressing to standard treatment [41]. Similarly, to the KEYNOTE 028 trial, the primary end-point here was the percentage of objective response. Differently from KEYNOTE 028, here, PD-L1 positivity was not an inclusion criterion, even though to enter the trial the collection of evaluable tumor samples was mandatory, in order to centrally test PD-L1 expression. One hundred and seven patients with ED-SCLC were included, and an ORR of 18.7% was registered. The percentage of responses was six times higher in PD-L1-positive compared to PD-L1-negative tumors (35.7% vs. 6.0%), and longer OS was observed in PD-L1-positive patients (14.6 vs. 7.7 months). A pooled analysis of the two studies, including only those patients who received two lines of chemotherapy (83/131), showed that 88% of responder patients had PD-L1-positive tumors, thus suggesting the importance of selecting patients according to PD-L1 expression [42].

Nivolumab was tested in the CheckMate 032 and CheckMate 331 trials.

The CheckMate 032 was a phase I/II study investigating the activity and safety of nivolumab as a monotherapy, or in combination with ipilimumab, in metastatic patients with different solid tumor types [43]. Two hundred and sixteen patients with LD or ED-SCLC progressing after one or more previous regimens were enrolled into four cohorts in a sequential manner. In each cohort, a different regimen was administered, including nivolumab 1 mg/kg + ipilimumab 1 mg/kg, nivolumab 1 mg/kg + ipilimumab 3 mg/kg, or nivolumab 3 mg/kg + ipilimumab 1 mg/kg. The combination was continued for four cycles, followed by nivolumab until progression or unacceptable toxicity. The percentage of objective response was the primary end-point of the trial. The ORR was 10% in patients receiving nivolumab, 23% in those included in the nivolumab 1 mg/kg + ipilimumab 3 mg/kg cohort, 19% in those receiving nivolumab 3 mg/kg + ipilimumab 1 mg/kg, and 33% in the group treated with nivolumab 1 mg/kg + ipilimumab 1 mg/kg. Tissue was available for PD-L1 assessment in 69% of cases. Conversely from what was observed with pembrolizumab, tumor responses occurred independently of PD-L1 expression. Despite the limited number of patients enrolled, the preliminary analysis showed a similar efficacy between platinum-sensitive and -resistant patients, and between those previously treated with one, or two or more, lines of therapy [44]. To confirm these findings, the phase III CheckMate 331 trial was designed. However, the study did not reach the primary end-point of showing the improved OS of nivolumab over chemotherapy (topotecan or amrubicin) in 569 patients with SCLC previously treated with one line of platinum–etoposide [45].

Table 2. Clinical trials exploring immune checkpoint inhibitors in patients with ED-SCLC.

Author	Treatment	Setting	Primary End-Point	OS (m)	p	PFS (m)	p
Reck [32]	Phased I + PC Concurrent I + PC PC	I line	irPFS	12.5 9.1 10.5	0.13 0.41	6.4 5.6 5.2	0.03 0.11
Reck [33]	Ipilimumab + PE PE	I line	OS	11 10.9	0.37	4.6 4.4	-
Horn [34]	Atezolizumab + CE CE	I line	OS PFS	12.3 10.3	0.007	5.2 4.3	0.02
Goldman [35]	DPE PE DTPE	I line	OS	12.9 10.5 10.4	0.0032 0.0045	5.1 5.4 4.9	-
Rudin [36]	Pembrolizumab + PE PE	I line	OS PFS	10.8 9.7	0.0164	4.5 4.3	0.0023
Leal [37]	Nivolumab + PE PE	I line	PFS	11.3 9.3	0.14	5.5 4.6	0.012
Gadgeel [38]	Pembrolizumab	maintenance	PFS	9.6	-	1.4	-
Owonikoko [39]	Nivolumab Nivolumab + Ipilimumab	maintenance	OS	10.4 9.2	-	1.9 1.7	-
Ott [40]	Pembrolizumab	II/III line	ORR	9.7	-	1.9	-
Chung [41]	Pembrolizumab	II/III line	ORR	9.1	-	2.0	-
Antonia [43]	Nivolumab Nivolumab 1 mg/kg + Ipilimumab 1 mg/kg Nivolumab 1 mg/kg + Ipilimumab 3 mg/kg Nivolumab 3 mg/kg + Ipilimumab 1 mg/kg	II/III line	ORR	5.7 4.7 (#)	-	1.4 1.5 (#)	-
Reck [45]	Nivolumab Topotecan/amrubicine	II line	OS	7.5 8.4	0.11	1.4 3.8	-
Goldman [46]	Durvalumab	I/II line	safety	4.8	-	1.5	-
Pujol [47]	Atezolizumab Topotecan/PE	II line	ORR at 6 months	9.5 8.7	0.60	1.4 4.3	-

I: ipilimumab. PC: paclitaxel, carboplatin. CE: etoposide, carboplatin. DPE: durvalumab, platinum*, etoposide. DTPE: durvalumab, tremilimumab, platinum*, etoposide. * cisplatin or carboplatin was allowed according to investigators' choice. PFS: progression-free survival. ORR: objective response rate. (#): includes all the patients receiving nivolumab + ipilimumab irrespective of the schedule used.

The efficacy of durvalumab was evaluated in a phase I/II study, enrolling 21 patients with pretreated ES-SCLC [46], whose primary objective was to determine the safety profile of durvalumab. An ORR of only 9.5% was registered.

Finally, atezolizumab did not demonstrate any advantage over topotecan or re-induction of chemotherapy in 73 patients with pretreated ED-SCLC, enrolled in the phase II IFCT-1603 trial [47].

In conclusion, immune checkpoint inhibitors have not shown a significant advantage in relapsing patients with ED-SCLC, despite the fact that a subgroup of them might experience a durable clinical benefit. Biomarkers able to select those patients who benefit more have not been identified yet, despite results from the KEYNOTE 028 and the KEYNOTE 058 studies suggesting that PD-L1 expression could be considered. However, these findings were not confirmed in the studies testing nivolumab, where the activity was observed irrespective of PD-L1 status. Finally, in the trials evaluating durvalumab and atezolizumab, patients were not selected according to PD-L1 expression, and no definitive conclusions could be drawn [48].

4. Second Line and Beyond

Those patients relapsing or progressing during first-line treatment are classified as refractory. In the case of progression within 3 months, they are considered platinum-resistant. If relapse is observed after 3 months (the last cycle of first-line chemotherapy), they are considered platinum-sensitive.

According to ESMO guidelines, in sensitive patients, a rechallenge with drugs used in first-line therapy is allowed. However, the lack of PFS and OS benefit was observed in a retrospective analysis, including data from 65 patients with sensitive ED-SCLC [49]. On the other hand, a systematic analysis, including data from 1692 sensitive and refractory patients with SCLC, showed higher ORR and longer OS in sensitive patients [50].

Different compounds have been tested as therapeutic strategies in refractory patients with ED-SCLC (Table 3).

Table 3. Clinical trials exploring second-line therapies in patients with ED-SCLC.

Author	Regimen	Primary End-Point	OS (m)	ORR %	PFS (m)
von Pawel [51]	Topotecan	PFS	25.0	24.3	3.3
	CAV		24.7	18.3	3.0.
Jotte [52]	Topotecan	ORR	7.8	15	3.3
	Amrubicin		7.5	44	4.5
Gregorc [53]	NGR-hTNF + Doxorubicin	PFS	13.1	25	3.2

PFS: progression-free survival. ORR: objective response rate.

Among these, topotecan failed to demonstrate improved efficacy in terms of ORR over CAV in a randomized trial enrolling 211 relapsing patients with ED-SCLC. No significant difference was observed in terms of ORR, PFS or OS between the two arms, although a greater proportion of patients in the topotecan group showed improved symptoms [51]. Thanks to these findings, topotecan was approved for the second-line treatment of sensitive SCLC patients.

The efficacy of topotecan was compared to amrubicin in a phase II trial enrolling 76 patients with ED-SCLC who were sensitive to previous first-line platinum-based chemotherapy [52]. ORR was the primary end-point of the study. The results showed significantly higher ORR with amrubicin, and longer, but non-statistically significant, OS. The limited number of patients enrolled in the phase II study and the lack of independent confirmation of responses might have influenced the final results. A phase III trial is currently ongoing to confirm (or not) these data.

The promising results from a phase II study with lurbinectedin in 105 refractory patients with SCLC, showing an ORR of 35% with a median response duration of 5.3 months [54], secured lurbinectedin the accelerated approval of the FDA for patients with metastatic SCLC previously treated with platinum-based chemotherapy. However, the phase III ATLANTIS trial, comparing lurbinectedin in combination with doxorubicin versus the physician's choice of topotecan or CAV, failed to demonstrate an OS improvement in 613 patients with SCLC progressing to one previous line of platinum-based chemotherapy.

Alternative strategies to chemotherapy and immune check point inhibitors, including compounds targeting angiogenesis, have been tested. Among these, a single-arm phase II trial safely combined NGR-hTNF, a vascular-targeting agent (0.8 µg/m^2), which increases intra-tumoral chemotherapy penetration and T-lymphocyte infiltration [55], with doxorubicin (75 mg/m^2 every 3 weeks), showing manageable toxicity and promising activity in unselected platinum-resistant or platinum-sensitive patients with relapsed ED-SCLC. The primary end-point was PFS. Safety, ORR and OS were the secondary end-points. The median PFS was longer in platinum-sensitive compared to platinum-resistant patients (4.1 vs. 2.7 months, respectively). Prolonged OS was observed in those patients with increased lymphocyte counts [53]. The preclinical data indicate that NGR-hTNF modifies the composition of the tumor microenvironment, including the infiltration of CD8+ T cells, and favors the secretion of cytokines and chemokines [55], thus suggesting that NGR-hTNF might enhance the efficacy of immune checkpoint inhibitors [56]. NGR-hTNF combined with immunotherapy might represent a strategy to be evaluated in patients with relapsed SCLC.

All the agents tested have shown modest activity. To date, topotecan represents the only approved drug for the second-line treatment of patients with ED-SCLC.

5. Discussion and Future Directions

SCLC remains the most aggressive form of neuroendocrine tumor of the lung, for which treatment options remain limited. The characterization of the tumor biology of SCLC has been challenging, mainly due to the limited availability of tumor tissue, since surgery represents an option confined to a small number of cases. The high number of somatic mutations, generally including loss of function mutations or deletions in tumor suppressor genes, have further increased the difficulty of developing selected targeted therapies. Alterations in the genes involved in cell cycle regulation or DNA damage response, including RB transcriptional corepressor 1 (RB1) and tumor protein p53 (TP53), are commonly observed in SCLC [57]. The amplification of the chromosomal regions, including L-myc [58] or C-myc [59], the overexpression of the cyclin D1 [57], the alteration of PTEN [60] or of genes involved in transcriptional regulation and chromatin modification, the presence of inactivating mutations in NOTCH, and the overexpression of genes responsible for DNA damage response, represent some of the molecular aberrations characterizing the genomic landscape of SCLC [61]. To date, the majority of the trials investigating a molecular approach have provided disappointing results, mainly because the patients enrolled were not selected according to specific driver molecular alterations. The introduction of immune checkpoint inhibitors has improved systemic treatments after decades (Figure 1). However, patients' prognoses remain dismal, and new therapeutic approaches are required. Tissue collection is strongly advocated to gain new insights into the biology of this complex disease. The implementation of non-invasive methods, including the analysis of circulating tumor DNA and the use of circulating tumor cells (CTC), might become tools to overcome the inadequate amounts of tumor samples, in order to dissect the pathogenesis of SCLC and discover new targetable molecular alterations. Preclinical studies using CTC-derived explants (CDX) might be useful to identify the bypass signaling of acquired resistance, and design combinatorial strategies to overcome these pathways.

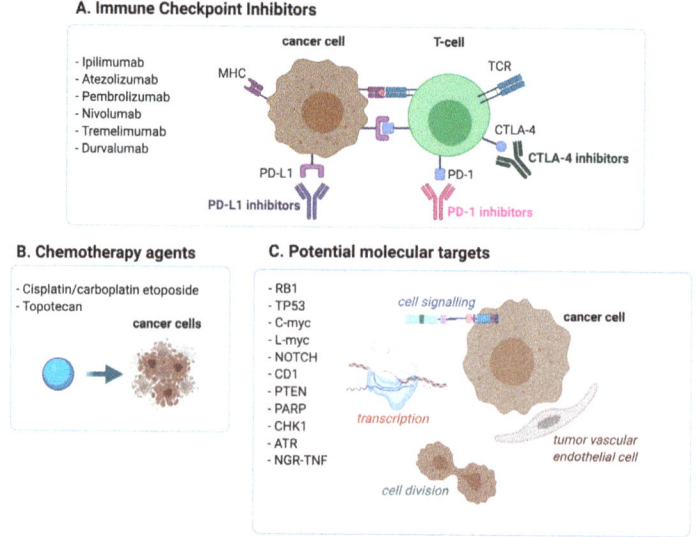

Figure 1. (**A**) Immunotherapy treatment strategies currently approved or tested in patients with ED-SCLC. (**B**) Approved chemotherapy treatments for patients with ED-SCLC. (**C**) Potentially targetable and identified molecular pathways in ED-SCLC.

Author Contributions: Conception: V.G.; collection and assembly of data: C.L. and A.M.; manuscript writing: all authors; (VII) final approval of manuscript: all authors. Image: S.I. All authors have read and agreed to the published version of the manuscript.

Funding: This research received no external funding.

Institutional Review Board Statement: N/A.

Informed Consent Statement: N/A.

Data Availability Statement: N/A.

Acknowledgments: Alliance Against Cancer.

Conflicts of Interest: The authors declare no conflict of interest.

References

1. Shepherd, F.A.; Crowley, J.; Van Houtte, P.; Postmus, P.E.; Carney, D.; Chansky, K.; Shaikh, Z.; Goldstraw, P. International Association for the Study of Lung Cancer International Staging Committee and Participating Institutions The International Association for the Study of Lung Cancer Lung Cancer Staging Project: Proposals Regarding the Clinical Staging of Small Cell Lung Cancer in the Forthcoming (Seventh) Edition of the Tumor, Node, Metastasis Classification for Lung Cancer. *J. Thorac Oncol.* **2007**, *2*, 1067–1077. [CrossRef]
2. Nicholson, A.G.; Chansky, K.; Crowley, J.; Beyruti, R.; Kubota, K.; Turrisi, A.; Eberhardt, W.E.E.; van Meerbeeck, J.; Rami-Porta, R.; Staging and Prognostic Factors Committee, Advisory Boards, and Participating Institutions; et al. The International Association for the Study of Lung Cancer Lung Cancer Staging Project: Proposals for the Revision of the Clinical and Pathologic Staging of Small Cell Lung Cancer in the Forthcoming Eighth Edition of the TNM Classification for Lung Cancer. *J. Thorac Oncol.* **2016**, *11*, 300–311. [CrossRef] [PubMed]
3. Kalemkerian, G.P.; Akerley, W.; Bogner, P.; Borghaei, H.; Chow, L.Q.; Downey, R.J.; Gandhi, L.; Ganti, A.K.P.; Govindan, R.; Grecula, J.C.; et al. Small Cell Lung Cancer. *J. Natl. Compr. Canc. Netw.* **2013**, *11*, 78–98. [CrossRef] [PubMed]
4. Wang, S.; Tang, J.; Sun, T.; Zheng, X.; Li, J.; Sun, H.; Zhou, X.; Zhou, C.; Zhang, H.; Cheng, Z.; et al. Survival Changes in Patients with Small Cell Lung Cancer and Disparities between Different Sexes, Socioeconomic Statuses and Ages. *Sci. Rep.* **2017**, *7*, 1339. [CrossRef]
5. Byers, L.A.; Rudin, C.M. Small Cell Lung Cancer: Where Do We Go from Here? *Cancer* **2015**, *121*, 664–672. [CrossRef]
6. Roth, B.J.; Johnson, D.H.; Einhorn, L.H.; Schacter, L.P.; Cherng, N.C.; Cohen, H.J.; Crawford, J.; Randolph, J.A.; Goodlow, J.L.; Broun, G.O. Randomized Study of Cyclophosphamide, Doxorubicin, and Vincristine versus Etoposide and Cisplatin versus Alternation of These Two Regimens in Extensive Small-Cell Lung Cancer: A Phase III Trial of the Southeastern Cancer Study Group. *J. Clin. Oncol.* **1992**, *10*, 282–291. [CrossRef] [PubMed]
7. Mascaux, C.; Paesmans, M.; Berghmans, T.; Branle, F.; Lafitte, J.J.; Lemaitre, F.; Meert, A.P.; Vermylen, P.; Sculier, J.P. European Lung Cancer Working Party (ELCWP) A Systematic Review of the Role of Etoposide and Cisplatin in the Chemotherapy of Small Cell Lung Cancer with Methodology Assessment and Meta-Analysis. *Lung Cancer* **2000**, *30*, 23–36. [CrossRef]
8. Rossi, A.; Di Maio, M.; Chiodini, P.; Rudd, R.M.; Okamoto, H.; Skarlos, D.V.; Früh, M.; Qian, W.; Tamura, T.; Samantas, E.; et al. Carboplatin- or Cisplatin-Based Chemotherapy in First-Line Treatment of Small-Cell Lung Cancer: The COCIS Meta-Analysis of Individual Patient Data. *J. Clin. Oncol.* **2012**, *30*, 1692–1698. [CrossRef] [PubMed]
9. Morabito, A.; Carillio, G.; Daniele, G.; Piccirillo, M.C.; Montanino, A.; Costanzo, R.; Sandomenico, C.; Giordano, P.; Normanno, N.; Perrone, F.; et al. Treatment of Small Cell Lung Cancer. *Crit. Rev. Oncol. Hematol.* **2014**, *91*, 257–270. [CrossRef]
10. Loehrer, P.J.; Ansari, R.; Gonin, R.; Monaco, F.; Fisher, W.; Sandler, A.; Einhorn, L.H. Cisplatin plus Etoposide with and without Ifosfamide in Extensive Small-Cell Lung Cancer: A Hoosier Oncology Group Study. *J. Clin. Oncol.* **1995**, *13*, 2594–2599. [CrossRef]
11. Pujol, J.L.; Daurès, J.P.; Rivière, A.; Quoix, E.; Westeel, V.; Quantin, X.; Breton, J.L.; Lemarié, E.; Poudenx, M.; Milleron, B.; et al. Etoposide plus Cisplatin with or without the Combination of 4′-Epidoxorubicin plus Cyclophosphamide in Treatment of Extensive Small-Cell Lung Cancer: A French Federation of Cancer Institutes Multicenter Phase III Randomized Study. *J. Natl. Cancer Inst.* **2001**, *93*, 300–308. [CrossRef]
12. Ihde, D.C.; Mulshine, J.L.; Kramer, B.S.; Steinberg, S.M.; Linnoila, R.I.; Gazdar, A.F.; Edison, M.; Phelps, R.M.; Lesar, M.; Phares, J.C. Prospective Randomized Comparison of High-Dose and Standard-Dose Etoposide and Cisplatin Chemotherapy in Patients with Extensive-Stage Small-Cell Lung Cancer. *J. Clin. Oncol.* **1994**, *12*, 2022–2034. [CrossRef]
13. Reck, M.; von Pawel, J.; Macha, H.-N.; Kaukel, E.; Deppermann, K.-M.; Bonnet, R.; Ulm, K.; Hessler, S.; Gatzemeier, U. Randomized Phase III Trial of Paclitaxel, Etoposide, and Carboplatin versus Carboplatin, Etoposide, and Vincristine in Patients with Small-Cell Lung Cancer. *J. Natl. Cancer Inst.* **2003**, *95*, 1118–1127. [CrossRef] [PubMed]
14. Masuda, N.; Fukuoka, M.; Kusunoki, Y.; Matsui, K.; Takifuji, N.; Kudoh, S.; Negoro, S.; Nishioka, M.; Nakagawa, K.; Takada, M. CPT-11: A New Derivative of Camptothecin for the Treatment of Refractory or Relapsed Small-Cell Lung Cancer. *J. Clin. Oncol.* **1992**, *10*, 1225–1229. [CrossRef]

15. Kudoh, S.; Fujiwara, Y.; Takada, Y.; Yamamoto, H.; Kinoshita, A.; Ariyoshi, Y.; Furuse, K.; Fukuoka, M. Phase II Study of Irinotecan Combined with Cisplatin in Patients with Previously Untreated Small-Cell Lung Cancer. West Japan Lung Cancer Group. *J. Clin. Oncol.* **1998**, *16*, 1068–1074. [CrossRef] [PubMed]
16. Noda, K.; Nishiwaki, Y.; Kawahara, M.; Negoro, S.; Sugiura, T.; Yokoyama, A.; Fukuoka, M.; Mori, K.; Watanabe, K.; Tamura, T.; et al. Irinotecan plus Cisplatin Compared with Etoposide plus Cisplatin for Extensive Small-Cell Lung Cancer. *New Engl. J. Med.* **2002**, *346*, 85–91. [CrossRef] [PubMed]
17. Hanna, N.; Bunn, P.A.; Langer, C.; Einhorn, L.; Guthrie, T.; Beck, T.; Ansari, R.; Ellis, P.; Byrne, M.; Morrison, M.; et al. Randomized Phase III Trial Comparing Irinotecan/Cisplatin with Etoposide/Cisplatin in Patients with Previously Untreated Extensive-Stage Disease Small-Cell Lung Cancer. *J. Clin. Oncol.* **2006**, *24*, 2038–2043. [CrossRef] [PubMed]
18. Lara, P.N.; Natale, R.; Crowley, J.; Lenz, H.J.; Redman, M.W.; Carleton, J.E.; Jett, J.; Langer, C.J.; Kuebler, J.P.; Dakhil, S.R.; et al. Phase III Trial of Irinotecan/Cisplatin Compared with Etoposide/Cisplatin in Extensive-Stage Small-Cell Lung Cancer: Clinical and Pharmacogenomic Results from SWOG S0124. *J. Clin. Oncol.* **2009**, *27*, 2530–2535. [CrossRef]
19. Hermes, A.; Bergman, B.; Bremnes, R.; Ek, L.; Fluge, S.; Sederholm, C.; Sundstrøm, S.; Thaning, L.; Vilsvik, J.; Aasebø, U.; et al. Irinotecan plus Carboplatin versus Oral Etoposide plus Carboplatin in Extensive Small-Cell Lung Cancer: A Randomized Phase III Trial. *J. Clin. Oncol.* **2008**, *26*, 4261–4267. [CrossRef]
20. Jiang, J.; Liang, X.; Zhou, X.; Huang, L.; Huang, R.; Chu, Z.; Zhan, Q. *A Meta-Analysis of Randomized Controlled Trials Comparing Irinotecan/Platinum with Etoposide/Platinum in Patients with Previously Untreated Extensive-Stage Small Cell Lung Cancer*; Centre for Reviews and Dissemination: UK, 2010.
21. Fink, T.H.; Huber, R.M.; Heigener, D.F.; Eschbach, C.; Waller, C.; Steinhauer, E.U.; Virchow, J.C.; Eberhardt, F.; Schweisfurth, H.; Schroeder, M.; et al. Topotecan/Cisplatin Compared with Cisplatin/Etoposide as First-Line Treatment for Patients with Extensive Disease Small-Cell Lung Cancer: Final Results of a Randomized Phase III Trial. *J. Thorac Oncol.* **2012**, *7*, 1432–1439. [CrossRef]
22. Sun, Y.; Cheng, Y.; Hao, X.; Wang, J.; Hu, C.; Han, B.; Liu, X.; Zhang, L.; Wan, H.; Xia, Z.; et al. Randomized Phase III Trial of Amrubicin/Cisplatin versus Etoposide/Cisplatin as First-Line Treatment for Extensive Small-Cell Lung Cancer. *BMC Cancer* **2016**, *16*, 265. [CrossRef] [PubMed]
23. Alexandrov, L.B.; Nik-Zainal, S.; Wedge, D.C.; Aparicio, S.A.J.R.; Behjati, S.; Biankin, A.V.; Bignell, G.R.; Bolli, N.; Borg, A.; Børresen-Dale, A.-L.; et al. Signatures of Mutational Processes in Human Cancer. *Nature* **2013**, *500*, 415–421. [CrossRef] [PubMed]
24. Tani, T.; Tanaka, K.; Idezuka, J.; Nishizawa, M. Regulatory T Cells in Paraneoplastic Neurological Syndromes. *J. Neuroimmunol.* **2008**, *196*, 166–169. [CrossRef] [PubMed]
25. Remon, J.; Passiglia, F.; Ahn, M.-J.; Barlesi, F.; Forde, P.M.; Garon, E.B.; Gettinger, S.; Goldberg, S.B.; Herbst, R.S.; Horn, L.; et al. Immune Checkpoint Inhibitors in Thoracic Malignancies: Review of the Existing Evidence by an IASLC Expert Panel and Recommendations. *J. Thorac Oncol.* **2020**, *15*, 914–947. [CrossRef]
26. Hato, S.V.; Khong, A.; de Vries, I.J.M.; Lesterhuis, W.J. Molecular Pathways: The Immunogenic Effects of Platinum-Based Chemotherapeutics. *Clin. Cancer Res.* **2014**, *20*, 2831–2837. [CrossRef]
27. Peng, J.; Hamanishi, J.; Matsumura, N.; Abiko, K.; Murat, K.; Baba, T.; Yamaguchi, K.; Horikawa, N.; Hosoe, Y.; Murphy, S.K.; et al. Chemotherapy Induces Programmed Cell Death-Ligand 1 Overexpression via the Nuclear Factor-KB to Foster an Immunosuppressive Tumor Microenvironment in Ovarian Cancer. *Cancer Res.* **2015**, *75*, 5034–5045. [CrossRef]
28. Qiao, M.; Jiang, T.; Ren, S.; Zhou, C. Combination Strategies on the Basis of Immune Checkpoint Inhibitors in Non-Small-Cell Lung Cancer: Where Do We Stand? *Clin. Lung Cancer* **2018**, *19*, 1–11. [CrossRef]
29. Liu, W.M.; Fowler, D.W.; Smith, P.; Dalgleish, A.G. Pre-Treatment with Chemotherapy Can Enhance the Antigenicity and Immunogenicity of Tumours by Promoting Adaptive Immune Responses. *Br. J. Cancer* **2010**, *102*, 115–123. [CrossRef]
30. Suzuki, E.; Kapoor, V.; Jassar, A.S.; Kaiser, L.R.; Albelda, S.M. Gemcitabine Selectively Eliminates Splenic Gr-1+/CD11b+ Myeloid Suppressor Cells in Tumor-Bearing Animals and Enhances Antitumor Immune Activity. *Clin. Cancer Res.* **2005**, *11*, 6713–6721. [CrossRef]
31. Lazzari, C.; Karachaliou, N.; Bulotta, A.; Viganó, M.; Mirabile, A.; Brioschi, E.; Santarpia, M.; Gianni, L.; Rosell, R.; Gregorc, V. Combination of Immunotherapy with Chemotherapy and Radiotherapy in Lung Cancer: Is This the Beginning of the End for Cancer? *Ther. Adv. Med. Oncol.* **2018**, *10*. [CrossRef]
32. Reck, M.; Bondarenko, I.; Luft, A.; Serwatowski, P.; Barlesi, F.; Chacko, R.; Sebastian, M.; Lu, H.; Cuillerot, J.-M.; Lynch, T.J. Ipilimumab in Combination with Paclitaxel and Carboplatin as First-Line Therapy in Extensive-Disease-Small-Cell Lung Cancer: Results from a Randomized, Double-Blind, Multicenter Phase 2 Trial. *Ann. Oncol.* **2013**, *24*, 75–83. [CrossRef]
33. Reck, M.; Luft, A.; Szczesna, A.; Havel, L.; Kim, S.-W.; Akerley, W.; Pietanza, M.C.; Wu, Y.-L.; Zielinski, C.; Thomas, M.; et al. Phase III Randomized Trial of Ipilimumab Plus Etoposide and Platinum Versus Placebo Plus Etoposide and Platinum in Extensive-Stage Small-Cell Lung Cancer. *J. Clin. Oncol.* **2016**, *34*, 3740–3748. [CrossRef]
34. Horn, L.; Mansfield, A.S.; Szczęsna, A.; Havel, L.; Krzakowski, M.; Hochmair, M.J.; Huemer, F.; Losonczy, G.; Johnson, M.L.; Nishio, M.; et al. First-Line Atezolizumab plus Chemotherapy in Extensive-Stage Small-Cell Lung Cancer. *N. Engl. J. Med.* **2018**, *379*, 2220–2229. [CrossRef]
35. Goldman, J.W.; Dvorkin, M.; Chen, Y.; Reinmuth, N.; Hotta, K.; Trukhin, D.; Statsenko, G.; Hochmair, M.J.; Özgüroğlu, M.; Ji, J.H.; et al. Durvalumab, with or without Tremelimumab, plus Platinum-Etoposide versus Platinum-Etoposide Alone in First-Line Treatment of Extensive-Stage Small-Cell Lung Cancer (CASPIAN): Updated Results from a Randomised, Controlled, Open-Label, Phase 3 Trial. *Lancet Oncol.* **2021**, *22*, 51–65. [CrossRef]

36. Rudin, C.M.; Awad, M.M.; Navarro, A.; Gottfried, M.; Peters, S.; Csőszi, T.; Cheema, P.K.; Rodriguez-Abreu, D.; Wollner, M.; Yang, J.C.-H.; et al. Pembrolizumab or Placebo Plus Etoposide and Platinum as First-Line Therapy for Extensive-Stage Small-Cell Lung Cancer: Randomized, Double-Blind, Phase III KEYNOTE-604 Study. *J. Clin. Oncol.* **2020**, *38*, 2369–2379. [CrossRef] [PubMed]
37. Leal, T.; Wang, Y.; Dowlati, A.; Lewis, D.A.; Chen, Y.; Mohindra, A.R.; Razaq, M.; Ahuja, H.G.; Liu, J.; King, D.M.; et al. Randomized Phase II Clinical Trial of Cisplatin/Carboplatin and Etoposide (CE) Alone or in Combination with Nivolumab as Frontline Therapy for Extensive-Stage Small Cell Lung Cancer (ES-SCLC): ECOG-ACRIN EA5161. *JCO* **2020**, *38*, 9000. [CrossRef]
38. Gadgeel, S.M.; Pennell, N.A.; Fidler, M.J.; Halmos, B.; Bonomi, P.; Stevenson, J.; Schneider, B.; Sukari, A.; Ventimiglia, J.; Chen, W.; et al. Phase II Study of Maintenance Pembrolizumab in Patients with Extensive-Stage Small Cell Lung Cancer (SCLC). *J. Thorac Oncol.* **2018**, *13*, 1393–1399. [CrossRef] [PubMed]
39. Owonikoko, T.K.; Kim, H.R.; Govindan, R.; Ready, N.; Reck, M.; Peters, S.; Dakhil, S.R.; Navarro, A.; Rodriguez-Cid, J.; Schenker, M.; et al. Nivolumab (Nivo) plus Ipilimumab (Ipi), Nivo, or Placebo (Pbo) as Maintenance Therapy in Patients (Pts) with Extensive Disease Small Cell Lung Cancer (ED-SCLC) after First-Line (1L) Platinum-Based Chemotherapy (Chemo): Results from the Double-Blind, Randomized Phase III CheckMate 451 Study. *Ann. Oncol.* **2019**, *30*, ii77. [CrossRef]
40. Ott, P.A.; Elez, E.; Hiret, S.; Kim, D.-W.; Morosky, A.; Saraf, S.; Piperdi, B.; Mehnert, J.M. Pembrolizumab in Patients With Extensive-Stage Small-Cell Lung Cancer: Results From the Phase Ib KEYNOTE-028 Study. *J. Clin. Oncol.* **2017**, *35*, 3823–3829. [CrossRef]
41. Chung, H.C.; Lopez-Martin, J.A.; Kao, S.C.-H.; Miller, W.H.; Ros, W.; Gao, B.; Marabelle, A.; Gottfried, M.; Zer, A.; Delord, J.-P.; et al. Phase 2 Study of Pembrolizumab in Advanced Small-Cell Lung Cancer (SCLC): KEYNOTE-158. *JCO* **2018**, *36*, 8506. [CrossRef]
42. Chung, H.C.; Piha-Paul, S.A.; Lopez-Martin, J.; Schellens, J.H.M.; Kao, S.; Miller, W.H.; Delord, J.-P.; Gao, B.; Planchard, D.; Gottfried, M.; et al. Pembrolizumab After Two or More Lines of Previous Therapy in Patients With Recurrent or Metastatic SCLC: Results From the KEYNOTE-028 and KEYNOTE-158 Studies. *J. Thorac Oncol.* **2020**, *15*, 618–627. [CrossRef]
43. Antonia, S.J.; López-Martin, J.A.; Bendell, J.; Ott, P.A.; Taylor, M.; Eder, J.P.; Jäger, D.; Pietanza, M.C.; Le, D.T.; de Braud, F.; et al. Nivolumab Alone and Nivolumab plus Ipilimumab in Recurrent Small-Cell Lung Cancer (CheckMate 032): A Multicentre, Open-Label, Phase 1/2 Trial. *Lancet Oncol.* **2016**, *17*, 883–895. [CrossRef]
44. Ready, N.; Farago, A.F.; de Braud, F.; Atmaca, A.; Hellmann, M.D.; Schneider, J.G.; Spigel, D.R.; Moreno, V.; Chau, I.; Hann, C.L.; et al. Third-Line Nivolumab Monotherapy in Recurrent SCLC: CheckMate 032. *J. Thorac Oncol.* **2019**, *14*, 237–244. [CrossRef]
45. Reck, M.; Vicente, D.; Ciuleanu, T.; Gettinger, S.; Peters, S.; Horn, L.; Audigier-Valette, C.; Pardo, N.; Juan-Vidal, O.; Cheng, Y.; et al. Efficacy and Safety of Nivolumab (Nivo) Monotherapy versus Chemotherapy (Chemo) in Recurrent Small Cell Lung Cancer (SCLC): Results from CheckMate 331. *Ann. Oncol.* **2018**, *29*, x43. [CrossRef]
46. Goldman, J.W.; Dowlati, A.; Antonia, S.J.; Nemunaitis, J.J.; Butler, M.O.; Segal, N.H.; Smith, P.A.; Weiss, J.; Zandberg, D.P.; Xiao, F.; et al. Safety and Antitumor Activity of Durvalumab Monotherapy in Patients with Pretreated Extensive Disease Small-Cell Lung Cancer (ED-SCLC). *JCO* **2018**, *36*, 8518. [CrossRef]
47. Pujol, J.-L.; Greillier, L.; Audigier-Valette, C.; Moro-Sibilot, D.; Uwer, L.; Hureaux, J.; Guisier, F.; Carmier, D.; Madelaine, J.; Otto, J.; et al. A Randomized Non-Comparative Phase II Study of Anti-Programmed Cell Death-Ligand 1 Atezolizumab or Chemotherapy as Second-Line Therapy in Patients With Small Cell Lung Cancer: Results From the IFCT-1603 Trial. *J. Thorac Oncol.* **2019**, *14*, 903–913. [CrossRef] [PubMed]
48. Poirier, J.T.; George, J.; Owonikoko, T.K.; Berns, A.; Brambilla, E.; Byers, L.A.; Carbone, D.; Chen, H.J.; Christensen, C.L.; Dive, C.; et al. New Approaches to SCLC Therapy: From the Laboratory to the Clinic. *J. Thorac Oncol.* **2020**, *15*, 520–540. [CrossRef]
49. Wakuda, K.; Kenmotsu, H.; Naito, T.; Akamatsu, H.; Ono, A.; Shukuya, T.; Nakamura, Y.; Tsuya, A.; Murakami, H.; Takahashi, T.; et al. Efficacy of Rechallenge Chemotherapy in Patients with Sensitive Relapsed Small Cell Lung Cancer. *Am. J. Clin. Oncol.* **2015**, *38*, 28–32. [CrossRef]
50. Owonikoko, T.K.; Behera, M.; Chen, Z.; Bhimani, C.; Curran, W.J.; Khuri, F.R.; Ramalingam, S.S. A Systematic Analysis of Efficacy of Second-Line Chemotherapy in Sensitive and Refractory Small-Cell Lung Cancer. *J. Thorac Oncol.* **2012**, *7*, 866–872. [CrossRef]
51. von Pawel, J.; Schiller, J.H.; Shepherd, F.A.; Fields, S.Z.; Kleisbauer, J.P.; Chrysson, N.G.; Stewart, D.J.; Clark, P.I.; Palmer, M.C.; Depierre, A.; et al. Topotecan versus Cyclophosphamide, Doxorubicin, and Vincristine for the Treatment of Recurrent Small-Cell Lung Cancer. *J. Clin. Oncol.* **1999**, *17*, 658–667. [CrossRef]
52. Jotte, R.; Conkling, P.; Reynolds, C.; Galsky, M.D.; Klein, L.; Fitzgibbons, J.F.; McNally, R.; Renschler, M.F.; Oliver, J.W. Randomized Phase II Trial of Single-Agent Amrubicin or Topotecan as Second-Line Treatment in Patients with Small-Cell Lung Cancer Sensitive to First-Line Platinum-Based Chemotherapy. *J. Clin. Oncol.* **2011**, *29*, 287–293. [CrossRef]
53. Gregorc, V.; Cavina, R.; Novello, S.; Grossi, F.; Lazzari, C.; Capelletto, E.; Genova, C.; Salini, G.; Lambiase, A.; Santoro, A. NGR-HTNF and Doxorubicin as Second-Line Treatment of Patients with Small Cell Lung Cancer. *Oncologist* **2018**, *23*, 1133-e112. [CrossRef] [PubMed]
54. Trigo, J.; Subbiah, V.; Besse, B.; Moreno, V.; López, R.; Sala, M.A.; Peters, S.; Ponce, S.; Fernández, C.; Alfaro, V.; et al. Lurbinectedin as Second-Line Treatment for Patients with Small-Cell Lung Cancer: A Single-Arm, Open-Label, Phase 2 Basket Trial. *Lancet Oncol.* **2020**, *21*, 645–654. [CrossRef]
55. Calcinotto, A.; Grioni, M.; Jachetti, E.; Curnis, F.; Mondino, A.; Parmiani, G.; Corti, A.; Bellone, M. Targeting TNF-α to Neoangiogenic Vessels Enhances Lymphocyte Infiltration in Tumors and Increases the Therapeutic Potential of Immunotherapy. *J. Immunol.* **2012**, *188*, 2687–2694. [CrossRef] [PubMed]

56. Tang, H.; Wang, Y.; Chlewicki, L.K.; Zhang, Y.; Guo, J.; Liang, W.; Wang, J.; Wang, X.; Fu, Y.-X. Facilitating T Cell Infiltration in Tumor Microenvironment Overcomes Resistance to PD-L1 Blockade. *Cancer Cell* **2016**, *29*, 285–296. [CrossRef] [PubMed]
57. George, J.; Lim, J.S.; Jang, S.J.; Cun, Y.; Ozretić, L.; Kong, G.; Leenders, F.; Lu, X.; Fernández-Cuesta, L.; Bosco, G.; et al. Comprehensive Genomic Profiles of Small Cell Lung Cancer. *Nature* **2015**, *524*, 47–53. [CrossRef]
58. Nau, M.M.; Brooks, B.J.; Battey, J.; Sausville, E.; Gazdar, A.F.; Kirsch, I.R.; McBride, O.W.; Bertness, V.; Hollis, G.F.; Minna, J.D. L-Myc, a New Myc-Related Gene Amplified and Expressed in Human Small Cell Lung Cancer. *Nature* **1985**, *318*, 69–73. [CrossRef] [PubMed]
59. Johnson, B.E.; Makuch, R.W.; Simmons, A.D.; Gazdar, A.F.; Burch, D.; Cashell, A.W. Myc Family DNA Amplification in Small Cell Lung Cancer Patients' Tumors and Corresponding Cell Lines. *Cancer Res.* **1988**, *48*, 5163–5166.
60. Yokomizo, A.; Tindall, D.J.; Drabkin, H.; Gemmill, R.; Franklin, W.; Yang, P.; Sugio, K.; Smith, D.I.; Liu, W. PTEN/MMAC1 Mutations Identified in Small Cell, but Not in Non-Small Cell Lung Cancers. *Oncogene* **1998**, *17*, 475–479. [CrossRef]
61. Karachaliou, N.; Pilotto, S.; Lazzari, C.; Bria, E.; de Marinis, F.; Rosell, R. Cellular and Molecular Biology of Small Cell Lung Cancer: An Overview. *Transl. Lung Cancer Res.* **2016**, *5*, 2–15. [CrossRef]

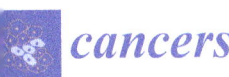

Review

Pathology and Classification of SCLC

Maria Gabriela Raso *, Neus Bota-Rabassedas and Ignacio I. Wistuba *

Department of Translational Molecular Pathology, The University of Texas MD Anderson Cancer Center, Houston, TX 77030, USA; mbota@mdanderson.org
* Correspondence: graso@mdanderson.org (M.G.R.); iiwistuba@mdanderson.org (I.I.W.); Tel.: +1-713-834-6026 (M.G.R.); +1-713-563-9184 (I.I.W.)

Simple Summary: Small cell lung carcinoma (SCLC), is a high-grade neuroendocrine carcinoma defined by its aggressiveness, poor differentiation, and somber prognosis. This review highlights current pathological concepts including classification, immunohistochemistry features, and differential diagnosis. Additionally, we summarize the current knowledge of the immune tumor microenvironment, tumor heterogeneity, and genetic variations of SCLC. Recent comprehensive genomic research has improved our understanding of the diverse biological processes that occur in this tumor type, suggesting that a new era of molecular-driven treatment decisions is finally foreseeable for SCLC patients.

Abstract: Lung cancer is consistently the leading cause of cancer-related death worldwide, and it ranks as the second most frequent type of new cancer cases diagnosed in the United States, both in males and females. One subtype of lung cancer, small cell lung carcinoma (SCLC), is an aggressive, poorly differentiated, and high-grade neuroendocrine carcinoma that accounts for 13% of all lung carcinomas. SCLC is the most frequent neuroendocrine lung tumor, and it is commonly presented as an advanced stage disease in heavy smokers. Due to its clinical presentation, it is typically diagnosed in small biopsies or cytology specimens, with routine immunostaining only. However, immunohistochemistry markers are extremely valuable in demonstrating neuroendocrine features of SCLC and supporting its differential diagnosis. The 2015 WHO classification grouped all pulmonary neuroendocrine carcinomas in one category and maintained the SCLC combined variant that was previously recognized. In this review, we explore multiple aspects of the pathologic features of this entity, as well as clinically relevant immunohistochemistry markers expression and its molecular characteristics. In addition, we will focus on characteristics of the tumor microenvironment, and the latest pathogenesis findings to better understand the new therapeutic options in the current era of personalized therapy.

Keywords: pathology and classification of SCLC; biology of SCLC; immune-checkpoint inhibitors in SCLC

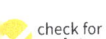

Citation: Raso, M.G.; Bota-Rabassedas, N.; Wistuba, I.I. Pathology and Classification of SCLC. *Cancers* **2021**, *13*, 820. https://doi.org/10.3390/cancers13040820

Academic Editors: Alessandro Morabito and Christian Rolfo
Received: 21 December 2020
Accepted: 10 February 2021
Published: 16 February 2021

Publisher's Note: MDPI stays neutral with regard to jurisdictional claims in published maps and institutional affiliations.

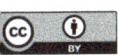

Copyright: © 2021 by the authors. Licensee MDPI, Basel, Switzerland. This article is an open access article distributed under the terms and conditions of the Creative Commons Attribution (CC BY) license (https://creativecommons.org/licenses/by/4.0/).

1. Introduction

Lung carcinoma has consistently remained the leading cause of cancer-related death worldwide [1,2]. Currently, in the United States, it ranks as the second most frequent type of new cancer case, both in males and females, accounting for more than 228,800 new cases in 2020 and 12.7% of all new cancer cases [3,4]. Small cell lung carcinoma (SCLC) is a very aggressive, poorly differentiated, and high-grade neuroendocrine carcinoma representing approximately 13% of all lung carcinomas. Most commonly seen in heavy smokers as an advanced stage disease, it clinically presents with early metastatic spread and good responsiveness to initial therapy, and in most patients, it is consistently followed by relapse with a chemo resistant disease [5].

Remarkably, no preneoplastic lesions have been identified in SCLC [6]. This is in stark contrast with the recognition of the diffuse idiopathic pulmonary neuroendocrine cell hyperplasia (DIPNECH) as the precursor lesion for neuroendocrine carcinoids of the lung [7,8], pulmonary neuroendocrine cells (PNECs) are considered putative precursors of small cell lung cancer [9], while the expression of ASCL1 (both in tumors and cell lines) confirms SCLC neuroendocrine lineage [10,11]. However, this concept was challenged with the identification of a distinctive tuft cell variant, showing high POU2F3 expression while lacking neuroendocrine markers, postulating a SCLC-P entity distinctive from the classical neuroendocrine variants, and strongly suggesting a distinct cell-of-origin for this subtype [12]. Alternatively, trans-differentiation towards a tuft cell expression profile from a cell of origin shared with other subtypes remains an alternative explanation. Data from genetically engineered mouse models and human tumors have revealed multiple levels of heterogeneity in SCLC. Additionally, using genetically defined mouse models of SCLC, investigators have uncovered distinct metastatic programs attributable to the cell-of-origin cell-type, concluding that intra-tumoral heterogeneity is influenced by the cell of origin and proposing that SCLC can arise from molecularly distinctive cells.

2. Pathological Classification of SCLC

SCLC was first described in 1879 by Harting and Hesse and classified as a lymphosarcoma [13]; later, in 1926, it was classified as small 'oat cell' carcinomas of the lung [14]. From that point forward, it has been historically known as oat cell carcinoma [15,16], and belongs to the neuroendocrine lung tumors group defined in the last WHO Classification of Lung Tumors [17]. In 2015, the World Health Organization (WHO) Classification of Tumors of the Lung, Pleura, Thymus, and Heart was published with numerous important changes from the previous 2004 publication. One of the most significant changes in this edition involves the inclusion of neuroendocrine tumors (NE) grouped together in one category, recognizing four major NE tumors: typical carcinoid tumor (TC), atypical carcinoid tumor (AC), SCLC, and large cell NE carcinoma (LCNEC) [17]. The current sub-classification recognizes two subtypes: pure SCLC and combined SCLC, the latter is determined by the presence of features of a different histological carcinoma, non-small cell lung carcinoma (NSCLC), variant or at least containing 10% of large cell carcinoma component. Up to 28% of surgically resected SCLC tumors are combined SCLC, and of these, 16% belong to the large cell carcinoma variant [18,19].

3. Macroscopic Features of SCLC

As a highly aggressive disease, SCLC is found disseminated in the initial clinical presentation in the majority of cases, and surgery is limited to a small subgroup of patients with confined disease [20]. Usually, these tumors undergo surgical resection only when diagnosis of SCLC has not been previously established, and it is from those infrequent surgical specimens that a macroscopic description of SCLC tumors is described. These tumors are grossly identifiable as fleshy, ranging from a white and grayish to a light tan color, soft and friable irregular masses, with necrotic cut surface areas. The majority of them are situated in hilar or perihilar areas, with less than 5% of the cases presenting in peripheral locations. Invasion into the peribronchial tissue and lymph node is often grossly identifiable, typically spreading in circumferentially along the submucosa of the bronchi.

4. Microscopic Features of SCLC

4.1. Cytological Features

Cytology is a very reliable method to establish a SCLC diagnosis and often a valuable complement to bronchial biopsies where crush artifacts may hamper a definitive diagnosis. The most common cytologic feature is highly cellular aspirates with presence of small blue cells with very scant or null cytoplasm, loosely arranged or in a syncytial pattern (Figure 1). Within tightly cohesive sheets, nuclear molding is well developed. Additionally, a background of single cells, doublets, triplets, and small cell cords with extensive necrosis are characteristic of this entity. The mitotic rate is usually very high (10 mitosis per 10 high power fields) and chromatin smearing is very frequent. Well-preserved cells show the characteristic "salt and pepper" chromatin patter, while less well-preserved cells show dark blue chromatin. Cytoplasmic globules, also named paranuclear blue bodies, are considered distinctive of a SCLC diagnosis [21,22].

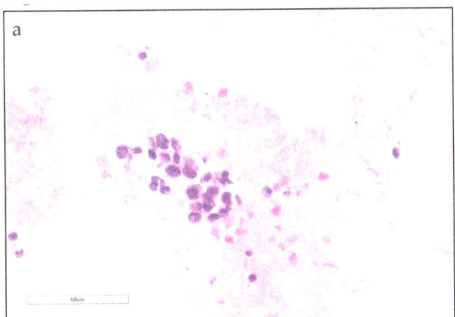 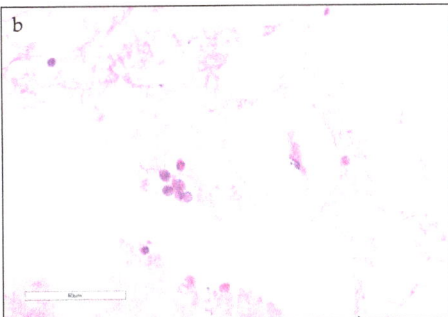

Figure 1. Small cell lung carcinoma (SCLC) cytological and histological characteristics. (**a,b**) High power field view of SCLC in cellular aspirates. Loosely arranged small blue cells with scant cytoplasm and fine chromatin features (arrow).

4.2. Histopathological Features

Hematoxylin and eosin (H&E) assessment of a SCLC tumor under a light microscope main features is defined by the presence of diffuse sheets of small round to fusiform cells, with scant cytoplasm, and inconspicuous or absent nucleoli with finely granular nuclear chromatin (Figure 2). Nuclear chromatin smearing, also called crushed artifact, is a common feature together with nuclear molding (Figures 2 and 3). Extensive intratumoral necrosis is often recognized, as well as the high mitotic index that defines the tumor (average of 40 mitosis/mm^2 area) [18,23,24] (Figure 2). In addition to the common diffuse sheet-like growth pattern, SCLC tumor can demonstrate other growth features as peripheral palisading, streams, ribbons, organoid nesting, and rosettes [18,23]. Another characteristic feature is the frequent basophilic nuclear debris encrustation of the blood vessel wall, widely known as Azzopardi effect (Figure 4) [25,26]. Larger specimens may present a variety of cellular characteristics like larger cells, pleomorphic cells, giant tumor cells, and dispersed chromatin with prominent nucleoli, among others.

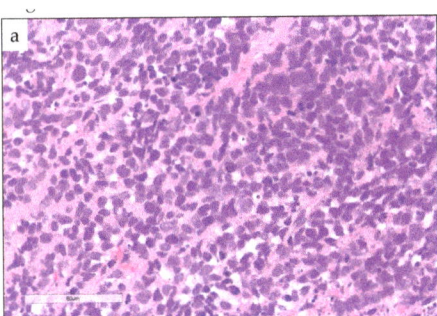 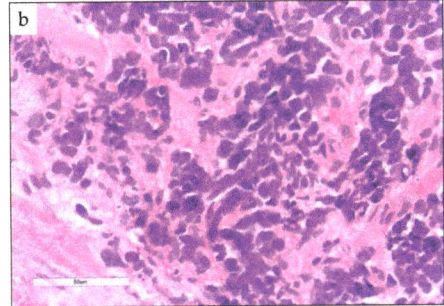

Figure 2. Small cell lung carcinoma (SCLC) cytological and histological characteristics. High power field view of a formalin fixed paraffin embedded tissue H&E stained slide showing in (**a**). sheets of small cells with scant cytoplasm and nuclear molding and (**b**). Sheets of tightly packed small cells and intratumoral necrosis.

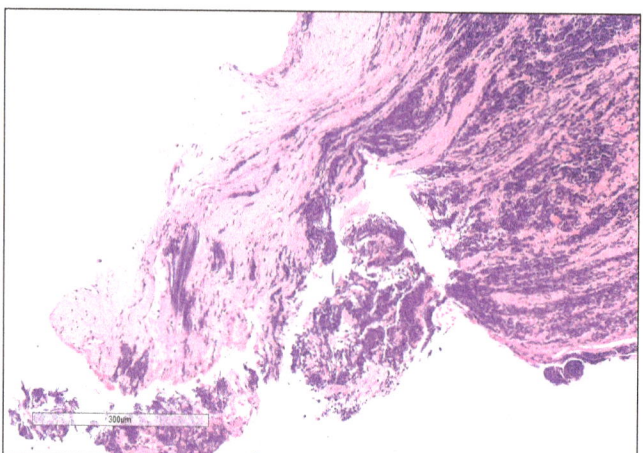

Figure 3. Chromatin smearing "crush artifact". High magnification showing Small cell lung carcinoma (SCLC) with extensive chromatin smearing "crush artifact".

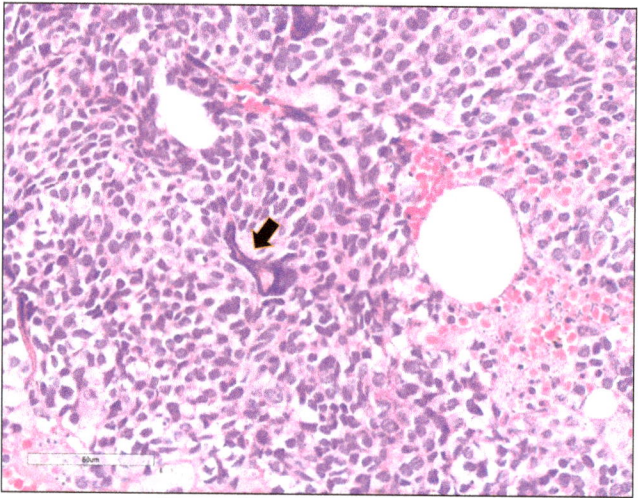

Figure 4. Azzopardi phenomenon. High magnification showing Small cell lung carcinoma (SCLC) with basophilic nuclear debris encrustation of the blood vessel wall (arrow).

SCLC can be observed as a pure SCLC histology or combined with NSCLC histology features. The latter refers to the admixture of NSCLC elements; where adenocarcinoma, squamous cell carcinoma (SCC), and large cell carcinoma can be seen, as well as, although at a lower frequency, giant cell carcinoma and spindle cell carcinoma [17]. To establish a diagnosis of combined SCLC and large cell carcinoma, large cells have to constitute at least 10% of the tumor; however, no assessment of the percentage of the secondary histology is necessary to render a combined SCLC diagnosis for other NSCLC histologies [19].

4.3. Immunohistochemistry

The histopathological diagnosis is based on light microscopy using routine H&E stained slides, as stated in the current 2015 WHO classification. Immunohistochemistry (IHC) assays are required when confirmation of equivocal features is necessary or when a differential diagnosis must be addressed, especially in small biopsies with crush artifacts (Table 1).

Table 1. Immunohistochemistry (IHC) markers and immunohistochemical characteristics of SCLC.

Marker	Stain	Comments
Keratin (MW^{low})	+	Paranuclear/Cytoplasmatic diffuse
Keratin (MW^{high})	-	Not expressed in SCLC
Ki67	+	At high levels, hallmark of SCLC vs NE tumors
NCAM/CD56	+	Variable/Lower compared to other NE tumors
Chromogranin	+	Variable/Lower compared to other NE tumors
Synaptophysin	+	Variable/Lower compared to other NE tumors
INSM1	+	Variable/Lower compared to other NE tumors
Napsin A	-	Presence of this marker favors LCNEC diagnosis
TTF-1	+	Useful SCLC diagnosis vs NE tumors not originated in the lung
BCL-2	+	Often expressed in SCLC
P16	+	Expressed in >95% of SCLC
CD117/KIT	+	Expressed in 60% of SCLC
P-RB	-	Never expressed in SCLC
OTP	-	Never expressed in SCLC

SCLC stains positively for low molecular weight keratins, showing a dot-like paranuclear or diffuse cytoplasmic staining, and is negative for high molecular weight keratins. SCLC shows a variable expression of neuroendocrine differentiation markers such as neural cell adhesion molecule (NCAM/CD56), chromogranin, synaptophysin, and insulinoma-associated protein 1 (INSM1), and usually presents lower protein levels than low-to-intermediate grade neuroendocrine tumors. It is important to note that a minority of SCLCs are negative for all standard neuroendocrine markers. Importantly, immunohistochemistry has only a limited role in distinguishing LCNEC and SCLC. One potentially helpful, although with low-sensitivity, feature is focal and weak napsin A immunoreactivity, which can be seen in up to 15% of LCNEC [27] while SCLC is consistently negative for this marker. Thus, when present, weak napsin A labeling in a high-grade NE carcinoma may favor the diagnosis towards LCNEC. Thyroid transcription factor-1 (TTF-1) is a homeodomain-containing transcription factor selectively expressed in pulmonary adenocarcinomas, thyroid tumors, and small cell carcinomas. Interestingly, TTF-1 is expressed in close to 90% of SCLC, which can be useful for differentiating SCLC from neuroendocrine cancers not originating from the lung.

High Ki67 (MIB-1) labeling index (>50%, usually 70–100%) is a hallmark of SCLC, helping in distinguishing it from low- and intermediate-grade neuroendocrine cancers [28]. Other markers used to characterize SCLC are: B-cell lymphoma 2 (BCL2; expressed often), P16 nuclear staining (expressed in 95–100% of cases), tyrosine-protein kinase KIT (CD117/c-KIT; expressed in about 60% of cases, retinoblastoma protein (P-RB; always negative), and homeobox protein orthopedia (OTP, always negative) [29].

5. Differential Diagnosis of SCLC

Although SCLC has a very well-defined diagnostic criteria, sampling issues, fixation artifacts, and the morphologic variability of pure SCLC tumor cells, can all potentially make the diagnosis of SCLC challenging.

The current WHO classification of lung cancer recognizes four neuroendocrine tumors, namely typical carcinoid tumor (TC), atypical carcinoid tumor (AC), SCLC, and large cell NE carcinoma (LCNEC). Neuroendocrine tumors have a wide differential diagnosis based on their mitotic rate and necrosis extension. Other histologies, such as basaloid squamous cell carcinoma, small round cell sarcoma, metastatic breast carcinoma, and non-Hodgkin's lymphoma, may be considered in the differential diagnosis of SCLC. In these cases, it is important to perform IHC in order to confirm its neuroendocrine differentiation and epithelial nature, detect other differentiation markers, as well as to assess the site of origin and proliferation rate. As an example, p63 and TTF-1 expression is useful in distinguishing SCLC from poorly differentiated nonkeratinizing SCC: p63 positive and TTF-1 negative expression consequently indicates a poorly differentiated nonkeratinizing SCC, while an opposite immunostaining pattern identifies a SCLC diagnosis.

6. Landscape of the Immune Tumor Microenvironment in SCLC

Current evidence shows that the immune system is capable of generating antitumor responses against various tumors, including lung cancer, suggesting that immunotherapy may be a viable therapeutic approach for patients with SCLC [30]. Increasing evidence shows that the immune system is involved in the pathophysiology of SCLC [31]. Moreover confirmation that SCLC is immunogenic comes from the relationship between immune activity and prognosis. For instance, more infiltrating CD45+ T-cells in SCLC tumors were found to be a predictor of better OS, independently of stage and performance status. In addition, more effector T-cells were found in limited stage disease (LD) SCLC compared with extended stage disease (ED) SCLC cases, and higher effector-to-regulatory T-cell ratios were associated with longer survival [22,30,32].

As it is known, NSCLC patients with a high mutation burden have been shown to be particularly sensitive to immunotherapeutic agents that inhibit the PD-1 pathway [30,33,34], indicating that SCLC could potentially benefit from immunotherapy treatments, given its high mutation burden [35]. However, several mechanisms of immune resistance have been identified in SCLC, such as downregulation of major histocompatibility complex (MHC) antigens I and II, low PD-L1 expression, increase in regulatory T-cells, and poor tumor infiltration of effector T-cells, partially due to a lack of vasculature surrounding the tumor [36]. These features likely diminish the response in SCLC compared to the observed immunotherapeutic response in NSCLC.

Immunotherapies targeted against programmed death ligand 1 (PD-L1) and its receptor (PD-1) have improved survival in a subset of NSCLC patients. PD-L1 protein expression has emerged as a biomarker that predicts which patients are more likely to respond to immunotherapy. Noticeably, PD-L1 expression has been demonstrated in SCLC, although at lower levels than NSCLC. In one retrospective study of 102 SCLC specimens, PD-L1 expression was observed in 72% of tumor cells and was associated with significantly longer overall survival (OS) [37]. In contrast, another study involving 94 clinical cases of small cell NE carcinoma found PD-L1 expression in 19% of cases, and only expressed in stromal cells [38]. Similarly, others have reported PD-L1 expression in tumor cells, ranging from 27% to 89% [39,40]. The inconsistency of these findings is most likely related to differences in PD-L1 detection methods, the utilization of different IHC platforms and antibodies, as well as the lack of standardized scoring methods [41].

Regulatory CD4$^+$ T-cells play a major role suppressing other immune cells, lessening the immune response. A study demonstrated the ability of SCLC cell lines to induce a de novo differentiation from activated CD4$^+$ T-cells to regulatory CD4$^+$ T-cells (FOXP3$^+$ T-cells), by secretion of IL-15 [42]. The same study, including data from a cohort of 65 SCLC patients, demonstrated the presence of IL-15 in SCLC biopsies, and a positive correlation between increase in tumor infiltration of FOXP3 T-cells and worse OS [42], opening new avenues for future immune therapies against SCLC.

MHC proteins are usually present at the cell surface of tumor cells, playing a central role in antigen presentation to activate cytotoxic T-cells and elicit antitumor immune response. Strikingly, it is another component of SCLC suppressed immunogenicity, as both MHC class I and II expression have been reported to be decreased in SCLC [43,44].

Overall, there is solid evidence that SCLC has the potential to be immunogenic. This could be achieved by counteracting the immunosuppressive nature of this tumor type, and for this purpose, further research is needed to understand the specific pathways that drive SCLC-mediated immunosuppression.

7. SCLC Tumor Heterogeneity

Evidence of intra-tumoral heterogeneity in SCLC was demonstrated many years ago by the diverse expression of antigens detectable with monoclonal antibodies [45]. Contemporary work from animal models such as genetically engineered mouse models (GEMMs) and patient-derived xenograft/cell-derived xenograft (PDX/CDX) models has shown new levels of cellular complexity in SCLC. The presence of several subpopulations of SCLC cells and their functional interactions may explain the outstanding plasticity of SCLC tumors and their striking metastatic potential [46,47]. Additionally, SCLC tumors that look similar at the histopathological level may represent distinct subtypes of tumors, and these differences have an impact on the response to specific therapeutic agents. A better understanding of genetic and cellular heterogeneity will guide the development of personalized approaches to help SCLC patients [46].

8. Genetic Variation of SCLC

SCLC is a molecularly complex disease comprising numerous genetic alterations, including variations in tumor suppressor genes, copy number variation, somatic mutations in transcription factors, chromatin modification, and receptor tyrosine kinases or their downstream signaling components [48] (Table 2). Notably, 95% of tumors reveal loss of *Retinoblastoma 1 (RB1)* and more than 65% present *TP53* mutations [49–53]. In addition, frequent allelic loss involving chromosome arm 3p deletion has been reported in 91% of SLCC tumors [54]. Mutations in *v-myc avian myelocytomatosis viral oncogene homolog (MYC)* family genes, *BCL2*, *Phosphatase and tensin homolog (PTEN)*, *Slit homolog 2 (SLIT2)*, *CREB binding protein (CREBBP)*, *Ephrin type-A receptor 7 (EPHA7)*, and *Fibroblast Growth Factor Receptor 1 (FGFR1)* mutations have been identified [35]. Other molecular abnormalities, such as increased expression of c-KIT, amplification of *MYC* family members (*MYC*, *MYC lung carcinoma-derived homolog 1 [MYCL1]*, *MYC neuroblastoma-derived homolog [MYCN]*), and loss of *PTEN* have also been described in subsets of SCLC [54–58].

Table 2. Genomic alterations and markers for Small cell lung carcinoma (SCLC).

Marker	Genetic Alteration	Comments
RB1	Loss	95% of SCLC
TP53	Mutation	65% of SCLC
Chromosome arm 3p	Deletion	91% of SCLC
MYC	Mutation	Variable
BCL2	Mutation	Variable
PTEN	Mutation	Variable
SLIT2	Mutation	Variable
CREBBP	Mutation	Variable
EPHA7	Mutation	Variable
FGFR1	Mutation	Variable
c-KIT	Increased Expression	Described in some SCLC subsets
MYC, MYCL1, MYCN	Amplification	Described in some SCLC subsets
PTEN	Loss	Described in some SCLC subsets

Recently, comprehensive genomic research studies with cell lines, GEMMs, and PDX models have revealed biologically heterogenous SCLC subtypes (Table 3), based on mRNA expression profiles defined by the differential expression of four key transcription regulators: *achaete-scute homologue 1 (ASCL1*; also known as *ASH1)*, *neurogenic differentiation factor 1 (NeuroD1)*, *yes-associated protein 1 (YAP1)*, and *POU class 2 homeobox 3 (POU2F3)*. As a result of such studies, recent consensus suggested grouping SCLC into four subtypes defined by mRNA expression of *ASCL1*, *NEUROD1*, *POU2F3*, and *YAP1*. Consequently, a working nomenclature for SCLC subtypes defined by the relative expression of these four factors was proposed, classifying cases as: ASCL1 high (SCLC-A), NEUROD1 high (SCLC-N), POU2F3 high (SCLC-P), and YAP1 high (SCLC-Y) [12,59–61]. SCLC-Y is characterized by WT *RB1* enrichment [62] and low or absent expression of *ASCL1*, *NEUROD1*, and other neuroendocrine markers, accounting for approximately 5% to 10% of SCLC tumors. In most instances of combined SCLC with NSCLC histologies, there is a strong evidence of clonality between SCLC and NSCLC components, likely indicating a common precursor cell in such cases [12,63]. When comparing the morphological features and considering the similar genetics and genomics characteristics between SCLC-Y (WT *RB1*) and LCNEC (WT *RB1*, WT *KEAP1*, WT *STK11*) subtypes, together with a low or absent expression of *ASCL1* and *NEUROD1*, it has been suggested that these two lung cancer subtypes belong to a single entity [62]; thus, implying potential impact in molecular classification and clinical implications. Recently, a first comprehensive IHC-based study in patient samples has confirmed highly distinct characteristics of SCLC tumors expressing *ASCL1* (SCLC-A) and/or *NEUROD1* (SCLC-N) (86%) compared to SCLC lacking these markers (14%) [59]. The former is associated with a high NE program (NE-markers high/TTF-1 high/DLL3 high) and a pure SCLC histology, whereas the latter exhibits an enrichment in a combined SCLC histology. The same study also confirmed a highly distinctive nature for *POU2F3*-expressing tumors (SCLC-P), which account for 7% of SCLC [59]. Using tumor expression data and non-negative matrix factorization, Gay et al. identified four SCLC subtypes defined largely by differential expression of transcription factors ASCL1, NEUROD1, and POU2F3 or low expression of all three transcription factor signatures accompanied by an Inflamed gene signature (SCLC-A, N, P, and I, respectively). Stating that the SCLC-I subgroup may benefit from the addition of immunotherapy to chemotherapy, while the other subtypes each have distinct vulnerabilities, including to inhibitors of PARP, Aurora kinases, or BCL-2 [64].

Table 3. Molecular classification of Small cell lung carcinoma (SCLC) subsets.

SCLC Subtype	Markers	Characteristics
SCLC-A	ASCL1	Pure SCLC histology; NE-markers^{high}/TTF-1^{high}/DLL3^{high}
SCLC-N	NEUROD1	Enrichment in combined SCLC histology; NE-markers^{high}/TTF-1^{high}/DLL3^{high}
SCLC-P	POU2F3	Low or absent expression of ASCL1 and NEUROD1, NE-markers^{low}/TTF-1^{low}/DLL3^{low}
SCLC-Y	YAP1	Low or absent expression of ASCL1 and NEUROD1; RB1^{wt}
SCLC-I	Inflamed Gene signature	Low expression of ASCL1, NEUROD1, and POU2F3

Albeit uncommon, transformation of NSCLC into SCLC has been observed as a resistance mechanism upon treatment of *EGFR*-mutated NSCLC with *EGFR* tyrosine kinase inhibitors (TKI) (3% to 10% of *EGFR*-TKI resistant cases) [65,66]. Interestingly, NSCLC to SCLC transformation is dependent on EGFR mutation, as only rare instances of such transformation have been reported in EGFR-WT NSCLC, and it is often accompanied by mutations in *TP53*, *Rb1*, and *PIK3CA* [66–70].

9. Conclusions

SCLC represents one of the most lethal forms of cancer, with limited successful therapeutic options and consequently presenting striking low survival rates in late stages. It is reckoned as a high-grade neuroendocrine lung carcinoma and it is classified as either pure SCLC or combined SCLC, the latter when a portion of the tumor shows NSCLC features. Although the histological diagnosis is based mostly in H&E specimens, IHC can prove very helpful in the differential diagnosis setting. Intratumoral heterogeneity is thought to be related with its remarkable plasticity and striking metastatic potential. Histologically similar SCLC tumors may actually represent distinct subtypes of tumors, linked to disparate response outcomes to specific therapeutic agents. Recent molecular classifications approaches are paving the way to a deeper understanding of this entity and to related potential treatment approaches. Further knowledge of this entity, including both its genetic features and cellular heterogeneity, as well as its tumor microenvironment, will guide the development of personalized therapeutic strategies for SCLC patients. In the authors opinion, an exciting new era of molecular driven treatment decisions is finally foreseeable in the near future for SCLC patients.

Funding: This work was funded by the Specialized Program of Research Excellence (SPORE) from the National Cancer Institute [Grant 1-P50-CA70907-01].

Conflicts of Interest: I.I.W. receives research funding from Genentech, Oncoplex, HTG Molecular, DepArray, Merck, Bristol-Myers Squibb, Medimmune, Adaptive, Adaptimmune, EMD Serono, Pfizer, Takeda, Amgen, Karus, Johnson & Johnson, Bayer, Iovance, 4D, Novartis, and Akoya. I.I.W. sits on the advisory board of the following companies: Genentech/Roche, Bayer, Bristol-Myers Squibb, Astra Zeneca/Medimmune, Pfizer, HTG Molecular, Asuragen, Merck, GlaxoSmithKline, Guardant Health, Oncocyte, and MSD. The funders had no role in the writing of the manuscript.

References

1. Bray, F.; Ferlay, J.; Soerjomataram, I.; Siegel, R.L.; Torre, L.A.; Jemal, A. Global cancer statistics 2018: GLOBOCAN estimates of incidence and mortality worldwide for 36 cancers in 185 countries. *CA Cancer J.Clin.* **2018**, *68*, 394–424. [CrossRef]
2. International Agency for Research on Cancer (WHO). Available online: https://gco.iarc.fr/today/home (accessed on 11 December 2020).
3. American Cancer Society. Key Statistics for Small Cell Lung Cancer. Available online: https://www.cancer.org/cancer/lung-cancer/about/key-statistics.html (accessed on 11 December 2020).
4. National Health Institute. Surveillance, Edipemiology, and End Results Program (SEER). Available online: https://seer.cancer.gov/statfacts/html/lungb.html (accessed on 11 December 2020).
5. Gibbons, D.L.; Byers, L.A.; Kurie, J.M. Smoking, p53 mutation, and lung cancer. *Mol. Cancer Res.* **2014**, *12*, 3–13. [CrossRef]
6. Kadara, H.; Scheet, P.; Wistuba, I.I.; Spira, A.E. Early events in the molecular pathogenesis of lung cancer. *Cancer Prev Res.* **2016**, *9*, 518–527. [CrossRef]
7. Carr, L.L.; Chung, J.H.; Duarte Achcar, R.; Lesic, Z.; Rho, J.Y.; Yagihashi, K.; Tate, R.M.; Swigris, J.J.; Kern, J.A. The clinical course of diffuse idiopathic pulmonary neuroendocrine cell hyperplasia. *Chest* **2015**, *147*, 415–422. [CrossRef]
8. Rossi, G.; Cavazza, A.; Spagnolo, P.; Sverzellati, N.; Longo, L.; Jukna, A.; Montanari, G.; Carbonelli, C.; Vincenzi, G.; Bogina, G.; et al. Diffuse idiopathic pulmonary neuroendocrine cell hyperplasia syndrome. *Eur. Respir. J.* **2016**, *47*, 1829–1841. [CrossRef] [PubMed]
9. Chen, H.J.; Poran, A.; Unni, A.M.; Huang, S.X.; Elemento, O.; Snoeck, H.W.; Varmus, H. Generation of pulmonary neuroendocrine cells and SCLC-like tumors from human embryonic stem cells. *J. Exp. Med.* **2019**, *216*, 674–687. [CrossRef]
10. Augustyn, A.; Borromeo, M.; Wang, T.; Fujimoto, J.; Shao, C.; Dospoy, P.D.; Lee, V.; Tan, C.; Sullivan, J.P.; Larsen, J.E.; et al. ASCL1 is a lineage oncogene providing therapeutic targets for high-grade neuroendocrine lung cancers. *Proc. Natl. Acad. Sci. USA* **2014**, *111*, 14788–14793. [CrossRef] [PubMed]
11. Borromeo, M.D.; Savage, T.K.; Kollipara, R.K.; He, M.; Augustyn, A.; Osborne, J.K.; Girard, L.; Minna, J.D.; Gazdar, A.F.; Cobb, M.H.; et al. ASCL1 and NEUROD1 Reveal heterogeneity in pulmonary neuroendocrine tumors and regulate distinct genetic programs. *Cell Rep.* **2016**, *16*, 1259–1272. [CrossRef]
12. Huang, Y.H.; Klingbeil, O.; He, X.Y.; Wu, X.S.; Arun, G.; Lu, B.; Somerville, T.D.D.; Milazzo, J.P.; Wilkinson, J.E.; Demerdash, O.E.; et al. POU2F3 is a master regulator of a tuft cell-like variant of small cell lung cancer. *Genes Dev.* **2018**, *32*, 915–928. [CrossRef]
13. Härting, F.H.; Hesse, W. *Der Lungenkrebs, die Bergkrankheit in den Schneeberger Gruben*; Gedruckt bei, L., Ed.; Schumacher: Berlin, Germany, 1879.
14. Bernard, W.G. The nature of the 'oat-celled sarcoma' of the mediastinum. *J. Pathol. Bacteriol.* **1926**, *29*, 241–244. [CrossRef]
15. Azzopardi, J.G. Oat-cell carcinoma of the bronchus. *J. Pathol. Bacteriol.* **1959**, *78*, 513–519. [CrossRef] [PubMed]
16. Watson, W.L.; Berg, J.W. Oat cell lung cancer. *Cancer* **1962**, *15*, 759–768. [CrossRef]
17. Travis, W.D.; Brambilla, E.; Nicholson, A.G.; Yatabe, Y.; Austin, J.H.M.; Beasley, M.B.; Chirieac, L.R.; Dacic, S.; Duhig, E.; Flieder, D.B.; et al. The 2015 world health organization classification of lung tumors: Impact of genetic, clinical and radiologic advances since the 2004 classification. *J. Thorac. Oncol.* **2015**, *10*, 1243–1260. [CrossRef] [PubMed]
18. Nicholson, S.A.; Beasley, M.B.; Brambilla, E.; Hasleton, P.S.; Colby, T.V.; Sheppard, M.N.; Falk, R.; Travis, W.D. Small cell lung carcinoma (SCLC): A clinicopathologic study of 100 cases with surgical specimens. *Am. J. Surg. Pathol.* **2002**, *26*, 1184–1197. [CrossRef]
19. Travis, W.D. Update on small cell carcinoma and its differentiation from squamous cell carcinoma and other non-small cell carcinomas. *Mod. Pathol.* **2012**, *25*, S18–S30. [CrossRef]
20. Hamilton, G.; Rath, B. Mesenchymal-epithelial transition and circulating tumor cells in small cell lung cancer. *Adv. Exp. Med. Biol.* **2017**, *994*, 229–245. [CrossRef]
21. Mullins, R.K.; Thompson, S.K.; Coogan, P.S.; Shurbaji, M.S. Paranuclear blue inclusions: An aid in the cytopathologic diagnosis of primary and metastatic pulmonary small-cell carcinoma. *Diagn. Cytopathol.* **1994**, *10*, 332–335. [CrossRef]

22. Wang, W.; Hodkinson, P.; McLaren, F.; Mackean, M.J.; Williams, L.; Howie, S.E.M.; Wallace, W.A.H.; Sethi, T. Histologic assessment of tumor-associated CD45+ cell numbers is an independent predictor of prognosis in small cell lung cancer. *Chest* **2013**, *143*, 146–151. [CrossRef] [PubMed]
23. Travis, W.D. Lung tumours with neuroendocrine differentiation. *Eur. J. Cancer* **2009**, *45*, 251–266. [CrossRef]
24. Travis, W.D. Pathology of lung cancer. *Clin. Chest Med.* **2011**, *32*, 669–692. [CrossRef]
25. Moran, C.A.; Suster, S.; Coppola, D.; Wick, M.R. Neuroendocrine carcinomas of the lung: A critical analysis. *Am. J. Clin. Pathol.* **2009**, *131*, 206–221. [CrossRef] [PubMed]
26. Weissferdt, A. Neuroendocrine tumors of the lung. In *Diagnostic Thoracic Pathology*; Springer: Cham, Switzerland, 2020.
27. Baine, M.K.; Sinard, J.H.; Cai, G.; Homer, R.J. A semiquantitative scoring system may allow biopsy diagnosis of pulmonary large cell neuroendocrine carcinoma. *Am. J. Clin. Pathol* **2020**, *153*, 165–174. [CrossRef] [PubMed]
28. Zheng, M. Classification and pathology of lung cancer. *Surg. Oncol. Clin. N. Am.* **2016**, *25*, 447–468. [CrossRef]
29. Thunnissen, E.; Borczuk, A.C.; Flieder, D.B.; Witte, B.; Beasley, M.B.; Chung, J.H.; Dacic, S.; Lantuejoul, S.; Russell, P.A.; den Bakker, M.; et al. The use of immunohistochemistry improves the diagnosis of small cell lung cancer and its differential diagnosis. An international reproducibility study in a demanding set of cases. *J. Thorac. Oncol.* **2017**, *12*, 334–346. [CrossRef]
30. Horn, L.; Reck, M.; Spigel, D.R. The future of immunotherapy in the treatment of small cell lung cancer. *Oncologist* **2016**, *21*, 910–921. [CrossRef]
31. Tani, T.; Tanaka, K.; Idezuka, J.; Nishizawa, M. Regulatory T cells in paraneoplastic neurological syndromes. *J. Neuroimmunol.* **2008**, *196*, 166–169. [CrossRef]
32. Koyama, K.; Kagamu, H.; Miura, S.; Hiura, T.; Miyabayashi, T.; Itoh, R.; Kuriyama, H.; Tanaka, H.; Tanaka, J.; Yoshizawa, H.; et al. Reciprocal CD4+ T-cell balance of effector CD62L^{low} CD4+ and CD62L^{high}CD25+ CD4+ regulatory T cells in small cell lung cancer reflects disease stage. *Clin. Cancer Res.* **2008**, *14*, 6770–6779. [CrossRef]
33. Rizvi, N.A.; Hellmann, M.D.; Snyder, A.; Kvistborg, P.; Makarov, V.; Havel, J.J.; Lee, W.; Yuan, J.; Wong, P.; Ho, T.S.; et al. Mutational landscape determines sensitivity to PD-1 blockade in non–small cell lung cancer. *Science* **2015**, *348*, 124–128. [CrossRef] [PubMed]
34. Willis, C.; Fiander, M.; Tran, D.; Korytowsky, B.; Thomas, J.-M.; Calderon, E.; Zyczynski, T.M.; Brixner, D.; Stenehjem, D.D. Tumor mutational burden in lung cancer: A systematic literature review. *Oncotarget* **2019**, *10*, 6604–6622. [CrossRef]
35. Peifer, M.; Fernández-Cuesta, L.; Sos, M.L.; George, J.; Seidel, D.; Kasper, L.H.; Plenker, D.; Leenders, F.; Sun, R.; Zander, T.; et al. Integrative genome analyses identify key somatic driver mutations of small-cell lung cancer. *Nat. Genet.* **2012**, *44*, 1104–1110. [CrossRef]
36. Hamilton, G.; Rath, B. Immunotherapy for small cell lung cancer: Mechanisms of resistance. *Expert Opin. Biol. Ther.* **2019**, *19*, 423–432. [CrossRef]
37. Ishii, H.; Azuma, K.; Kawahara, A.; Yamada, K.; Imamura, Y.; Tokito, T.; Kinoshita, T.; Kage, M.; Hoshino, T. Significance of programmed cell death-ligand 1 expression and its association with survival in patients with small cell lung cancer. *J. Thorac. Oncol.* **2015**, *10*, 426–430. [CrossRef]
38. Schultheis, A.M.; Scheel, A.H.; Ozretić, L.; George, J.; Thomas, R.K.; Hagemann, T.; Zander, T.; Wolf, J.; Buettner, R. PD-L1 expression in small cell neuroendocrine carcinomas. *Eur. J. Cancer* **2015**, *51*, 421–426. [CrossRef] [PubMed]
39. Komiya, T.; Madan, R. PD-L1 expression in small cell lung cancer. *Eur. J. Cancer* **2015**, *51*, 1853–1855. [CrossRef] [PubMed]
40. Ott, P.A.; Fernandez, M.E.E.; Hiret, S.; Kim, D.-W.; Moss, R.A.; Winser, T.; Yuan, S.; Cheng, J.D.; Piperdi, B.; Mehnert, J.M. Pembrolizumab (MK-3475) in patients (pts) with extensive-stage small cell lung cancer (SCLC): Preliminary safety and efficacy results from KEYNOTE-028. *J. Clin. Oncol.* **2015**, *33*, 7502. [CrossRef]
41. Yu, H.; Boyle, T.A.; Zhou, C.; Rimm, D.L.; Hirsch, F.R. PD-L1 expression in lung cancer. *J. Thorac. Oncol.* **2016**, *11*, 964–975. [CrossRef]
42. Wang, W.; Hodkinson, P.; McLaren, F.; MacKinnon, A.; Wallace, W.; Howie, S.; Sethi, T. Small cell lung cancer tumour cells induce regulatory T lymphocytes, and patient survival correlates negatively with FOXP3+ cells in tumour infiltrate. *Int. J. Cancer* **2012**, *131*, E928–E937. [CrossRef]
43. Doyle, A.; Martin, W.J.; Funa, K.; Gazdar, A.; Carney, D.; Martin, S.E.; Linnoila, I.; Cuttitta, F.; Mulshine, J.; Bunn, P.; et al. Markedly decreased expression of class I histocompatibility antigens, protein, and mRNA in human small-cell lung cancer. *J. Exp. Med.* **1985**, *161*, 1135–1151. [CrossRef] [PubMed]
44. He, Y.; Rozeboom, L.; Rivard, C.J.; Ellison, K.; Dziadziuszko, R.; Yu, H.; Zhou, C.; Hirsch, F.R. MHC class II expression in lung cancer. *Lung Cancer* **2017**, *112*, 75–80. [CrossRef]
45. Fargion, S.; Carney, D.; Mulshine, J.; Rosen, S.; Bunn, P.; Jewett, P.; Cuttitta, F.; Gazdar, A.; Minna, J. Heterogeneity of cell surface antigen expression of human small cell lung cancer detected by monoclonal antibodies. *Cancer Res.* **1986**, *46*, 2633–2638.
46. Shue, Y.T.; Lim, J.S.; Sage, J. Tumor heterogeneity in small cell lung cancer defined and investigated in pre-clinical mouse models. *Transl. Lung Cancer Res.* **2018**, *7*, 21–31. [CrossRef] [PubMed]
47. Yang, D.; Denny, S.K.; Greenside, P.G.; Chaikovsky, A.C.; Brady, J.J.; Ouadah, Y.; Granja, J.M.; Jahchan, N.S.; Lim, J.S.; Kwok, S.; et al. Intertumoral heterogeneity in SCLC is influenced by the cell type of origin. *Cancer Discov.* **2018**, *8*, 1316–1331. [CrossRef]
48. Arcaro, A. Targeted therapies for small cell lung cancer: Where do we stand? *Crit. Rev. Oncol. Hematol.* **2015**, *95*, 154–164. [CrossRef] [PubMed]

49. D'Amico, D.; Carbone, D.; Mitsudomi, T.; Nau, M.; Fedorko, J.; Russell, E.; Johnson, B.; Buchhagen, D.; Bodner, S.; Phelps, R.; et al. High frequency of somatically acquired p53 mutations in small-cell lung cancer cell lines and tumors. *Oncogene* **1992**, *7*, 339–346.
50. Helin, K.; Holm, K.; Niebuhr, A.; Eiberg, H.; Tommerup, N.; Hougaard, S.; Poulsen, H.S.; Spang-Thomsen, M.; Norgaard, P. Loss of the retinoblastoma protein-related p130 protein in small cell lung carcinoma. *Proc. Natl. Acad. Sci. USA* **1997**, *94*, 6933–6938. [CrossRef] [PubMed]
51. George, J.; Lim, J.S.; Jang, S.J.; Cun, Y.; Ozretić, L.; Kong, G.; Leenders, F.; Lu, X.; Fernández-Cuesta, L.; Bosco, G.; et al. Comprehensive genomic profiles of small cell lung cancer. *Nature* **2015**, *524*, 47–53. [CrossRef]
52. Meder, L.; König, K.; Ozretić, L.; Schultheis, A.M.; Ueckeroth, F.; Ade, C.P.; Albus, K.; Boehm, D.; Rommerscheidt-Fuss, U.; Florin, A.; et al. NOTCH, ASCL1, p53 and RB alterations define an alternative pathway driving neuroendocrine and small cell lung carcinomas. *Int. J. Cancer* **2016**, *138*, 927–938. [CrossRef]
53. Rudin, C.M.; Durinck, S.; Stawiski, E.W.; Poirier, J.T.; Modrusan, Z.; Shames, D.S.; Bergbower, E.A.; Guan, Y.; Shin, J.; Guillory, J.; et al. Comprehensive genomic analysis identifies SOX2 as a frequently amplified gene in small-cell lung cancer. *Nat. Genet.* **2012**, *44*, 1111–1116. [CrossRef]
54. Wistuba, I.I.; Gazdar, A.F.; Minna, J.D. Molecular genetics of small cell lung carcinoma. *Semin. Oncol.* **2001**, *28*, 3–13. [CrossRef]
55. Byers, L.A.; Rudin, C.M. Small cell lung cancer: Where do we go from here? *Cancer* **2015**, *121*, 664–672. [CrossRef]
56. Minna, J.D.; Roth, J.A.; Gazdar, A.F. Focus on lung cancer. *Cancer Cell* **2002**, *1*, 49–52. [CrossRef]
57. Rohr, U.P.; Rehfeld, N.; Pflugfelder, L.; Geddert, H.; Müller, W.; Steidl, U.; Fenk, R.; Gräf, T.; Schott, M.; Thiele, K.P.; et al. Expression of the tyrosine kinase c-kit is an independent prognostic factor in patients with small cell lung cancer. *Int. J. Cancer* **2004**, *111*, 259–263. [CrossRef] [PubMed]
58. Tamborini, E.; Bonadiman, L.; Negri, T.; Greco, A.; Staurengo, S.; Bidoli, P.; Pastorino, U.; Pierotti, M.A.; Pilotti, S. Detection of overexpressed and phosphorylated wild-type kit receptor in surgical specimens of small cell lung cancer. *Clin. Cancer Res.* **2004**, *10*, 8214–8219. [CrossRef] [PubMed]
59. Baine, M.K.; Hsieh, M.S.; Lai, W.V.; Egger, J.V.; Jungbluth, A.; Daneshbod, Y.; Beras, A.; Spencer, R.; Lopardo, J.; Bodd, F.; et al. Small cell lung carcinoma subtypes defined by ASCL1, NEUROD1, POU2F3 and YAP1: Comprehensive immunohistochemical and histopathologic characterization. *J. Thorac. Oncol.* **2020**. [CrossRef]
60. Rudin, C.M.; Poirier, J.T.; Byers, L.A.; Dive, C.; Dowlati, A.; George, J.; Heymach, J.V.; Johnson, J.E.; Lehman, J.M.; MacPherson, D.; et al. Molecular subtypes of small cell lung cancer: A synthesis of human and mouse model data. *Nat. Rev. Cancer* **2019**, *19*, 289–297. [CrossRef]
61. McColl, K.; Wildey, G.; Sakre, N.; Lipka, M.B.; Behtaj, M.; Kresak, A.; Chen, Y.; Yang, M.; Velcheti, V.; Fu, P.; et al. Reciprocal expression of INSM1 and YAP1 defines subgroups in small cell lung cancer. *Oncotarget* **2017**, *8*, 73745–73756. [CrossRef]
62. Sonkin, D.; Thomas, A.; Teicher, B.A. Are neuroendocrine negative small cell lung cancer and large cell neuroendocrine carcinoma with WT RB1 two faces of the same entity? *Lung Cancer Manag.* **2019**, *8*, Lmt13. [CrossRef]
63. Wagner, P.L.; Kitabayashi, N.; Chen, Y.T.; Saqi, A. Combined small cell lung carcinomas: Genotypic and immunophenotypic analysis of the separate morphologic components. *Am. J. Clin. Pathol.* **2009**, *131*, 376–382. [CrossRef]
64. Gay, C.M.; Stewart, C.A.; Park, E.M.; Diao, L.; Groves, S.M.; Heeke, S.; Nabet, B.Y.; Fujimoto, J.; Solis, L.M.; Lu, W.; et al. Patterns of transcription factor programs and immune pathway activation define four major subtypes of SCLC with distinct therapeutic vulnerabilities. *Cancer Cell* **2021**. [CrossRef] [PubMed]
65. Yu, H.A.; Arcila, M.E.; Rekhtman, N.; Sima, C.S.; Zakowski, M.F.; Pao, W.; Kris, M.G.; Miller, V.A.; Ladanyi, M.; Riely, G.J. Analysis of tumor specimens at the time of acquired resistance to EGFR-TKI therapy in 155 patients with EGFR-mutant lung cancers. *Clin. Cancer Res.* **2013**, *19*, 2240–2247. [CrossRef] [PubMed]
66. Sequist, L.V.; Waltman, B.A.; Dias-Santagata, D.; Digumarthy, S.; Turke, A.B.; Fidias, P.; Bergethon, K.; Shaw, A.T.; Gettinger, S.; Cosper, A.K.; et al. Genotypic and histological evolution of lung cancers acquiring resistance to EGFR inhibitors. *Sci. Transl. Med.* **2011**, *3*, 75ra26. [CrossRef]
67. Marcoux, N.; Gettinger, S.N.; O'Kane, G.; Arbour, K.C.; Neal, J.W.; Husain, H.; Evans, T.L.; Brahmer, J.R.; Muzikansky, A.; Bonomi, P.D.; et al. EGFR-mutant adenocarcinomas that transform to small-cell lung cancer and other neuroendocrine carcinomas: Clinical outcomes. *J. Clin. Oncol.* **2019**, *37*, 278–285. [CrossRef] [PubMed]
68. Niederst, M.J.; Sequist, L.V.; Poirier, J.T.; Mermel, C.H.; Lockerman, E.L.; Garcia, A.R.; Katayama, R.; Costa, C.; Ross, K.N.; Moran, T.; et al. RB loss in resistant EGFR mutant lung adenocarcinomas that transform to small-cell lung cancer. *Nat. Commun.* **2015**, *6*, 6377. [CrossRef] [PubMed]
69. Offin, M.; Chan, J.M.; Tenet, M.; Rizvi, H.A.; Shen, R.; Riely, G.J.; Rekhtman, N.; Daneshbod, Y.; Quintanal-Villalonga, A.; Penson, A.; et al. Concurrent RB1 and TP53 alterations define a subset of EGFR-mutant lung cancers at risk for histologic transformation and inferior clinical outcomes. *J. Thorac. Oncol.* **2019**, *14*, 1784–1793. [CrossRef] [PubMed]
70. Iams, W.T.; Beckermann, K.E.; Almodovar, K.; Hernandez, J.; Vnencak-Jones, C.; Lim, L.P.; Raymond, C.K.; Horn, L.; Lovly, C.M. Small cell lung cancer transformation as a mechanism of resistance to PD-1 therapy in KRAS-mutant lung adenocarcinoma: A report of two cases. *J. Thorac. Oncol.* **2019**, *14*, e45–e48. [CrossRef] [PubMed]

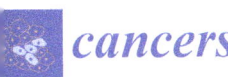

Review

PARP Inhibitors in Small-Cell Lung Cancer: Rational Combinations to Improve Responses

Erik H. Knelson [1], Shetal A. Patel [2] and Jacob M. Sands [1,*]

1. Dana-Farber Cancer Institute, Boston, MA 02215, USA; erik_knelson@dfci.harvard.edu
2. Department of Medicine, University of North Carolina School of Medicine, Chapel Hill, NC 27599, USA; shetal_patel@med.unc.edu
* Correspondence: jacob_sands@dfci.harvard.edu

Simple Summary: Small-cell lung cancer carries a dismal prognosis with few long-term treatment options. The enzyme poly-(ADP)-ribose polymerase (PARP), which functions to repair DNA breaks, has emerged as a promising therapeutic target, with modest response rates in early clinical trials prompting investigation of predictive biomarkers and therapeutic combinations. This review summarizes the development and testing of PARP inhibitors in small-cell lung cancer with an emphasis on developing treatment combinations. These combinations can be divided into three categories: (1) contributing to DNA damage; (2) inhibiting the DNA damage response; and (3) activating the immune system. An evolving classification of small-cell lung cancer subtypes and gene expression patterns will guide PARP inhibitor biomarker identification to improve treatments for this challenging cancer.

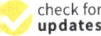

Citation: Knelson, E.H.; Patel, S.A.; Sands, J.M. PARP Inhibitors in Small-Cell Lung Cancer: Rational Combinations to Improve Responses. *Cancers* 2021, 13, 727. https://doi.org/10.3390/cancers13040727

Academic Editors: Alessandro Morabito and Christian Rolfo

Received: 2 January 2021
Accepted: 8 February 2021
Published: 10 February 2021

Publisher's Note: MDPI stays neutral with regard to jurisdictional claims in published maps and institutional affiliations.

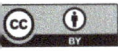

Copyright: © 2021 by the authors. Licensee MDPI, Basel, Switzerland. This article is an open access article distributed under the terms and conditions of the Creative Commons Attribution (CC BY) license (https://creativecommons.org/licenses/by/4.0/).

Abstract: Despite recent advances in first-line treatment for small-cell lung cancer (SCLC), durable responses remain rare. The DNA repair enzyme poly-(ADP-ribose) polymerase (PARP) was identified as a therapeutic target in SCLC using unbiased preclinical screens and confirmed in human and mouse models. Early trials of PARP inhibitors, either alone or in combination with chemotherapy, showed promising but limited responses, suggesting that selecting patient subsets and treatment combinations will prove critical to further clinical development. Expression of SLFN11 and other components of the DNA damage response (DDR) pathway appears to select for improved responses. Combining PARP inhibitors with agents that damage DNA and inhibit DDR appears particularly effective in preclinical and early trial data, as well as strategies that enhance antitumor immunity downstream of DNA damage. A robust understanding of the mechanisms of DDR in SCLC, which exhibits intrinsic replication stress, will improve selection of agents and predictive biomarkers. The most effective combinations will target multiple nodes in the DNA damage/DDR/immune activation cascade to minimize toxicity from synthetic lethality.

Keywords: SCLC; PARP; DDR; ICB; synthetic lethality; SLFN11; STING

1. Introduction

Small-cell lung cancer (SCLC) is a high-grade neuroendocrine malignancy with a poor prognosis that accounts for 13% of all lung cancer diagnoses [1,2]. First-line treatment for extensive-stage SCLC (ES-SCLC) is often effective, with a response rate of more than 60% to platinum-based chemotherapy, but prior to recent first-line advances, median overall survival was less than 11 months [2,3]. Immune checkpoint blockade (ICB) using inhibitors of the programmed cell death protein and its ligand (PD-1/PD-L1) initially showed promise in the third-line setting, and inclusion into first-line platinum-based therapy has demonstrated an overall survival benefit, becoming the new standard of care [4–7] with particular improvement in durable responses. Until recently, topotecan has been the only option approved by the United States Food and Drug Administration (FDA) in the second-line setting but has not been widely utilized due to concerns about toxicity and only modest efficacy [8–10]. Despite this, multiple randomized studies with a topotecan control arm have been negative, highlighting the resistant disease state [11–13] after prior platinum-based therapy. One of the negative studies that failed to meet its primary overall survival endpoint was a recent combination of lurbinectedin and doxorubicin compared to a control arm of either topotecan or CAV (cyclophosphamide, doxorubicin, vincristine) [14] which followed prior accelerated FDA approval of single-agent lurbinectedin based upon impressive data in small-cell lung cancer from a basket trial [15]. National Comprehensive Cancer Network guidelines include multiple regimens that may be considered in the second-line setting and beyond, but clinical trial is one of the three preferred regimens, highlighting the need for more effective treatments [16].

SCLC is a transcriptionally active disease with common (up to 90%) loss-of-function genomic alterations in the tumor suppressor genes *TP53* and *RB1*, creating further genomic instability by preventing arrest of the cell cycle for important DNA repair [17–20]. This suggests the potential for synergy with treatments that disrupt replication enough to halt the process and lead to apoptosis. One such approach, poly-(ADP)-ribose polymerase (PARP) inhibitors, have been a compelling class of drugs in the ongoing efforts to improve outcomes in this cancer that has been so resistant to other treatment options. Overexpression of PARP1 in SCLC further suggests therapeutic potential for PARP inhibitors [21].

Recurrent, targetable genomic alterations have not been identified in SCLC, but epigenetic and gene expression studies have led to the description of four distinct molecular subtypes defined by transcriptional regulators [22]. Subtyping of SCLC may offer an opportunity for better identification of treatment options with a higher likelihood of generating durable responses and will likely be an important component of prospective studies, including those evaluating PARP inhibitors and combinations.

PARP inhibitors represent a therapeutic class that has become an important treatment option for multiple tumor types. Although there is evidence of response, PARP inhibitors are not currently part of the treatment armamentarium for SCLC, and single-agent efficacy is limited. There is substantial ongoing investigation incorporating PARP inhibitors into the treatment of SCLC, and the following sections outline the mechanisms and rationale for these promising therapeutic combinations.

2. PARP Inhibitor Mechanism of Action

Recognition and repair of DNA damage form an essential cellular function mediated by a number of interconnected pathways termed the DNA damage response (DDR; Figure 1). PARP enzymes are a family of proteins that function in recognition and repair of DNA breaks, chromatin remodeling, and transcriptional regulation [23]. PARP 1 and 2 enzymatic function is activated by binding single-strand DNA breaks (SSB) and involves poly-ADP ribosylation (PARylation) of various substrates and recruitment of proteins that mediate DNA repair (Figure 1). PAR groups are subsequently metabolized by Poly-(ADP)-ribose glycohydrolase (PARG) and other enzymes as part of coordinated dePARylation critical to effective DNA repair [23]. In the absence of SSB repair by PARP1, the replication fork stalls and double strand breaks occur prompting repair via homologous recombination (HR) or non-homologous end joining (NHEJ). If DSBs are not correctly repaired, replication aberrancies such as mutations, deletions, chromosomal translocations, and amplifications can occur resulting in cell death, senescence or malignant transformation. PARP inhibitors were initially developed to sensitize tumor cells to standard treatments such as chemotherapy or radiation, which induce DNA damage [24]. However, the observation that tumor cells with defects in HR are highly sensitive to single-agent PARP inhibition accelerated their clinical development [25,26]. The activity of PARP inhibitors in patients with *BRCA1* or *BRCA2* mutant cancers was the first clinical demonstration of synthetic lethality for cancer therapy [27]. In this setting, by inhibiting PARP catalytic activity and trapping PARP on DNA, PARP inhibitors stall replication machinery leading to DNA double strand breaks (DSB). In the absence of BRCA1 or BRCA2, these breaks cannot be repaired by HR (Figure 1). Several PARP inhibitors are currently approved or in clinical trials. In addition to differences in their selectivity for PARP 1/2, these agents differ in their PARP trapping function, with talazoparib being the most potent [28]. Further studies in tumors without HR deficiency suggest that PARP inhibitors could have a broader role in cancer therapy [29].

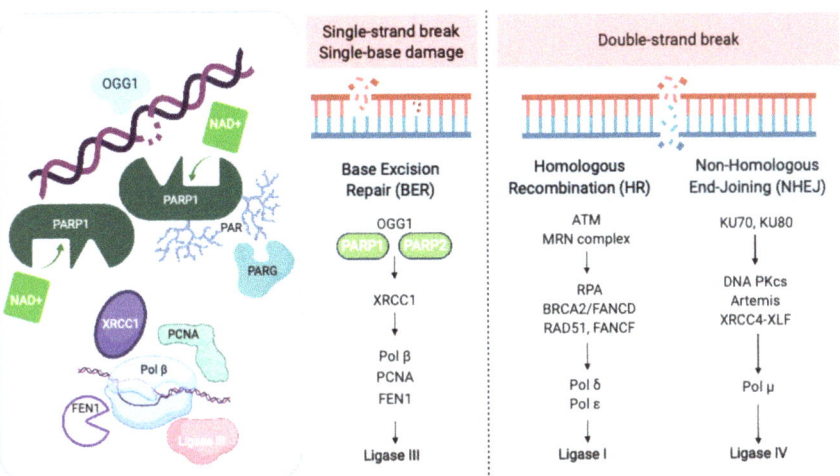

Figure 1. The Role of PARP in the DNA Damage Response. PARP = poly-(ADP)-ribose polymerase, OGG1 = 8-oxoguanine glycosylase, XRCC1 = X-ray repair cross-complementing protein 1, Pol β = DNA polymerase beta, PCNA = proliferating cell nuclear antigen, FEN1 = flap endonuclease 1, ATM = ataxia telangiectasia, mutated, MRN complex = Mre11 + RAD50 + NBS1/nibrin, RPA = replication protein A, BRCA2 = FANCD1 breast cancer susceptibility gene and DNA repair enzyme, Pol δ = DNA polymerase delta, Pol ε = DNA polymerase sigma, KU70/80 = lupus Ku autoantigen protein p70/p80, DNA PKcs = DNA-dependent protein kinase, catalytic subunit, XRCC4 = X-ray repair cross-complementing protein 4, XLF = XRCC4-like factor, and Pol μ = DNA polymerase mu. Created with BioRender.com; accessed on 21 January 2021.

PARP was initially identified as a potential therapeutic target in SCLC through seminal work by Byers et al., who performed unbiased proteomic analysis of cell lines using reverse-phase protein arrays (RPPA) to identify proteins that were differentially expressed in SCLC compared with non-small-cell lung carcinoma (NSCLC) [21]. PARP1 transcript and protein levels were significantly elevated in SCLC cell lines compared to NSCLC. Increased PARP1 protein expression was also confirmed by immunohistochemical (IHC) analysis of tissue microarrays. Notably, several other components of the DDR pathway were increased in SCLC, including the checkpoint kinases CHK1 and CHK2, the ataxia telangiectasia related protein ATR, and the DNA-dependent protein kinase catalytic subunit DNA PK$_{cs}$, which may be important to maintain cell viability in light of high replication stress (Figure 1). Treatment of a series of lung cancer cell lines with AZD2281 (olaparib) demonstrated that SCLC lines were significantly more sensitive to PARP inhibition than other histologic subtypes of lung cancer. Combining PARP inhibition with chemotherapy further decreased tumor cell viability.

These observations led to the initial studies of PARP inhibitors in SCLC as single agents (Table 1). In a phase I trial of talazoparib, 23 patients with SCLC were treated at the recommended phase II dose of 1.0 mg daily [30]. Two patients had a partial response, for an objective response rate (ORR) of 9% with a duration of response of 12.0 and 15.3 weeks. Both patients with an objective response had a platinum-free interval of 6 months or less. An additional four patients had stable disease, for a clinical benefit rate of 26% at 16 weeks. The UK STOMP trial examined the role of olaparib in the maintenance setting, but failed to show an improvement in progression-free survival (PFS) [31].

Table 1. Studies including PARP inhibitors in SCLC with outcomes data.

Study Population	Drug(s)	Response Rate	PFS (Months)	OS (Months)	Unique Trial Data
Patients with ≤1 prior treatment regimen[30]	Talazoparib	9%	11.1 weeks		
First-line ES-SCLC[32]	CE + veliparib vs. CE + placebo	71.9% vs. 65.6%	6.1 vs. 5.5	10.3 vs. 8.9	Elevated LDH and male gender correlated with benefit
First-line ES-SCLC[45]	(A) CE+ veliparib -> veliparib (B) CE + veliparib -> placebo (C) CE + placebo -> placebo	77% 59.3% 63.9%	5.8 5.7 5.6	10.1 10.0 12.4	
Relapsed ES-SCLC[36]	TMZ + veliparib vs. TMZ + placebo	39% vs. 14%	3.8 vs. 2.0	8.2 vs. 7.0	SLFN11 positive tumors prolonged PFS and OS
Relapsed ES-SCLC[39]	TMZ + olaparib	41.7%	4.2	8.5	Co-clinical PDX trial
Relapsed ES-SCLC[65]	Durvalumab + olaparib	10.5%	1.8	4.1	Inflamed phenotype→ response
Relapsed ES-SCLC[66]	Durvalumab + olaparib	5.3%			Olaparib run in

PFS = progression-free survival, OS = overall survival, ES-SCLC = extensive-stage small-cell lung cancer, CE = cisplatin/etoposide, LDH = lactate dehydrogenase, TMZ = temozolamide, SLFN11 = schlafen family member 11, and PDX = patient-derived xenograft.

3. Biomarkers of Response to PARP Inhibitors in SCLC

Since only a subset of SCLC patients appears sensitive to PARP inhibition, identification of predictive biomarkers has been an important focus of translational research. Clinical trials have attempted to identify correlative markers of response. Based on their preclinical work Owonikoko et al. examined DNA-PKcs expression as a biomarker but did not observe a correlation with veliparib activity in their phase II trial [32]. Although elevated serum lactate dehydrogenase (LDH) levels and male gender are poor prognostic markers, in the veliparib arm, these correlated with improvement in PFS in multivariable analysis. Mutations in DNA damage response genes such as *BRCA1*, *BRCA2*, *ATM*, or *ATR* (Figure 1) are not frequently seen in SCLC. However, homologous recombination deficiency (HRD) assays have been used to identify *BRCA1/2* wildtype ovarian cancer patients with sensitivity to PARP inhibition. Using three different measures of HRD, Lok et al. analyzed a series of SCLC cell lines to determine if HRD predicted response to PARP inhibition [33]. While they did not observe any correlation between HRD scores and response to PARP inhibitors, gene expression analysis demonstrated that high levels of *schlafen family member 11* (*SLFN11*) transcript did correlate with PARP inhibitor sensitivity. SLFN11 has been identified as critical for SCLC cell line and patient-derived xenograft (PDX) response to chemotherapy [34,35], as well as a potential biomarker for PARP inhibitor response using unbiased screens in SCLC cell lines and PDXs [33,35]. SLFN11 is a protein that is recruited to sites of DNA damage, inhibits HR, and activates a replication-stress response. High levels of SLFN11 have been correlated with enhanced response to PARP inhibitors in many [33–37] but not all [38,39] SCLC trials and preclinical models. Furthermore, using clustered regularly interspaced short palindromic repeats (CRISPR) based gene editing, deletion of *SLFN11* was found to confer resistance to talazoparib [33]. Importantly for clinical translation, a SLFN11 IHC H-score predicted sensitivity of SCLC PDXs to PARP inhibition [34]. A bimodal expression pattern of *SLFN11* transcript levels was observed in SCLC from The Cancer Genome Atlas (TCGA) dataset [33].

Using the NCI-60 database to identify genomic correlates of sensitivity to talazoparib across multiple tumor types, Murai et al. also identified *SLFN11* among the top-ranking genes [37]. They observed that deletion of *SLFN11* conferred resistance to PARP inhibition but found that ATR inhibition could overcome this resistance. An integrated proteomic and transcriptomic analysis of SCLC PDX models also identified SLFN11 protein levels as predictive of response to PARP inhibition [40]. Additionally, low ATM and high E-cadherin expression correlated with sensitivity to PARP inhibition. Treatment with cisplatin or PARP inhibitors reduced SLFN11 expression in cell line models, raising the question of dynamic changes in this marker in response to prior therapy. Using gene expression derived from PDX models, Farago et al. identified an inflammatory gene signature (*CEACAM1*, TNFSF10, OAS1, TGIF1) that selected for sensitivity to olaparib + temozolamide. Markers of epithelial-to-mesenchymal transition (EMT) and high *MYC* target gene expression correlated with resistance. Collectively, these studies demonstrate that high SLFN11 expression is a promising biomarker for sensitivity to PARP inhibitor activity in SCLC, but prospective validation is needed and integration of multiple markers may improve predictive ability. SLFN11 expression is being studied prospectively as a biomarker in a randomized phase II clinical trial of talazoparib as maintenance therapy with atezolizumab in patients with ES-SCLC (SWOG1929, NCT04334941). Recent preclinical work argues that SCLC subtype can also influence response to PARP inhibitors, with expression of the transcription factor *POU2F3* sensitizing to PARP inhibitors [41].

4. PARP Inhibitors Combined with Chemotherapy

Given limited single-agent activity, a number of preclinical and clinical studies have examined combinations of PARP inhibitors with chemotherapy, radiation, and targeted therapies to enhance therapeutic benefit (Figure 2, Table 1). Several groups have demonstrated that PARP inhibition can potentiate the activity of platinum-based chemotherapy in SCLC cell lines and xenografts [21,42,43]. Owonikoko et al. tested the combination of veliparib with cisplatin (75 mg/m^2) and etoposide (100 mg/m^2 on days 1–3) in a phase I/II randomized clinical trial (ECOG-ACRIN 2511) in patients with ES-SCLC [32,44]. The recommended phase II dose for veliparib in combination with cisplatin and etoposide was determined to be 100 mg twice daily on days 1–7. Patients treated with veliparib had a median PFS of 6.1 months (95% CI, 5.9 to 6.7) relative to 5.5 months for placebo (95% CI, 5.0 to 6.1). Overall survival was 8.9 months (95% CI, 8.3 to 11.3) in patients receiving placebo relative to 10.3 months (95% CI 8.9 to 12.0) with the addition of veliparib (stratified HR, 0.83; 80% CI 0.64 to 1.07; p = 0.17). Patients were stratified by sex and serum LDH levels. Male patients with high LDH levels derived benefit in PFS (HR 0.34; 80% CI 0.22 to 0.51), but no difference in OS by strata was observed. The combination was tolerable, with higher rates of lymphopenia and grade 3 or 4 neutropenia seen with the addition of veliparib. The combination of veliparib with carboplatin (AUC = 5) and etoposide (100 mg/m^2 on days 1–3) has also been studied [45]. The recommended phase II dose for veliparib in this study was 240 mg twice daily for days 1–14, due to excess hematologic toxicity seen with continuous dosing. A randomized phase II study was performed with three arms: (A) carboplatin/etoposide + veliparib followed by veliparib, (B) carboplatin/etoposide + veliparib followed by placebo, and (C) carboplatin/etoposide + placebo followed by placebo. Median PFS in arm A was 5.8 months (80% CI 5.6 to 6.8), arm B 5.7 months (5.6 to 5.8) and 5.6 months (5.1 to 6.7) for arm C. Similarly, no significant differences in OS were observed.

PARP inhibitor and chemotherapy combinations have also been examined in patients with relapsed disease after platinum-based chemotherapy (Table 1). Temozolomide (TMZ) is an oral alkylating agent, previously demonstrated to have single-agent activity in SCLC [46]. TMZ methylates the O^6 position of guanine, ultimately leading to DSBs. O^6 methylguanine-DNA methyltransferase (MGMT) is involved in repair of these lesions; therefore, silencing of *MGMT* expression by promoter methylation has been correlated with improved clinical response to TMZ. Given that PARP proteins also have a role in repair of these lesions, it was hypothesized that the combination of PARP inhibitors and TMZ could have synergistic activity. Using talazoparib, Lok et al. evaluated the activity of TMZ and PARP inhibition in several SCLC models, demonstrating synergistic tumor growth inhibition, particularly in high *SLNF11*-expressing models [33]. *MGMT* expression did not correlate with sensitivity to TMZ + talazoparib. Murai et al. similarly observed synergistic activity for talazoparib and TMZ in SCLC models with high *SLFN11* expression [37]. Two phase II studies in relapsed SCLC patients have evaluated the combination of TMZ and PARP inhibition. Pietanza et al. performed a randomized, double-blind, placebo-controlled study of veliparib (40 mg twice daily, days 1 to 7) or placebo and TMZ (150–200 mg/m^2/day, days 1 to 5) on a 28-day cycle [36]. The primary endpoint of the study was 4-month PFS, with no significant differences observed between TMZ/veliparib (36%) and TMZ/placebo (27%, $p = 0.19$). Median PFS was 3.8 and 2.0 months (log-rank $p = 0.39$, HR 0.84; 95% CI 0.56 to 1.25) for the TMZ/veliparib and TMZ/placebo arms, respectively. OS was also similar between the 2 arms. ORR was higher for the combination of TMZ/veliparib (39%) versus TMZ/placebo (14%), in both platinum-sensitive and platinum-refractory patients Biomarker analysis was performed for PARP-1 and SLFN11 expression by IHC. No association with PARP-1 expression and clinical outcomes was observed. SLFN11-positive tumors (H-score cutoff ≥ 1) treated with TMZ/veliparib had improved PFS (5.7 vs. 3.6 months, $p = 0.009$) and OS (12.2 vs. 7.5 months; $p = 0.014$). Notably, the authors highlighted that a low dose of veliparib was used in this study and veliparib has lower PARP trapping activity, both of which could have contributed to limited efficacy.

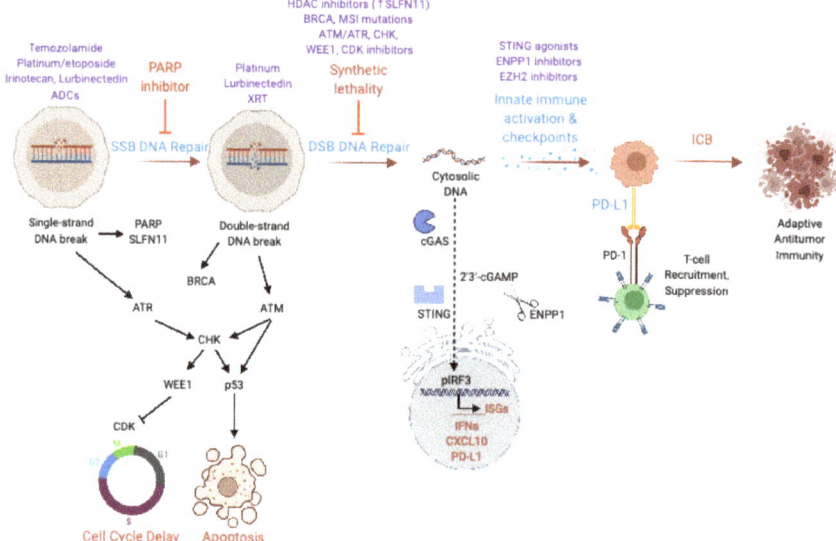

Figure 2. PARP Inhibitor Combinations: Enhancing Response in SCLC. PARP = poly-(ADP)-ribose polymerase, ADCs = antibody–drug conjugates, SSB = single-strand DNA break, DSB = double-strand DNA break, CDK = cyclin-dependent kinase, XRT = radiation therapy, HDAC = histone deacetylase, MSI = microsatellite instability, ssDNA = single-strand DNA, ISGs = Interferon-stimulated genes, and ICB = immune checkpoint blockade. Created with BioRender.com; accessed 29 on January 2021.

Using the more potent PARP inhibitor olaparib in combination with TMZ, Farago et al. performed a phase I/II study in relapsed SCLC [39]. To facilitate biomarker analysis and mechanistic studies, a co-clinical trial with PDXs was performed. At the recommended phase II dose of olaparib (200 mg twice daily, day 1–7) and TMZ (75 mg/m^2, day 1–7 of 21 days cycle), the ORR was 41%, with a median duration of response of 5.3 months. Across all dose levels, PFS was 4.2 months (95% CI, 2.8 to 5.7) with a median OS of 8.5 months (95% CI, 5.1 to 11.3). A phase II study of continuous talazoparib with intermittent low-dose TMZ (NCT03672773) in relapsed/refractory SCLC is ongoing. Additional studies are evaluating the combination of PARP inhibitors with agents that induce DNA damage such as pegylated SN-38, the active metabolite of irinotecan, an inhibitor of topoisomerase I activity (NCT04209595, Table 2).

Table 2. Ongoing studies in SCLC.

Study Population	Drug(s)	Phase	Unique Trial Data	Trial Number
ES-SCLC	Talazoparib + Atezolizumab maintenance	II	Prospective study of SLFN11 expression	NCT04334941
Relapsed/refractory ES-SCLC	Intermittent low-dose TMZ + continuous Talazoparib	II	Previous trials used intermittent talazoparib	NCT03672773
SCLC	PLX038 (Pegylated SN-38) + rucaparib	I/II	Potential enhancement in DNA damage from formulation of irinotecan metabolite	NCT04209595
ES-SCLC	Olaparib + low-dose radiotherapy	I	Maintenance therapy for stable disease after first-line chemotherapy	NCT03532880
ES-SCLC	Talazoparib + consolidative thoracic XRT	I	Maintenance therapy for stable disease after first-line chemotherapy	NCT04170946
Relapsed/refractory ES-SCLC	AZD1775 (WEE1)	II	Single-arm study	NCT02593019
Relapsed/refractory ES-SCLC	AZD1775 (WEE1)	II	Single-arm study; CDKN2A or MYC mutation required	NCT02688907
ES-SCLC	VX-970 (ATR) + CE or cisplatin (platinum resistant)	I	Flexible enrollment with first-line chemotherapy or relapsed/refractory disease	NCT02157792
Relapsed/refractory ES-SCLC	VX-970 (ATR) + topotecan	I/II		NCT02487095
Relapsed/refractory ES-SCLC	Prexasertib (CHK)	II		NCT02735980
Relapsed/refractory ES-SCLC	AZD1775 (WEE1) + olaparib	1b		NCT02511795
ES-SCLC	Rucaparib + nivolumab	II	Maintenance therapy for stable disease after first-line chemotherapy	NCT03958045
ES-SCLC	Thoracic radiation combined with durvalumab +/− (tremelimumab + olaparib)	I	Maintenance therapy for stable disease after first-line chemotherapy	NCT03923270
Relapsed/refractory ES-SCLC	BMS-986012 +/− nivolumab	I/II		NCT02247349
ES-SCLC	BMS-986012 + CE	I/II	First-line therapy	NCT02815592
Relapsed/refractory ES-SCLC	Olaparib + cediranib (VEGF)	II	Correlation with DNA repair gene expression	NCT02498613
Relapsed/refractory ES-SCLC	Vistusertib (mTOR) + Navitoclax (Bcl-2)	I/II	On treatment biopsy	NCT03366103

ES-SCLC = extensive-stage small-cell lung cancer, SLFN11 = schlafen family member 11, TMZ = temozolamide, and CE = cisplatin/etoposide.

Antibody–drug conjugates (ADCs) are another class of therapeutic that acts by inducing DNA damage selectively in tumor cells after targeting to tumor-specific antigens. The first ADC to enter clinical development for SCLC targeted the Notch inhibitory protein delta-like ligand 3 (DLL3), identified as enriched on SCLC cells with impaired Notch signaling [47]. The DLL3 ADC, Rovalpituzumab tesirine (Rova-T), showed promise in preclinical work and early trials [48], but ultimately failed to meet primary endpoints in phase II/III trials [12,49]. A phase I trial of an ADC targeting the tumor-associated calcium signal transducer Trop2 showed an acceptable safety profile and promising results with an ORR of 14% and clinical benefit in 34% of heavily pretreated patients with SCLC [50]. Further studies are ongoing, and ADCs may be of particular benefit in combination with other treatments including PARP inhibitors.

In addition to chemotherapy combinations, PARP inhibitors can also sensitize SCLC models to ionizing radiation [42,51]. Laird et al. noted that talazoparib is a more potent radiosensitizer than veliparib, suggesting that PARP trapping ability may play a role in sensitization to radiation. Talazoparib treatment led to increased DSBs compared to veliparib. Interestingly, radiosensitization was observed irrespective of SLFN11 expression. Several early phase trials are examining the combination of PARP inhibition and radiation in ES-SCLC (NCT03532880, NCT04170946, Table 2). Potential toxicity to normal tissues with these combinations is a concern and will be carefully evaluated in these studies.

5. Synthetic Lethality Downstream of PARP Inhibitors

In addition to synergy with chemotherapy and radiation, several preclinical studies have suggested that combinations with DDR inhibitors could enhance the therapeutic potential of PARP inhibitors in SCLC. These approaches aim to target multiple nodes of the DDR response to prevent resistance and promote synergistic antitumor activity. Since PARP inhibition prevents repair of single-strand DNA breaks, which subsequently progress to DSBs at stalled replication forks, PARP inhibitors are most effective when DSB repair is impaired. This strategy, referred to as synthetic lethality, was originally developed in the setting of *BRCA* germline mutations in ovarian cancer patients and holds particular appeal in SCLC, where defining mutations in *RB1* and *P53* combine with elevated tumor mutational burden from tobacco exposure to generate additional replication stress and dependence on DNA repair mechanisms [52,53]. SCLC is not associated with germline *BRCA* mutations, and global microsatellite instability in SCLC is rare. However, a "DNA-repair score" was shown to correlate with response to PARP inhibition in preclinical work using SCLC PDXs [54]. This prognostic score includes canonical DNA repair genes such as *PARP, BRCA, ATM, ATR, CHK, RAD50, 53BP1, MSH2,* and *FANC* (Figure 1) [54], several of which can also be inhibited pharmacologically (Figure 2). Early phase clinical trials have opened for SCLC patients targeting the DNA damage response (Table 2), including for AZD1775 targeting WEE1 (NCT02593019, NCT02688907), VX-970 targeting ATR (NCT02157792, NCT02487095), and Prexasertib targeting CHK (NCT02735980) [52]. While these specific trials do not include PARP inhibitors, combination studies with PARP inhibition are also being developed.

CHK1 is a protein kinase that plays an important role in DNA damage-dependent cell cycle arrest, particularly in TP53-deficient tumors. CHK1 protein expression is increased in SCLC patient tumors [21,55]. Combination therapy with the CHK1 inhibitor LY2606368 and cisplatin or olaparib enhanced tumor regression and survival in mouse SCLC models [55].

WEE1 is a kinase involved in S phase and G_2-M progression, by phosphorylating CDK1/2 and allowing for DNA repair prior to mitotic entry. Targeting WEE1 with inhibitors such as AZD1775 compromises DNA damage checkpoints, particularly in cancer cells that may be more dependent on the G_2-M checkpoint. Lallo et al. studied the combination of olaparib and AZD1775 in SCLC PDXs and observed activity in both chemotherapy sensitive and resistant models [56]. This combination is being evaluated in a trial for patients with refractory solid tumors, including SCLC (NCT02511795).

Preclinical work using cell lines and patient specimens suggests that treatment with histone deacetylase (HDAC) and enhancer of zeste homology 2 (EZH2) inhibitors can restore epigenetically suppressed SLFN11 expression [57], suggesting potential synergy with PARP inhibition. In the majority of SCLC with low SLFN11 expression, resistance to PARP inhibition may be overcome by pharmacologic ATR inhibition [37], further supporting the role for DDR synthetic lethality in enhancing response to PARP inhibitors in SCLC.

6. Combining PARP and Immune Checkpoint Inhibition

ICB has been incorporated into the first-line treatment of SCLC [6,7]. Combining ICB and PARP inhibitors may offer synergy because of molecular signaling pathways linking cytosolic DNA to PD-L1 expression. DNA-sensing pathways, which evolved to protect against bacteria and viruses, also recognize self-DNA released from the nucleus when DDR is suppressed [58]. Double-stranded DNA is recognized by the enzyme cyclic GMP-AMP synthase (cGAS), which produces the cyclic dinucleotide second messenger 2′3′-cGAMP, activating the Stimulator of Interferon Genes (STING) pathway, which upregulates interferon stimulated genes, including PD-L1. PARP inhibitors have been shown to activate STING and upregulate PD-L1 across cancer models regardless of *BRCA* mutation status, leading to synergy with PD-L1 inhibitors in preclinical mouse studies [59–63]. In SCLC, preclinical data suggest that synergy between PARP inhibitors and PD-L1 checkpoint inhibition may depend on intact tumor cell STING and innate immune activity downstream of cytosolic DNA released after PARP inhibition [64]. A phase II trial in relapsed SCLC combining durvalumab 1500 mg every 4 weeks with olaparib 300 mg twice a day showed an ORR of 10.5% (two patients out of nineteen) [65]. The treatment combination was well tolerated, with expected cytopenias from PARP inhibition but no evidence of overlapping toxicity. Of note, both responders exhibited an inflamed phenotype with CD8+ T cells contacting tumor cells in a pretreatment biopsy [65]. Co-mutation status and/or histology may influence response to combined PARP and immune checkpoint inhibition in SCLC, as one of the responders had a *BRCA* mutation that may have sensitized to PARP inhibition, and the other had *EGFR*-mutant transformed SCLC. Post-treatment biopsies confirmed increases in PD-L1 expression after PARP inhibition in 6/9 paired cases. However, these increases failed to correlate with T-cell infiltration. The disappointing response rates in this trial are similar to a previous phase II basket study including patients with relapsed SCLC that used the same doses of olaparib and durvalumab but with a 4-week olaparib run-in period [66]. These early results suggest that additional mechanisms suppress antitumor immunity in SCLC. The phase II trial of rucaparib + nivolumab in platinum-sensitive SCLC (NCT03958045) may identify a clinical context with residual disease where these agents are more effective [67].

Additional immune checkpoints, such as CTLA-4 (cytotoxic T-lymphocyte-associated protein 4), which binds to CD80/CD86, may suppress antitumor immunity downstream of PARP inhibition. A number of trials combining PARP and CTLA-4 inhibitors are currently underway, including a phase I trial of thoracic radiation combined with durvalumab +/− tremelimumab or olaparib in ES-SCLC after first-line chemotherapy (NCT03923270) [67]. Antibody dependent cellular cytotoxicity (ADCC) represents another promising approach to unleash antitumor immunity. Preclinical studies identified BMS-986012 as an antibody that can bind the tumor cell-specific ganglioside FucGM1, leading to ADCC [68]. This compound is currently being tested in phase I/II trials (NCT02247349, NCT02815592), either as part of first-line treatment for ES-SCLC alongside chemotherapy or in the relapsed setting alongside nivolumab. As the designs of these trials suggest, targeting multiple steps in DNA damage response concurrently (see Figure 2) may ultimately prove successful.

7. Restoring Tumor Cell Inflammatory Signaling to Enhance PARP Inhibitor Response

The majority of SCLC are "immune deserts" with minimal infiltration by CD8+ effector T cells [22]. However, a subset of non-neuroendocrine tumors demonstrates enhanced inflammatory infiltrates and markers of innate immunity including restored STING expression [69,70]. As suggested by the phase II data for durvalumab + olaparib [65], and confirmed in elegant preclinical work [41], the non-neuroendocrine inflamed subtype may represent a biomarker for response to this combination. To expand the patient population that can benefit from the combination of DDR inhibition and ICB, novel approaches to restore tumor cell inflammatory pathways are sorely needed. The neuroendocrine stress response inhibits inflammation, so strategies that target neuroendocrine lineage commitment could elicit antitumor immunity. Reversing EZH2 epigenetic programing to de-repress antigen presentation and tumor cell STING expression represents one promising approach [70,71]. Indeed, EZH2 levels are higher in SCLC than any other tumor type in TCGA [72], and EZH2 inhibitors can restore *SLFN11* expression to potentially improve response to PARP inhibitors [34]. The combination of EZH2 and PARP inhibitors was effective in preclinical models of ovarian cancer [73], and is being developed in SCLC, where both approaches have shown promise as monotherapies [21,74]. Restoring tumor suppressive *NOTCH1* or inhibiting the Notch suppressive protein DLL3 to alter neuroendocrine differentiation could have similar effects, as recent evidence suggests that phenotype switching can uncover therapeutic vulnerabilities [41]. Targeting negative regulators of DNA-sensing including ectonucleotide pyrophosphatase/phosphodiesterase family member 1 (ENPP1), the enzyme that cleaves the STING second messenger 2′3′-cGAMP [75], may also potentiate the effects of DDR inhibition. ENPP1 can also metabolize PAR downstream of PARP in the DNA damage response [76]. While inhibiting PARylation and dePARylation simultaneously may seem counterproductive, both processes cooperate in DNA damage repair, and their concurrent inhibition shows promise in preclinical cancer models [77]. Combinations that disrupt coordinated DNA damage repair are more likely to stimulate innate antitumor immunity and response to immune checkpoint blockade.

8. Orthogonal Approaches

The past decade has seen many advances in SCLC management, culminating in the adoption of ICB into first-line treatment [6]. Previously, second-line treatment was limited to topoisomerase inhibitors, but this has recently been expanded to include lurbinectedin and a host of promising clinical trials [78]. Many of these trials include PARP inhibitors, either alone or in combination as outlined in prior sections. Investigational targets outside of DNA damage, repair, and antitumor immunity include receptor tyrosine kinases (RTKs) and their ligands, which can be inhibited with monoclonal antibodies or tyrosine kinase inhibitors (TKIs). Disrupting tumor angiogenesis by targeting the vascular endothelial growth factor (VEGF) has proven effective in other cancers but failed in clinical trials for SCLC [79]. Preclinical work suggests combining VEGF monoclonal antibodies with checkpoint blockade in SCLC [80], and there is also interest in inhibiting VEGF alongside PARP [28]. A phase II trial evaluating olaparib in combination with the VEGF TKI cediranib has enrolled patients with SCLC (NCT02498613). This combination previously proved successful in extending PFS from PARP inhibition in recurrent platinum-sensitive ovarian cancer [81]. Preclinical studies have also identified fibroblast growth factors (FGF) and their receptors as therapeutic targets in SCLC, where approximately 6% of patients harbor amplifications in FGFR1 [53]. Signaling pathways downstream of RTKs offer additional targets. Preclinical data demonstrate an increase in PI3K/mTOR activity following PARP inhibition in SCLC models, providing rationale for combination therapy with PARP inhibitors plus PI3K/mTOR inhibitors [82]. A phase I/II trial is currently underway evaluating the mTOR inhibitor vistusertib in combination with the Bcl-2 inhibitor navitoclax in relapsed SCLC (NCT03366103). In theory, combined inhibition of growth factor signaling and PARP could enhance clinical response [28,78].

9. Conclusions

PARP inhibitors are a compelling class of drugs in the treatment of SCLC, with a mechanism of action that takes advantage of genomic instability and loss-of-function *TP53/RB* genomic alterations that challenge the cells' ability to repair DNA. Single-agent trials have demonstrated only modest results that do not yet warrant a role in the treatment armamentarium. Combination therapy such as temozolomide + olaparib has improved outcomes, and many other combinations are in progress or development. Biomarkers to identify patient subsets likely to respond to PARP inhibitors and/or combinations with synergistic mechanisms of action are required in the further development of PARP inhibitors as effective treatments for SCLC. SLFN11 and other components of the DDR pathway, perhaps combined in an expression signature, represent putative predictive biomarkers for PARP inhibitors, though prospective validation will be required.

SCLC subtyping provides a framework for future drug development. As new therapeutic options are prospectively evaluated within the context of identified subtypes of SCLC, an increasing opportunity exists to further define predictive biomarkers. For example, *POU2F3* expression may be as valuable in identifying tumors susceptible to PARP inhibition as *SLFN11* expression [41,83]. The emerging "inflamed" subtype may also demonstrate improved responses to PARP inhibitors in combination with ICB [41,65,84], since preclinical data suggest that downstream DNA-sensing pathways remain intact in some tumors [70] and could amplify the effects of impaired DDR. Epigenetic strategies to reverse subtype-specific gene expression patterns may also uncover vulnerability to PARP inhibitors. HDAC inhibitors to increase *SLFN11* expression [57] and EZH2 inhibitors to reverse neuroendocrine immunosuppression [71] are two notable examples.

Multiple compounds are in development to synergize with PARP inhibitors. In this review, we organized PARP combinations by mechanism of synergy (Figure 2): DNA damage, repair of DNA breaks/synthetic lethality, and immune activation. We predict that the most successful combinations will include compounds from multiple categories, analogous to vertical pathway inhibition downstream of RTKs. However, unlike combinations of TKIs, PARP inhibitor combinations may prove more tolerable for patients since toxicities are less likely to overlap and synergy will be most pronounced in SCLC cells with impaired DDR, allowing for dose decreases to minimize side effects. Though SCLC prognosis remains grave, clinical and translational advances in recent years offer hope of combining PARP inhibitors with agents that impair DDR and activate antitumor immunity to improve response rates and survival. Enthusiasm for PARP inhibitor combinations raises hopes that synthetic lethality and restored antitumor immunity, therapeutic strategies with great success in other cancers, can benefit patients with SCLC.

Author Contributions: Conceptualization, J.M.S. and E.H.K.; literature survey, E.H.K., S.A.P. and J.M.S.; writing—original draft preparation, E.H.K., S.A.P. and J.M.S.; writing—review and editing, E.H.K., S.A.P. and J.M.S.; supervision, J.M.S. All authors have read and agreed to the published version of the manuscript.

Funding: This research received no external funding.

Conflicts of Interest: E.H.K. reports a Sponsored Research Agreement with Takeda Pharmaceuticals. S.A.P. reports research funding to institution from AstraZeneca, Shattuck Labs, and Dracen Pharmaceuticals. J.M.S. reports honoraria for consulting/advisory board from AstraZeneca, Boehringer Ingelheim, Eli Lilly, Loxo, Merck, Genentech, Jazz Pharmaceuticals, Pharma Mar, and Takeda.

References

1. Jemal, A.; Bray, F.; Center, M.M.; Ferlay, J.; Ward, E.; Forman, D. Global cancer statistics. *CA Cancer J. Clin.* **2011**, *61*, 69–90. [CrossRef] [PubMed]
2. Socinski, M.A.; Smit, E.F.; Lorigan, P.; Konduri, K.; Reck, M.; Szczesna, A.; Blakely, J.; Serwatowski, P.; Karaseva, N.A.; Ciuleanu, T.; et al. Phase III study of pemetrexed plus carboplatin compared with etoposide plus carboplatin in chemotherapy-naive patients with extensive-stage small-cell lung cancer. *J. Clin. Oncol.* **2009**, *27*, 4787–4792. [CrossRef] [PubMed]
3. Spigel, D.R.; Townley, P.M.; Waterhouse, D.M.; Fang, L.; Adiguzel, I.; Huang, J.E.; Karlin, D.A.; Faoro, L.; Scappaticci, F.A.; Socinski, M.A. Randomized phase II study of bevacizumab in combination with chemotherapy in previously untreated extensive-stage small-cell lung cancer: Results from the SALUTE trial. *J. Clin. Oncol.* **2011**, *29*, 2215–2222. [CrossRef]
4. Chung, H.C.; Piha-Paul, S.A.; Lopez-Martin, J.; Schellens, J.H.M.; Kao, S.; Miller, W.H., Jr.; Delord, J.P.; Gao, B.; Planchard, D.; Gottfried, M.; et al. Pembrolizumab After Two or More Lines of Previous Therapy in Patients With Recurrent or Metastatic SCLC: Results From the KEYNOTE-028 and KEYNOTE-158 Studies. *J. Thorac. Oncol.* **2020**, *15*, 618–627. [CrossRef] [PubMed]
5. Ready, N.E.; Ott, P.A.; Hellmann, M.D.; Zugazagoitia, J.; Hann, C.L.; de Braud, F.; Antonia, S.J.; Ascierto, P.A.; Moreno, V.; Atmaca, A.; et al. Nivolumab Monotherapy and Nivolumab Plus Ipilimumab in Recurrent Small Cell Lung Cancer: Results From the CheckMate 032 Randomized Cohort. *J. Thorac. Oncol.* **2020**, *15*, 426–435. [CrossRef] [PubMed]
6. Horn, L.; Mansfield, A.S.; Szczesna, A.; Havel, L.; Krzakowski, M.; Hochmair, M.J.; Huemer, F.; Losonczy, G.; Johnson, M.L.; Nishio, M.; et al. First-Line Atezolizumab plus Chemotherapy in Extensive-Stage Small-Cell Lung Cancer. *N. Engl. J. Med.* **2018**, *379*, 2220–2229. [CrossRef]

7. Paz-Ares, L.; Dvorkin, M.; Chen, Y.; Reinmuth, N.; Hotta, K.; Trukhin, D.; Statsenko, G.; Hochmair, M.J.; Ozguroglu, M.; Ji, J.H.; et al. Durvalumab plus platinum-etoposide versus platinum-etoposide in first-line treatment of extensive-stage small-cell lung cancer (CASPIAN): A randomised, controlled, open-label, phase 3 trial. *Lancet* **2019**. [CrossRef]
8. O'Brien, M.E.; Ciuleanu, T.E.; Tsekov, H.; Shparyk, Y.; Cucevia, B.; Juhasz, G.; Thatcher, N.; Ross, G.A.; Dane, G.C.; Crofts, T. Phase III trial comparing supportive care alone with supportive care with oral topotecan in patients with relapsed small-cell lung cancer. *J. Clin. Oncol.* **2006**, *24*, 5441–5447. [CrossRef]
9. Von Pawel, J.; Schiller, J.H.; Shepherd, F.A.; Fields, S.Z.; Kleisbauer, J.P.; Chrysson, N.G.; Stewart, D.J.; Clark, P.I.; Palmer, M.C.; Depierre, A.; et al. Topotecan versus cyclophosphamide, doxorubicin, and vincristine for the treatment of recurrent small-cell lung cancer. *J. Clin. Oncol.* **1999**, *17*, 658–667. [CrossRef] [PubMed]
10. Eckardt, J.R.; von Pawel, J.; Pujol, J.L.; Papai, Z.; Quoix, E.; Ardizzoni, A.; Poulin, R.; Preston, A.J.; Dane, G.; Ross, G. Phase III study of oral compared with intravenous topotecan as second-line therapy in small-cell lung cancer. *J. Clin. Oncol.* **2007**, *25*, 2086–2092. [CrossRef]
11. Pujol, J.L.; Greillier, L.; Audigier-Valette, C.; Moro-Sibilot, D.; Uwer, L.; Hureaux, J.; Guisier, F.; Carmier, D.; Madelaine, J.; Otto, J.; et al. A Randomized Non-Comparative Phase II Study of Anti-Programmed Cell Death-Ligand 1 Atezolizumab or Chemotherapy as Second-Line Therapy in Patients With Small Cell Lung Cancer: Results From the IFCT-1603 Trial. *J. Thorac. Oncol.* **2019**, *14*, 903–913. [CrossRef] [PubMed]
12. Morgensztern, D.; Besse, B.; Greillier, L.; Santana-Davila, R.; Ready, N.; Hann, C.L.; Glisson, B.S.; Farago, A.F.; Dowlati, A.; Rudin, C.M.; et al. Efficacy and Safety of Rovalpituzumab Tesirine in Third-Line and Beyond Patients with DLL3-Expressing, Relapsed/Refractory Small-Cell Lung Cancer: Results From the Phase II TRINITY Study. *Clin. Cancer Res.* **2019**, *25*, 6958–6966. [CrossRef]
13. Reck, M.; Vicente, D.; Ciuleanu, T.; Gettinger, S.; Peters, S.; Horn, L.; Audigier-Valette, C.; Pardo, N.; Juan-Vidal, O.; Cheng, Y.; et al. Efficacy and safety of nivolumab (nivo) monotherapy versus chemotherapy (chemo) in recurrent small cell lung cancer (SCLC): Results from CheckMate 331. *Ann. Oncol.* **2018**, *29*, 43. [CrossRef]
14. Cision PR Newswire. *Jazz Pharmaceuticals and PharmaMar Announce Results of ATLANTIS Phase 3 Study Evaluating Zepzelca™ in Combination with Doxorubicin for Patients with Small Cell Lung Cancer Following One Prior Platinum-containing Line*; News Release; Jazz Pharmaceuticals: Dublin, Ireland, 2020.
15. Trigo, J.; Subbiah, V.; Besse, B.; Moreno, V.; Lopez, R.; Sala, M.A.; Peters, S.; Ponce, S.; Fernandez, C.; Alfaro, V.; et al. Lurbinectedin as second-line treatment for patients with small-cell lung cancer: A single-arm, open-label, phase 2 basket trial. *Lancet Oncol.* **2020**, *21*, 645–654. [CrossRef]
16. NCCN Clinical Practice Guidelines in Oncology: Small Cell Lung Cancer V1.2021-11 August. Available online: https://www.nccn.org (accessed on 29 January 2021).
17. Takahashi, T.; Nau, M.M.; Chiba, I.; Birrer, M.J.; Rosenberg, R.K.; Vinocour, M.; Levitt, M.; Pass, H.; Gazdar, A.F.; Minna, J.D. p53: A frequent target for genetic abnormalities in lung cancer. *Science* **1989**, *246*, 491–494. [CrossRef]
18. Hensel, C.H.; Hsieh, C.L.; Gazdar, A.F.; Johnson, B.E.; Sakaguchi, A.Y.; Naylor, S.L.; Lee, W.H.; Lee, E.Y. Altered structure and expression of the human retinoblastoma susceptibility gene in small cell lung cancer. *Cancer Res.* **1990**, *50*, 3067–3072. [PubMed]
19. Sherr, C.J.; McCormick, F. The RB and p53 pathways in cancer. *Cancer Cell* **2002**, *2*, 103–112. [CrossRef]
20. Zilfou, J.T.; Lowe, S.W. Tumor suppressive functions of p53. *Cold Spring Harb. Perspect. Biol.* **2009**, *1*, a001883. [CrossRef]
21. Byers, L.A.; Wang, J.; Nilsson, M.B.; Fujimoto, J.; Saintigny, P.; Yordy, J.; Giri, U.; Peyton, M.; Fan, Y.H.; Diao, L.; et al. Proteomic profiling identifies dysregulated pathways in small cell lung cancer and novel therapeutic targets including PARP1. *Cancer Discov.* **2012**, *2*, 798–811. [CrossRef]
22. Rudin, C.M.; Poirier, J.T.; Byers, L.A.; Dive, C.; Dowlati, A.; George, J.; Heymach, J.V.; Johnson, J.E.; Lehman, J.M.; MacPherson, D.; et al. Molecular subtypes of small cell lung cancer: A synthesis of human and mouse model data. *Nat. Rev. Cancer* **2019**, *19*, 289–297. [CrossRef]
23. Slade, D. PARP and PARG inhibitors in cancer treatment. *Genes Dev.* **2020**, *34*, 360–394. [CrossRef]
24. Lord, C.J.; Ashworth, A. PARP inhibitors: Synthetic lethality in the clinic. *Science* **2017**, *355*, 1152–1158. [CrossRef]
25. Bryant, H.E.; Schultz, N.; Thomas, H.D.; Parker, K.M.; Flower, D.; Lopez, E.; Kyle, S.; Meuth, M.; Curtin, N.J.; Helleday, T. Specific killing of BRCA2-deficient tumours with inhibitors of poly(ADP-ribose) polymerase. *Nature* **2005**, *434*, 913–917. [CrossRef] [PubMed]
26. Farmer, H.; McCabe, N.; Lord, C.J.; Tutt, A.N.; Johnson, D.A.; Richardson, T.B.; Santarosa, M.; Dillon, K.J.; Hickson, I.; Knights, C.; et al. Targeting the DNA repair defect in BRCA mutant cells as a therapeutic strategy. *Nature* **2005**, *434*, 917–921. [CrossRef]
27. Fong, P.C.; Boss, D.S.; Yap, T.A.; Tutt, A.; Wu, P.; Mergui-Roelvink, M.; Mortimer, P.; Swaisland, H.; Lau, A.; O'Connor, M.J.; et al. Inhibition of poly(ADP-ribose) polymerase in tumors from BRCA mutation carriers. *N. Engl. J. Med.* **2009**, *361*, 123–134. [CrossRef] [PubMed]
28. Barayan, R.; Ran, X.; Lok, B.H. PARP inhibitors for small cell lung cancer and their potential for integration into current treatment approaches. *J. Thorac. Dis.* **2020**, *12*, 6240–6252. [CrossRef] [PubMed]
29. Pilie, P.G.; Gay, C.M.; Byers, L.A.; O'Connor, M.J.; Yap, T.A. PARP Inhibitors: Extending Benefit Beyond BRCA-Mutant Cancers. *Clin. Cancer Res.* **2019**, *25*, 3759–3771. [CrossRef] [PubMed]

30. De Bono, J.; Ramanathan, R.K.; Mina, L.; Chugh, R.; Glaspy, J.; Rafii, S.; Kaye, S.; Sachdev, J.; Heymach, J.; Smith, D.C.; et al. Phase I, Dose-Escalation, Two-Part Trial of the PARP Inhibitor Talazoparib in Patients with Advanced Germline BRCA1/2 Mutations and Selected Sporadic Cancers. *Cancer Discov.* **2017**, *7*, 620–629. [CrossRef]
31. Woll, P.; Gaunt, P.; Steele, N.; Ahmed, S.; Mulatero, C.; Shah, R. P1.07–015 STOMP: A UK National Cancer Research Network randomised, double blind, multicentre phase II trial of olaparib as maintenance therapy in SCLC. *J. Thorac. Oncol.* **2017**, *12*, S704–S705. [CrossRef]
32. Owonikoko, T.K.; Dahlberg, S.E.; Sica, G.L.; Wagner, L.I.; Wade, J.L., 3rd; Srkalovic, G.; Lash, B.W.; Leach, J.W.; Leal, T.B.; Aggarwal, C.; et al. Randomized Phase II Trial of Cisplatin and Etoposide in Combination With Veliparib or Placebo for Extensive-Stage Small-Cell Lung Cancer: ECOG-ACRIN 2511 Study. *J. Clin. Oncol.* **2019**, *37*, 222–229. [CrossRef]
33. Lok, B.H.; Gardner, E.E.; Schneeberger, V.E.; Ni, A.; Desmeules, P.; Rekhtman, N.; de Stanchina, E.; Teicher, B.A.; Riaz, N.; Powell, S.N.; et al. PARP Inhibitor Activity Correlates with SLFN11 Expression and Demonstrates Synergy with Temozolomide in Small Cell Lung Cancer. *Clin. Cancer Res.* **2017**, *23*, 523–535. [CrossRef] [PubMed]
34. Gardner, E.E.; Lok, B.H.; Schneeberger, V.E.; Desmeules, P.; Miles, L.A.; Arnold, P.K.; Ni, A.; Khodos, I.; de Stanchina, E.; Nguyen, T.; et al. Chemosensitive Relapse in Small Cell Lung Cancer Proceeds through an EZH2-SLFN11 Axis. *Cancer Cell* **2017**, *31*, 286–299. [CrossRef]
35. Polley, E.; Kunkel, M.; Evans, D.; Silvers, T.; Delosh, R.; Laudeman, J.; Ogle, C.; Reinhart, R.; Selby, M.; Connelly, J.; et al. Small Cell Lung Cancer Screen of Oncology Drugs, Investigational Agents, and Gene and microRNA Expression. *J. Natl. Cancer Inst.* **2016**, *108*. [CrossRef] [PubMed]
36. Pietanza, M.C.; Waqar, S.N.; Krug, L.M.; Dowlati, A.; Hann, C.L.; Chiappori, A.; Owonikoko, T.K.; Woo, K.M.; Cardnell, R.J.; Fujimoto, J.; et al. Randomized, Double-Blind, Phase II Study of Temozolomide in Combination With Either Veliparib or Placebo in Patients With Relapsed-Sensitive or Refractory Small-Cell Lung Cancer. *J. Clin. Oncol.* **2018**, *36*, 2386–2394. [CrossRef]
37. Murai, J.; Feng, Y.; Yu, G.K.; Ru, Y.; Tang, S.W.; Shen, Y.; Pommier, Y. Resistance to PARP inhibitors by SLFN11 inactivation can be overcome by ATR inhibition. *Oncotarget* **2016**, *7*, 76534–76550. [CrossRef]
38. Drapkin, B.J.; George, J.; Christensen, C.L.; Mino-Kenudson, M.; Dries, R.; Sundaresan, T.; Phat, S.; Myers, D.T.; Zhong, J.; Igo, P.; et al. Genomic and Functional Fidelity of Small Cell Lung Cancer Patient-Derived Xenografts. *Cancer Discov.* **2018**, *8*, 600–615. [CrossRef]
39. Farago, A.F.; Yeap, B.Y.; Stanzione, M.; Hung, Y.P.; Heist, R.S.; Marcoux, J.P.; Zhong, J.; Rangachari, D.; Barbie, D.A.; Phat, S.; et al. Combination Olaparib and Temozolomide in Relapsed Small-Cell Lung Cancer. *Cancer Discov.* **2019**, *9*, 1372–1387. [CrossRef]
40. Stewart, C.A.; Tong, P.; Cardnell, R.J.; Sen, T.; Li, L.; Gay, C.M.; Masrorpour, F.; Fan, Y.; Bara, R.O.; Feng, Y.; et al. Dynamic variations in epithelial-to-mesenchymal transition (EMT), ATM, and SLFN11 govern response to PARP inhibitors and cisplatin in small cell lung cancer. *Oncotarget* **2017**, *8*, 28575–28587. [CrossRef] [PubMed]
41. Gay, C.M.; Stewart, C.A.; Park, E.M.; Diao, L.; Groves, S.M.; Heeke, S.; Nabet, B.Y.; Fujimoto, J.; Solis, L.M.; Lu, W.; et al. Patterns of transcription factor programs and immune pathway activation define four major subtypes of SCLC with distinct therapeutic vulnerabilities. *Cancer Cell* **2021**. [CrossRef]
42. Owonikoko, T.K.; Zhang, G.; Deng, X.; Rossi, M.R.; Switchenko, J.M.; Doho, G.H.; Chen, Z.; Kim, S.; Strychor, S.; Christner, S.M.; et al. Poly (ADP) ribose polymerase enzyme inhibitor, veliparib, potentiates chemotherapy and radiation in vitro and in vivo in small cell lung cancer. *Cancer Med.* **2014**, *3*, 1579–1594. [CrossRef] [PubMed]
43. Teicher, B.A.; Silvers, T.; Selby, M.; Delosh, R.; Laudeman, J.; Ogle, C.; Reinhart, R.; Parchment, R.; Krushkal, J.; Sonkin, D.; et al. Small cell lung carcinoma cell line screen of etoposide/carboplatin plus a third agent. *Cancer Med.* **2017**, *6*, 1952–1964. [CrossRef] [PubMed]
44. Owonikoko, T.K.; Dahlberg, S.E.; Khan, S.A.; Gerber, D.E.; Dowell, J.; Moss, R.A.; Belani, C.P.; Hann, C.L.; Aggarwal, C.; Ramalingam, S.S. A phase 1 safety study of veliparib combined with cisplatin and etoposide in extensive stage small cell lung cancer: A trial of the ECOG-ACRIN Cancer Research Group (E2511). *Lung Cancer* **2015**, *89*, 66–70. [CrossRef] [PubMed]
45. Atrafi, F.; Groen, H.J.M.; Byers, L.A.; Garralda, E.; Lolkema, M.P.; Sangha, R.S.; Viteri, S.; Chae, Y.K.; Camidge, D.R.; Gabrail, N.Y.; et al. A Phase I Dose-Escalation Study of Veliparib Combined with Carboplatin and Etoposide in Patients with Extensive-Stage Small Cell Lung Cancer and Other Solid Tumors. *Clin. Cancer Res.* **2019**, *25*, 496–505. [CrossRef]
46. Pietanza, M.C.; Kadota, K.; Huberman, K.; Sima, C.S.; Fiore, J.J.; Sumner, D.K.; Travis, W.D.; Heguy, A.; Ginsberg, M.S.; Holodny, A.I.; et al. Phase II trial of temozolomide in patients with relapsed sensitive or refractory small cell lung cancer, with assessment of methylguanine-DNA methyltransferase as a potential biomarker. *Clin. Cancer Res.* **2012**, *18*, 1138–1145. [CrossRef] [PubMed]
47. Saunders, L.R.; Bankovich, A.J.; Anderson, W.C.; Aujay, M.A.; Bheddah, S.; Black, K.; Desai, R.; Escarpe, P.A.; Hampl, J.; Laysang, A.; et al. A DLL3-targeted antibody-drug conjugate eradicates high-grade pulmonary neuroendocrine tumor-initiating cells in vivo. *Sci. Transl. Med.* **2015**, *7*, 302ra136. [CrossRef]
48. Rudin, C.M.; Pietanza, M.C.; Bauer, T.M.; Ready, N.; Morgensztern, D.; Glisson, B.S.; Byers, L.A.; Johnson, M.L.; Burris, H.A., 3rd; Robert, F.; et al. Rovalpituzumab tesirine, a DLL3-targeted antibody-drug conjugate, in recurrent small-cell lung cancer: A first-in-human, first-in-class, open-label, phase 1 study. *Lancet Oncol.* **2017**, *18*, 42–51. [CrossRef]
49. Schulze, A.B.; Evers, G.; Kerkhoff, A.; Mohr, M.; Schliemann, C.; Berdel, W.E.; Schmidt, L.H. Future Options of Molecular-Targeted Therapy in Small Cell Lung Cancer. *Cancers* **2019**, *11*, 690. [CrossRef]

50. Gray, J.E.; Heist, R.S.; Starodub, A.N.; Camidge, D.R.; Kio, E.A.; Masters, G.A.; Purcell, W.T.; Guarino, M.J.; Misleh, J. Schneider, C.J.; et al. Therapy of Small Cell Lung Cancer (SCLC) with a Topoisomerase-I-inhibiting Antibody-Drug Conjugate (ADC) Targeting Trop-2, Sacituzumab Govitecan. *Clin. Cancer Res.* **2017**, *23*, 5711–5719. [CrossRef]
51. Laird, J.H.; Lok, B.H.; Ma, J.; Bell, A.; de Stanchina, E.; Poirier, J.T.; Rudin, C.M. Talazoparib Is a Potent Radiosensitizer in Small Cell Lung Cancer Cell Lines and Xenografts. *Clin. Cancer Res.* **2018**, *24*, 5143–5152. [CrossRef]
52. Foy, V.; Schenk, M.W.; Baker, K.; Gomes, F.; Lallo, A.; Frese, K.K.; Forster, M.; Dive, C.; Blackhall, F. Targeting DNA damage in SCLC. *Lung Cancer* **2017**, *114*, 12–22. [CrossRef]
53. George, J.; Lim, J.S.; Jang, S.J.; Cun, Y.; Ozretic, L.; Kong, G.; Leenders, F.; Lu, X.; Fernandez-Cuesta, L.; Bosco, G.; et al. Comprehensive genomic profiles of small cell lung cancer. *Nature* **2015**, *524*, 47–53. [CrossRef]
54. Cardnell, R.J.; Feng, Y.; Diao, L.; Fan, Y.H.; Masrorpour, F.; Wang, J.; Shen, Y.; Mills, G.B.; Minna, J.D.; Heymach, J.V.; et al. Proteomic markers of DNA repair and PI3K pathway activation predict response to the PARP inhibitor BMN 673 in small cell lung cancer. *Clin. Cancer Res.* **2013**, *19*, 6322–6328. [CrossRef]
55. Sen, T.; Tong, P.; Stewart, C.A.; Cristea, S.; Valliani, A.; Shames, D.S.; Redwood, A.B.; Fan, Y.H.; Li, L.; Glisson, B.S.; et al. CHK1 Inhibition in Small-Cell Lung Cancer Produces Single-Agent Activity in Biomarker-Defined Disease Subsets and Combination Activity with Cisplatin or Olaparib. *Cancer Res.* **2017**, *77*, 3870–3884. [CrossRef]
56. Lallo, A.; Frese, K.K.; Morrow, C.J.; Sloane, R.; Gulati, S.; Schenk, M.W.; Trapani, F.; Simms, N.; Galvin, M.; Brown, S.; et al. The Combination of the PARP Inhibitor Olaparib and the WEE1 Inhibitor AZD1775 as a New Therapeutic Option for Small Cell Lung Cancer. *Clin. Cancer Res.* **2018**, *24*, 5153–5164. [CrossRef]
57. Tang, S.W.; Thomas, A.; Murai, J.; Trepel, J.B.; Bates, S.E.; Rajapakse, V.N.; Pommier, Y. Overcoming Resistance to DNA-Targeted Agents by Epigenetic Activation of Schlafen 11 (SLFN11) Expression with Class I Histone Deacetylase Inhibitors. *Clin. Cancer Res.* **2018**, *24*, 1944–1953. [CrossRef]
58. Wang, Y.; Luo, J.; Alu, A.; Han, X.; Wei, Y.; Wei, X. cGAS-STING pathway in cancer biotherapy. *Mol. Cancer* **2020**, *19*, 136. [CrossRef] [PubMed]
59. Shen, J.; Zhao, W.; Ju, Z.; Wang, L.; Peng, Y.; Labrie, M.; Yap, T.A.; Mills, G.B.; Peng, G. PARPi Triggers the STING-Dependent Immune Response and Enhances the Therapeutic Efficacy of Immune Checkpoint Blockade Independent of BRCAness. *Cancer Res.* **2019**, *79*, 311–319. [CrossRef]
60. Sato, H.; Niimi, A.; Yasuhara, T.; Permata, T.B.M.; Hagiwara, Y.; Isono, M.; Nuryadi, E.; Sekine, R.; Oike, T.; Kakoti, S.; et al. DNA double-strand break repair pathway regulates PD-L1 expression in cancer cells. *Nat. Commun.* **2017**, *8*, 1751. [CrossRef] [PubMed]
61. Jiao, S.; Xia, W.; Yamaguchi, H.; Wei, Y.; Chen, M.K.; Hsu, J.M.; Hsu, J.L.; Yu, W.H.; Du, Y.; Lee, H.H.; et al. PARP Inhibitor Upregulates PD-L1 Expression and Enhances Cancer-Associated Immunosuppression. *Clin. Cancer Res.* **2017**, *23*, 3711–3720. [CrossRef] [PubMed]
62. Chabanon, R.M.; Muirhead, G.; Krastev, D.B.; Adam, J.; Morel, D.; Garrido, M.; Lamb, A.; Henon, C.; Dorvault, N.; Rouanne, M.; et al. PARP inhibition enhances tumor cell-intrinsic immunity in ERCC1-deficient non-small cell lung cancer. *J. Clin. Investig.* **2019**, *129*, 1211–1228. [CrossRef] [PubMed]
63. Ding, L.; Kim, H.J.; Wang, Q.; Kearns, M.; Jiang, T.; Ohlson, C.E.; Li, B.B.; Xie, S.; Liu, J.F.; Stover, E.H.; et al. PARP Inhibition Elicits STING-Dependent Antitumor Immunity in Brca1-Deficient Ovarian Cancer. *Cell Rep.* **2018**, *25*, 2972–2980.e2975. [CrossRef]
64. Sen, T.; Rodriguez, B.L.; Chen, L.; Corte, C.M.D.; Morikawa, N.; Fujimoto, J.; Cristea, S.; Nguyen, T.; Diao, L.; Li, L.; et al. Targeting DNA Damage Response Promotes Antitumor Immunity through STING-Mediated T-cell Activation in Small Cell Lung Cancer. *Cancer Discov.* **2019**, *9*, 646–661. [CrossRef] [PubMed]
65. Thomas, A.; Vilimas, R.; Trindade, C.; Erwin-Cohen, R.; Roper, N.; Xi, L.; Krishnasamy, V.; Levy, E.; Mammen, A.; Nichols, S.; et al. Durvalumab in Combination with Olaparib in Patients with Relapsed SCLC: Results from a Phase II Study. *J. Thorac. Oncol.* **2019**, *14*, 1447–1457. [CrossRef]
66. Krebs, M.; Ross, K.; Kim, S.; De Jonge, M.; Barlesi, F.; Postel-Vinay, S.; Domchek, S.; Lee, J.; Angell, H.; Bui, K.; et al. P1.15-004 An Open-Label, Multitumor Phase II Basket Study of Olaparib and Durvalumab (MEDIOLA): Results in Patients with Relapsed SCLC. *J. Thorac. Oncol.* **2017**, *12*, S2044–S2045. [CrossRef]
67. Peyraud, F.; Italiano, A. Combined PARP Inhibition and Immune Checkpoint Therapy in Solid Tumors. *Cancers* **2020**, *12*, 1502. [CrossRef]
68. Ponath, P.; Menezes, D.; Pan, C.; Chen, B.; Oyasu, M.; Strachan, D.; LeBlanc, H.; Sun, H.; Wang, X.T.; Rangan, V.S.; et al. A Novel, Fully Human Anti-fucosyl-GM1 Antibody Demonstrates Potent In Vitro and In Vivo Antitumor Activity in Preclinical Models of Small Cell Lung Cancer. *Clin. Cancer Res.* **2018**, *24*, 5178–5189. [CrossRef]
69. Dora, D.; Rivard, C.; Yu, H.; Bunn, P.; Suda, K.; Ren, S.; Pickard, S.L.; Laszlo, V.; Harko, T.; Megyesfalvi, Z.; et al. Neuroendocrine subtypes of small cell lung cancer differ in terms of immune microenvironment and checkpoint molecule distribution. *Mol. Oncol.* **2020**, *14*, 1947–1965. [CrossRef] [PubMed]
70. Canadas, I.; Thummalapalli, R.; Kim, J.W.; Kitajima, S.; Jenkins, R.W.; Christensen, C.L.; Campisi, M.; Kuang, Y.; Zhang, Y.; Gjini, E.; et al. Tumor innate immunity primed by specific interferon-stimulated endogenous retroviruses. *Nat. Med.* **2018**, *24*, 1143–1150. [CrossRef]
71. Burr, M.L.; Sparbier, C.E.; Chan, K.L.; Chan, Y.C.; Kersbergen, A.; Lam, E.Y.N.; Azidis-Yates, E.; Vassiliadis, D.; Bell, C.C.; Gilan, O.; et al. An Evolutionarily Conserved Function of Polycomb Silences the MHC Class I Antigen Presentation Pathway and Enables Immune Evasion in Cancer. *Cancer Cell* **2019**, *36*, 385–401.e388. [CrossRef]

72. Poirier, J.T.; Gardner, E.E.; Connis, N.; Moreira, A.L.; de Stanchina, E.; Hann, C.L.; Rudin, C.M. DNA methylation in small cell lung cancer defines distinct disease subtypes and correlates with high expression of EZH2. *Oncogene* **2015**, *34*, 5869–5878. [CrossRef]
73. Karakashev, S.; Fukumoto, T.; Zhao, B.; Lin, J.; Wu, S.; Fatkhutdinov, N.; Park, P.H.; Semenova, G.; Jean, S.; Cadungog, M.G.; et al. EZH2 Inhibition Sensitizes CARM1-High, Homologous Recombination Proficient Ovarian Cancers to PARP Inhibition. *Cancer Cell* **2020**, *37*, 157–167.e156. [CrossRef]
74. Drapkin, B.J.; Rudin, C.M. Advances in Small-Cell Lung Cancer (SCLC) Translational Research. *Cold Spring Harb. Perspect. Med.* **2020**. [CrossRef] [PubMed]
75. Li, L.; Yin, Q.; Kuss, P.; Maliga, Z.; Millan, J.L.; Wu, H.; Mitchison, T.J. Hydrolysis of 2′3′-cGAMP by ENPP1 and design of nonhydrolyzable analogs. *Nat. Chem. Biol.* **2014**, *10*, 1043–1048. [CrossRef] [PubMed]
76. Palazzo, L.; Daniels, C.M.; Nettleship, J.E.; Rahman, N.; McPherson, R.L.; Ong, S.E.; Kato, K.; Nureki, O.; Leung, A.K.; Ahel, I. ENPP1 processes protein ADP-ribosylation in vitro. *FEBS J.* **2016**, *283*, 3371–3388. [CrossRef]
77. Kassab, M.A.; Yu, L.L.; Yu, X. Targeting dePARylation for cancer therapy. *Cell Biosci.* **2020**, *10*, 7. [CrossRef]
78. Poirier, J.T.; George, J.; Owonikoko, T.K.; Berns, A.; Brambilla, E.; Byers, L.A.; Carbone, D.; Chen, H.J.; Christensen, C.L.; Dive, C.; et al. New Approaches to SCLC Therapy: From the Laboratory to the Clinic. *J. Thorac. Oncol.* **2020**, *15*, 520–540. [CrossRef] [PubMed]
79. Stratigos, M.; Matikas, A.; Voutsina, A.; Mavroudis, D.; Georgoulias, V. Targeting angiogenesis in small cell lung cancer. *Transl. Lung Cancer Res.* **2016**, *5*, 389–400. [CrossRef]
80. Meder, L.; Schuldt, P.; Thelen, M.; Schmitt, A.; Dietlein, F.; Klein, S.; Borchmann, S.; Wennhold, K.; Vlasic, I.; Oberbeck, S.; et al. Combined VEGF and PD-L1 Blockade Displays Synergistic Treatment Effects in an Autochthonous Mouse Model of Small Cell Lung Cancer. *Cancer Res.* **2018**, *78*, 4270–4281. [CrossRef]
81. Liu, J.F.; Barry, W.T.; Birrer, M.; Lee, J.M.; Buckanovich, R.J.; Fleming, G.F.; Rimel, B.; Buss, M.K.; Nattam, S.; Hurteau, J.; et al. Combination cediranib and olaparib versus olaparib alone for women with recurrent platinum-sensitive ovarian cancer: A randomised phase 2 study. *Lancet Oncol.* **2014**, *15*, 1207–1214. [CrossRef]
82. Cardnell, R.J.; Feng, Y.; Mukherjee, S.; Diao, L.; Tong, P.; Stewart, C.A.; Masrorpour, F.; Fan, Y.; Nilsson, M.; Shen, Y.; et al. Activation of the PI3K/mTOR Pathway following PARP Inhibition in Small Cell Lung Cancer. *PLoS ONE* **2016**, *11*, e0152584. [CrossRef]
83. Gay, C.M.; Diao, L.; Stewart, C.A.; Xi, Y.; Cardnell, R.J.; Swisher, S.G.; Roth, J.A.; Glisson, B.S.; Wang, J.; Heymach, J.V.; et al. Abstract 3772: Inter- and intra-tumoral variations in ASCL1, NEUROD1, and POU2F3 transcriptional programs underlie three distinct molecular subtypes of small cell lung cancers. *Cancer Res.* **2019**, *79*, 3772. [CrossRef]
84. Gay, C.M.; Byers, L.A. PARP Inhibition Combined with Immune Checkpoint Blockade in SCLC: Oasis in an Immune Desert or Mirage? *J. Thorac. Oncol.* **2019**, *14*, 1323–1326. [CrossRef] [PubMed]

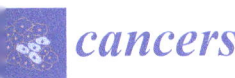

Review

Front Line Applications and Future Directions of Immunotherapy in Small-Cell Lung Cancer

Selina K. Wong [1,2] and Wade T. Iams [1,2,*]

1. Department of Medicine, Division of Hematology and Oncology, Nashville, TN 37232, USA; selina.wong@vumc.org
2. Vanderbilt-Ingram Cancer Center, Vanderbilt University Medical Center, Nashville, TN 37232, USA
* Correspondence: wade.t.iams@vumc.org; Tel.: +1-615-936-2511

Simple Summary: Small-cell lung cancer (SCLC) is an aggressive malignancy with a high risk of recurrence and poor prognosis despite aggressive treatment. The use of immunotherapy has revolutionized the therapeutic landscape of SCLC with the introduction of novel, effective treatment options. Immune checkpoint inhibitors (ICIs) are the primary type of immunotherapy that have been used, first in the extensive-stage setting and now under investigation in the limited-stage setting. Here, we review the use of ICIs in SCLC as well as other emerging immunotherapy strategies.

Abstract: After being stagnant for decades, there has finally been a paradigm shift in the treatment of small-cell lung cancer (SCLC) with the emergence and application of immune checkpoint inhibitors (ICIs). Multiple trials of first-line ICI-chemotherapy combinations have demonstrated survival benefit compared to chemotherapy alone in patients with extensive-stage SCLC, establishing this as the new standard of care. ICIs are now being applied in the potentially curative limited-stage setting, actively being investigated as concurrent treatment with chemoradiation and as adjuvant treatment following completion of chemoradiation. This review highlights the evidence behind the practice-changing addition of ICIs in the first-line setting of extensive-stage SCLC, the potentially practice-changing immunotherapy trials that are currently underway in the limited-stage setting, and alternate immunotherapeutic strategies being studied in the treatment of SCLC.

Keywords: small-cell lung cancer; immunotherapy; immune checkpoint inhibitors

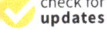

Citation: Wong, S.K.; Iams, W.T. Front Line Applications and Future Directions of Immunotherapy in Small-Cell Lung Cancer. *Cancers* **2021**, *13*, 506. https://doi.org/10.3390/cancers13030506

Academic Editors: Alessandro Morabito and Christian Rolfo
Received: 17 December 2020
Accepted: 26 January 2021
Published: 29 January 2021

Publisher's Note: MDPI stays neutral with regard to jurisdictional claims in published maps and institutional affiliations.

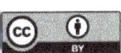

Copyright: © 2021 by the authors. Licensee MDPI, Basel, Switzerland. This article is an open access article distributed under the terms and conditions of the Creative Commons Attribution (CC BY) license (https://creativecommons.org/licenses/by/4.0/).

1. Introduction

Small-cell lung cancer (SCLC), which accounts for approximately 15% of lung cancers, is distinctive in its underlying biology, clinical course, and treatment approach. This aggressive malignancy exhibits rapid growth and early development of metastases, resulting in the majority of patients already having widespread, incurable disease at the time of presentation [1,2].

Early diagnosis and initiation of treatment is crucial in the management of SCLC. The Veteran's Administration Lung Cancer Study Group categorizes SCLC into limited-stage and extensive-stage, with the differentiating feature being whether disease is limited to one hemithorax and therefore encompassable within a feasible radiation field. In less than 5% of cases, SCLC may be diagnosed in very early stages, wherein guidelines recommend definitive surgical resection followed by platinum-based adjuvant chemotherapy for stage I and selected stage IIA patients [2,3]. Otherwise, the mainstay of treatment for limited-stage SCLC (LS-SCLC) is concurrent chemoradiation (CRT) and prophylactic cranial irradiation (PCI). In extensive-stage SCLC (ES-SCLC), systemic therapies remain the cornerstone of treatment. SCLC carries a high risk of recurrence and poor prognosis despite aggressive treatment, with a median survival of 15–20 months for limited-stage and 8–13 months for extensive-stage disease [1,4].

Before the addition of immunotherapy to the treatment algorithm of SCLC, the therapeutic landscape of this disease had been stagnant for decades and lacked meaningful advances in treatment [5,6]. As of 2019, the combination of immune checkpoint inhibitor (ICI) and chemotherapy has been established as the standard of care in the first-line setting of ES-SCLC [7,8]. With the successful application of ICIs in the extensive-stage, this immunotherapeutic strategy is now being applied within the potentially curative, limited-stage setting.

Immunotherapy with ICIs have transformed the therapeutic approach to SCLC and become a rapidly growing area of research. In this article, we review the rationale and data behind ICIs in ES-SCLC with a focus on the recent practice changing first line ICI use, and subsequently we detail the much-anticipated emerging data for ICIs in LS-SCLC. We also discuss the emerging studies evaluating novel immunologic strategies including chimeric antigen receptor (CAR) T cell therapy, vaccines, immunomodulators, and combination therapies. We will not explore the data for the use of ICIs in patients with relapsed SCLC in this review, rather we refer readers to previous reviews on the topic [9–11] and note that the directionality of the field of ICIs in SCLC is moving towards an emphasis on the front line setting. Of note, randomized trials have failed to demonstrate an overall survival (OS) benefit for ICIs compared to chemotherapy for relapsed SCLC [12,13] and the relapsed SCLC indication for nivolumab has been recently withdrawn (though this remains a category 3 treatment option in National Comprehensive Cancer Network guidelines) [14,15].

2. Rationale for Immunotherapy in Small-Cell Lung Cancer

The immune system plays a critical role in cancer pathogenesis. Normally, there exists a fine balance between the ability to recognize "self" to avoid autoimmunity and recognizing "non-self" to appropriately mount a response against foreign entities. By taking advantage of mechanisms utilized by the immune system to supress autoimmunity, cancer cells manage to establish sufficient immune tolerance so as to evade antitumor responses that would normally be activated against them [16,17].

High tumor mutational load is thought to facilitate the activation of the adaptive immune system through the production and subsequent presentation of tumor-specific neoantigens to T cells [18–20]. Although SCLC is characterized by high somatic mutational load [21,22], in part due to its strong association with tobacco exposure [23], there is accumulating evidence that SCLC exerts immunosuppressive effects. T cells, specifically effector T cells (Teffs) and regulatory T cells (Tregs), are key players in mediating the antigen-specific immune response pathway. Whereas the activation of Teffs leads to antitumor activity, Tregs act to downregulate immune responses as a means of preventing autoimmunity [24]. Abnormally high levels of Tregs relative to Teffs have been observed in the setting of cancer, hypothesized to be a means by which antitumor responses become downregulated [25,26]. Koyama et al. analyzed 35 peripheral blood samples of patients with SCLC, finding the Teffs to Tregs ratio to be prognostic. Not only did they observe significantly more Teffs in LS-SCLC and conversely more Tregs in ES-SCLC, but also that long-term survivors of SCLC maintained a high Teffs to Tregs ratio. On the other hand, this ratio was low among patients with recurrent disease [27].

Similarly, immune cell infiltration in the tumor microenvironment has demonstrated prognostic value in SCLC, with higher levels of T cells, CD8 cells, and CD45-positive T cells being detected in long-term survivors [28–30]. Most recently was a case-control study by Muppa et al., comparing resected tumors of 23 long-term SCLC survivors (>4 years) and 18 survivors with expected survival time of less than 2 years. Both the absolute number of tumor-infiltrating lymphocytes (TILs) and the ratio of these relative to immunosuppresive immune cells were found to be different in the two cohorts. Not only did long-term survivors have significantly more TILs, they notably also had higher numbers of suppressive cells (including monocytes, lymphocytes, and macrophages) albeit lower ratios of CD68-positive macrophages to CD3-positive T lymphocytes compared to those with less than 2 year survival [29]. Potential mechanisms by which SCLC is able to evade the immune system include decreased levels of TILs and loss of expression of major histocompatibility complex (MHC) class II [31,32].

The involvement of the immune system in the pathophysiology of SCLC is also evident in the association between occurrence of paraneoplastic syndromes (PNS), such as Lambert-Eaton myasthenic syndrome (LEMS), and long-term prognosis. Patients with SCLC who develop LEMS have a more favorable prognosis than those who do not develop the neurological illness [33]. A recent retrospective review of 145 SCLC patients demonstrated that those who developed a neurologic PNS were found to have both increased TILs and improved median overall survival (24 vs. 12 months) compared to those without PNS [34]. These accumulating data provide the basis for the application of immunotherapeutic strategies in SCLC.

3. Immune Checkpoint Inhibitors

The most extensively utilized type of immunotherapy has been ICIs, specifically those targeting the pathways involving programmed death-1 (PD-1) and cytotoxic T-lymphocyte associated protein 4 (CTLA-4). By expressing ligands that bind PD-1 or CTLA-4 receptors, tumors take advantage of the resulting negative co-stimulatory signals that inhibit T-cell activation and prevent downstream cell-mediated destruction. ICIs reinstitute appropriate antitumor response by inhibiting the binding of these receptors [35,36]

4. Extensive-Stage Small-Cell Lung Cancer

The benefit of combination ICI with chemotherapy in the first-line setting of ES-SCLC is well established and has been studied in four phase III trials (IMpower133, CASPIAN, KEYNOTE-604, and CA184-156) and more recently a phase II ECOG-ACRIN EA5161 trial (Table 1).

In the phase III, placebo-controlled, randomized IMpower133 trial, the anti-programmed death ligand 1 (PD-L1) agent atezolizumab or placebo was combined with the chemotherapy backbone of carboplatin and etoposide for four cycles, followed by either atezolizumab or placebo maintenance [7]. Testing for PD-L1 expression was not required nor were patients stratified, but exploratory analyses did include assessment of efficacy in relation to blood-based tumor mutational burden. A total of 403 previously untreated patients with ES-SCLC were enrolled, of which 201 patients received atezolizumab plus chemotherapy. Although PCI was permitted during the maintenance phase, consolidative thoracic radiotherapy was not. The two primary endpoints of the trial, progression-free survival (PFS) and OS, demonstrated statistical significance in favor of the atezolizumab plus chemotherapy cohort: PFS 5.2 months vs. 4.3 months (HR 0.77, 95% confidence interval [CI] 0.62–0.96, $p = 0.02$) and OS 12.3 months vs. 10.3 months (HR 0.70, 95% CI 0.54–0.91, $p = 0.007$). Incidence of grade 3 or 4 adverse events was balanced between the atezolizumab-containing (56.6%) and placebo (56.1%) arms. Though OS was already statistically significant at interim analysis, an updated exploratory OS analysis was presented at the 2019 European Society of Medical Oncology Congress. At a median follow-up of 22.9 months, improvement seen in the atezolizumab-containing arm persisted with 18-month OS of 24% vs. 21% [37].

Table 1. Summary of first-line ICI trials in ES-SCLC.

Trial	Phase	No. of Patients	Treatment	FDA Approval	Primary Endpoint(s) (Met?)	PFS	OS	ORR (%)	Grade 3/4 Adverse Events (%)
IMpower133 (Horn et al.)	III	403	Atezolizumab + carboplatin/etoposide vs. carboplatin/etoposide	Yes	OS (yes) PFS (yes)	5.2 vs. 4.3 months (HR 0.77, 95%CI 0.62–0.96, $p = 0.02$)	12.3 vs. 10.3 months (HR 0.70, 95%CI 0.54–0.91, $p = 0.007$)	60.2 vs. 64.4	56.6 vs. 56.1
CASPIAN * (Paz-Ares et al.)	III	805	Durvalumab + platinum/etoposide vs. platinum/etoposide	Yes	OS (yes)	5.1 vs. 5.4 months (HR 0.78, 95% CI 0.65–0.94)	13.0 vs. 10.3 months (HR 0.73, 95%CI 0.59–0.91, $p = 0.0047$)	79 vs. 70	62 vs. 62
ECOG-ACRIN EA5161 (Leal et al.)	II	160	Nivolumab + platinum/etoposide vs. platinum/etoposide	No	PFS (yes)	5.5 vs. 4.6 months (HR 0.65, 95%CI 0.46–0.91, $p = 0.012$)	11.3 vs. 8.5 months (HR 0.67, 95%CI 0.46–0.98, $p = 0.038$)	52.3 vs. 47.7	77 vs. 62
KEYNOTE-604 (Rudin et al.)	III	453	Pembrolizumab + platinum/etoposide vs. platinum/etoposide	No	OS (no) PFS (yes)	4.5 vs. 4.3 months (HR 0.75, 95% CI 0.61–0.91, $p = 0.0023$)	10.8 vs. 9.7 months (HR 0.80, 95%CI 0.64–0.98, $p = 0.0164$)	70.6 vs. 61.8	76.7 vs. 74.9
CA184-156 (Reck et al.)	III	1132	Ipilimumab + platinum/etoposide vs. platinum/etoposide	No	OS (no)	4.6 vs. 4.4 months (HR 0.85, 95%CI 0.75–0.97, $p = 0.0161$)	11.0 vs. 10.9 months (HR 0.94, 95%CI 0.81–1.09, $p = 0.3775$)	62 vs. 62	48 vs. 45

* treatment arm containing durvalumab plus tremelimumab plus platinum plus etoposide did not reach statistical significance.

The efficacy of combining durvalumab with or without tremelimumab with chemotherapy was investigated in the phase III trial CASPIAN [8]. Patients were randomized to receive durvalumab plus platinum-etoposide, durvalumab, tremelimumab (a CTLA-4 inhibitor) plus platinum-etoposide, or platinum-etoposide alone, followed by maintenance. PCI was permitted at the physician's discretion in the chemotherapy alone group only. At interim analysis in 2019, results were presented for the durvalumab plus platinum-etoposide vs. the platinum-etoposide only groups. The primary endpoint of OS had been met and was in favor of the durvalumab group: 13.0 months vs. 10.3 months, HR 0.73, 95% CI 0.59–0.91, p = 0.0047. PFS, a secondary endpoint, was 5.1 months in the durvalumab arm vs. 5.4 months in the chemotherapy only arm, HR 0.78, 95% CI 0.65–0.94. After a median follow up of 25.1 months, the updated efficacy analyses of durvalumab plus platinum-etoposide as well as the initial results of the tremelimumab-containing cohort were presented at the 2020 American Society of Clinical Oncology meeting [38]. The durvalumab-containing arm continued to demonstrate superior OS compared to platinum-etoposide alone, 12.9 months vs. 10.5 months, HR 0.75, 95% CI 0.62–0.91, p = 0.0032 and this benefit was seen regardless of whether carboplatin or cisplatin was used. On the other hand, the tremelimumab arm did not reach statistical significance with median OS of 10.4 months vs. 10.5 months with chemotherapy alone (HR 0.82, 95% CI 0.68–1.00, p = 0.0451). Two-year survival rates were 22.2% in the durvalumab arm, 23.4% in the tremelimumab arm, and 14.4% with platinum-etoposide alone. Occurrence of grade 3 or 4 adverse events was slightly higher with the dual ICI plus chemotherapy arm (70.3%), but was otherwise well balanced between the durvalumab and chemotherapy alone arms (62.3% and 62.8%, respectively).

At the 2020 American Society of Clinical Oncology meeting, the efficacy of nivolumab given in combination with platinum-etoposide vs. platinum-etoposide alone for first-line treatment of ES-SCLC was presented from the randomized phase II ECOG-ACRIN EA5161 trial [39]. The addition of nivolumab to chemotherapy, followed by nivolumab maintenance, improved both PFS (5.5 months vs. 4.6 months, HR 0.65, 95% CI 0.46–0.91, p = 0.012) and OS (11.3 months vs. 8.5 months, HR 0.67, 95% CI 0.46–0.98, p = 0.038). No new safety signals were observed, with the incidence of grade 3 or 4 adverse events 77% with nivolumab vs. 62%.

KEYNOTE-604 investigated the addition of pembrolizumab, an anti-PD-1 agent, to platinum-etoposide as first-line treatment of ES-SCLC [40]. Eligible patients received chemotherapy plus either pembrolizumab or placebo, followed by maintenance. Although the addition of pembrolizumab improved PFS (4.5 months vs. 4.3 months, HR 0.75, 95% CI 0.61–0.91, p = 0.0023), a statistically significant difference in OS was narrowly missed (10.8 months vs. 9.7 months, HR 0.80, 95% CI 0.64–0.98, p = 0.0164). Pembrolizumab was generally well tolerated, with a grade 3 or 4 adverse event rate of 76.7% with pembrolizumab vs. 74.9% with chemotherapy alone.

After promising results from a phase II trial wherein ipilimumab was administered in a phased approach after initial exposure to chemotherapy [41], Reck et al. undertook the multicenter, randomized, double-blinded phase III CA184-156 trial to explore the utility of adding an anti-CTLA-4 agent ipilimumab to platinum-etoposide, followed by ipilimumab or placebo maintenance [42]. During the induction phase (6 cycles), patients in both arms received platinum-etoposide throughout cycles 1 to 4. In cycles 3 and 4, patients were randomized to receive either the addition of ipilimumab or placebo. Patients then received only ipilimumab or placebo in the final cycles 5 and 6 of induction, followed by maintenance among patients who achieved either a complete or partial response. This study failed to meet its primary endpoint of OS: 11.0 months in the ipilimumab arm vs. 10.9 months in the placebo arm, HR 0.94, 95% CI 0.81–1.09, p = 0.3775.

5. Limited-Stage Small-Cell Lung Cancer

Having demonstrated benefit in the extensive-stage setting, ICIs are now under rigorous investigation in the limited-stage setting. Even after curative-intent treatment, there is a high recurrence risk of approximately 70% at 5 years [43]. Being that the primary treatment modality for LS-SCLC is concurrent CRT [44,45], the addition of ICIs is being investigated both in the concurrent setting with CRT and in the adjuvant setting after definitive CRT (Table 2).

In the concurrent setting, data from a single-center, open label, phase I/II trial of pembrolizumab given with concurrent chemoradiation in the treatment of LS-SCLC and other neuroendocrine tumors was recently published [46]. The primary endpoint was safety (dose-limiting toxicities) and secondary endpoints included PFS, OS, and tumor response. Pembrolizumab was started concurrently with CRT (45Gy radiotherapy and platinum-etoposide chemotherapy) and continued for up to 16 cycles. PCI was permitted at the physician's discretion, with a total of 27 (61%) patients who underwent PCI. A total of 40 patients were treated with at least one cycle of pembrolizumab: median PFS was 19.7 months (95% CI 8.8–30.5) and OS was 39.5 months (95% CI 8.0–71.0). At the median follow-up time of 23.1 months, 20 (50%) patients had developed disease progression. Thirty-three of the 40 patients were evaluable for response and had an ORR of 79%. Three patients experienced grade 4 toxicities (2 neutropenia and 1 respiratory failure) while the most common grade 3 toxicities were neutropenia (5 patients) and anemia (5 patients). A pneumonitis rate of 15% was seen (three grade 2 and three grade 3). The authors concluded that this regimen not only yielded favorable outcomes, but was also well tolerated. The safety of combination immunotherapy and radiation in this trial was comparable to that of the CONVERT trial of once-daily vs. twice-daily chemoradiation in LS-SCLC: pneumonitis 15% vs. 21% in CONVERT and esophagitis 42.5% vs. 81% in CONVERT [43]. Given these results from the first prospective trial of concurrent ICI and CRT in LS-SCLC, the results of an ongoing phase II/III trial LU005 (NCT03811002) of atezolizumab plus CRT vs. CRT alone in LS-SCLC are much anticipated.

In the adjuvant setting where ICIs are given as maintenance following curative CRT, multiple trials are underway including the phase II ACHILES (NCT03540420), phase III ADRIATIC (NCT03703297), and phase II STIMULI (NCT02046733) trials. Respectively, these trials are investigating the efficacy of maintenance atezolizumab, durvalumab and/or tremelimumab, and nivolumab plus ipilimumab following completion of chemoradiation (Table 2). Given the practice-changing findings from the PACIFIC trial of maintenance durvalumab after definitive CRT in unresectable stage III non-small cell lung cancer (NSCLC) [47,48], the results of these SCLC trials are eagerly awaited.

Table 2. Summary of ICI trials in LS-SCLC.

Trial	Phase	Status	Setting	Treatment	Primary Endpoint(s)	Target Enrolment	Start Date–Estimated Completion Date
Welsh et al. 2020	I/II	Complete	Concurrent with CRT	Pembrolizumab + concurrent CRT	Safety: no grade 5 toxicity, pneumonitis 15%, esophagitis 42.5% * PFS was 19.7 months (95% CI 8.8–30.5) * OS was 39.5 months (95% CI 8.0–71.0) * ORR of 79%	40	Completed
LU-005 (NCT03811002)	II/III	Ongoing	Concurrent with CRT	Atezolizumab + concurrent CRT vs. CRT	OS, PFS	506	28 May 2019–28 December 2026
ACHILES (NCT03540420)	II	Ongoing	Maintenance after CRT	Atezolizumab vs. observation	2-year survival	212	31 July 2018–December 2026
ADRIATIC (NCT03703297)	III	Ongoing	Maintenance after CRT	Durvalumab vs. durvalumab + tremelimumab vs. placebo	OS, PFS	724	27 September 2018–10 May 2024
STIMULI (NCT02046733)	II	Ongoing	Maintenance after CRT	Nivolumab + ipilimumab vs. observation	OS, PFS	174	28 July 2014–January 2022

* Secondary outcomes.

6. Predictive Biomarkers

Unlike in NSCLC where PD-L1 expression is used to guide first-line treatment with ICI monotherapy [49], an equivalent predictive biomarker to inform the use of ICIs in SCLC remains elusive. PD-L1 expression is evaluated by immunohistochemistry, with multiple clinical trial validated assays that have been approved as companion diagnostics. There are inherent limitations of this biomarker [50], including its heterogeneity both temporally and spatially (intratumoral and intertumoral), inter-assay variability, and potential discordance between surgical resected and matched biopsy specimens [51–53]. Furthermore, PD-L1 expression may vary depending on whether expression is determined on tumor cells, immune cells, and/or stroma.

In the first-line setting, IMpower133, CASPIAN, and KEYNOTE-604 did not demonstrate a strong association between PD-L1 expression and ICI efficacy. IMpower133 included an exploratory analysis of PD-L1 expression (on immune or tumor cells) and survival. The PD-L1 evaluable population comprised 34% (137/403 patients) of the intention-to-treat population, with efficacy analyses conducted using PD-L1 cut-offs of 1% and 5%. An OS benefit favoring the addition of atezolizumab to chemotherapy was seen in the PD-L1 < 1% cohort (10.2 months vs. 8.3 months), but not in the PD-L1 $\geq$ 1% and $\geq$5% cohorts [37,51–53]. In the CASPIAN trial, only 5% of patients had PD-L1 expression $\geq$1% in tumor cells and 22% of patients with PD-L1 expression $\geq$1% in immune cells. The investigators evaluated PD-L1 expression as a continuous variable and did not observe any impact on ORR, PFS, or OS between treatment arms [54]. KEYNOTE-604 measured PD-L1 expression using the combined positive score (CPS), which takes into account both tumors cells and tumor-infiltrating cells. Similarly, no differences in PFS or OS were observed based on PD-L1 expression [40].

Some evidence has suggested that the expression of PD-L1 in the tumor microenvironment, specifically on host cells as opposed to tumors cells, may in fact be a better predictor of response to ICIs [55,56]. Schultheis et al. examined 94 cases of SCLC, among which none of them demonstrated PD-L1 expression on tumor cells but 17 (18%) of them expressed PD-L1 within the stroma [57]. The importance of the PD-1/PD-L1 pathway in the tumor microenvironment was also demonstrated in a study of 193 patients with large cell neuroendocrine carcinoma or SCLC examined for PD-L1 expression on tumor cells and tumor-infiltrating immune cells. No correlation was seen between PD-L1 expression on tumor cells and that on immune cells. Patients with PD-L1 expression on immune cells had significantly longer PFS than those without (11.3 months vs. 7.0 months, $p = 0.02$) and notably, this correlation with survival was not demonstrated with PD-L1 expression on tumor cells [58].

Tumor mutational burden (TMB), a measure of non-synonymous somatic mutations, has been shown across multiple cancer types to be associated with improved OS after treatment with ICIs [59]. Its utility in guiding the treatment of SCLC has proven to be inconclusive, similar to PD-L1 expression. High TMB is thought to result in a higher neoantigen load which allows for T cell activation and downstream antitumor effects [60]. Ricciuti et al. collected data from 52 patients with relapsed or refractory SCLC who went on to receive treatment with an ICI. Patients with high TMB (above 50th percentile) achieved significantly longer PFS and OS compared to their low TMB (below 50th percentile) counterparts: median PFS 3.3 months vs. 1.2 months and OS 10.4 months vs. 2.5 months [61]. Based on findings by Gandara et al. showing the ability of blood-based TMB (bTMB) to identify patients who derive clinically significant improvements in PFS from atezolizumab in second-line or later advanced NSCLC [62], the utility of bTMB as a predictive biomarker was an exploratory analysis in IMpower133. Blood-based TMB analyses with cut-off values of 10 and 16 mutations per megabase (Mb) were possible in 351 of the 403 patients (93.8%). Consistent OS and PFS benefits were demonstrated across all subgroups in favor of atezolizumab plus chemotherapy, although the <10 mutations/Mb and $\geq$16 mutations/Mb subgroups did not reach statistical significance [7].

7. Other Immunotherapeutic Approaches

Apart from ICIs, there are a variety of different mechanisms by which the immune system can be harnessed to mount an antitumor response. These include CAR T cell therapy, bispecific T cell engagers (BiTEs), antibody-drug conjugates, and immunomodulators (Table 3).

Table 3. Overview of other immunotherapeutic approaches, used alone or in combination with ICIs, in the treatment of SCLC.

Type	Examples
CAR T cell therapy	AMG 119 (targeting DLL-3)
Bispecific T cell engager	AMG 757 (targeting DLL-3)
Antibody-drug conjugate	Rovalpituzumab tesirine (targeting DLL-3)
Immunomodulators	Interleukin-2 Interferon Lefitolimod (TLR9 agonist) N-803 (interleukin-15 agonist) BNT411 (TLR7 agonist)
Vaccine	Fucosyl GM-1 GD3 ganglioside Polysialic acid Dendritic cell-based p53
Immune checkpoint	TIM-3 LAG-3 TIGIT
Small molecule	CDK4/6 inhibitor PARP inhibitor
Alkylating agent	Lurbinectedin
Other	Lutetium-labeled somatostatin analog

While endogenous T cell activation is dependent on antigen presentation by MHC class I, T cell-based therapy is an MHC-independent therapeutic strategy. Chimeric antigen receptors are recombinant receptors for tumor-specific antigens, which then become engineered into T cells to enable expression, expansion, and anti-tumor specificity [63]. Multiple cell surface molecules have emerged as potential therapeutic targets, including CD56 [64] and CD47 [65], both of which are highly expressed on the surface of SCLC cells. Similarly, delta-like ligand 3 (DLL3) is an inhibitory Notch pathway ligand that is upregulated and overexpressed in high-grade neuroendocrine tumors [66]. While it is expressed in over 80% of SCLC, there is little to no expression on normal lung tissue, therefore making it an attractive therapeutic target [67,68]. DLL3-targeted CAR T cell-based therapy, AMG 119, is being studied in an ongoing phase I trial of patients with relapsed/refractory SCLC (NCT03392064). Another DLL-3 targeted immunotherapy that has been developed is the BiTE, AMG 757. BiTEs are recombinant bispecific proteins that simultaneously target a T-cell surface molecule (such as CD3) and a tumor-specific surface antigen, thereby facilitating T cell adherence and antitumor response independent of MHC [69]. AMG 757 alone and in combination with pembrolizumab is currently being evaluated in a phase I trial (NCT03319940). Rovalpituzumab tesirine (Rova-T), a DLL3-targeted antibody-drug conjugate [70], has failed to establish a role in the treatment of SCLC after limited activity was demonstrated in the third-line (phase II single-arm TRINITY), second-line (phase III TAHOE), and first-line maintenance following platinum-based chemotherapy (phase III MERU) [71,72].

Vaccines are a potentially promising strategy in the management of SCLC and remain under investigation. Vaccines are designed with the intent of exposing host cells to tumor antigens, thereby potentiating an adaptive immune response. Multiple vaccines have been studied thus far, including fucosyl GM-1, GD3 ganglioside, polysialic acid, and dendritic cell-based p53 [9,73,74].

The utility of immunomodulatory agents such as interleukin-2 and interferon has been studied and failed to demonstrate benefit [74]. Most recently, the efficacy of lefitolimod as maintenance therapy after first-line chemotherapy was investigated in phase II trial IMPULSE. The mechanism of action for lefitolimod, a toll-like receptor (TLR) 9 agonist, is the activation of innate immunity via stimulation of cytokine production [75]. IMPULSE failed to demonstrate an OS benefit in the intention-to-treat population, although a subgroup analysis of patients with a low frequency of activated CD86+ B cell revealed an OS benefit signal, HR 0.53, 95% CI 0.26–1.08 [76].

Multiple novel immunotherapeutic strategies are emerging to investigate combination approaches with ICIs (Table 3). TIM-3 and LAG-3 are two immune checkpoint molecules that contribute to immune tolerance. Their upregulation has been observed and implicated in the development of resistance to PD-1 blockade [77,78]. Anti-TIM-3 agents are being investigated as monotherapy, in combination with anti-PD-1/anti-CTLA-4 agents, and dual blockade using bispecific antibodies [79]. A phase II trial of anti-PD-1 agent, spartalizumab, and anti-LAG-3 agent, LAG525, reported preliminary efficacy analyses across seven tumor types including SCLC. Promising activity in SCLC was reported, although final results have yet to be presented [80]. T cell immunoreceptor with immunoglobulin and ITIM domains (TIGIT) and its ligands CD155 and CD112, is another immune checkpoint pathway being targeted for anticancer therapy [81]. In ES-SCLC, the SKYSCRAPER-02 (NCT04256421) is a phase III, randomized, double-blind, placebo-controlled trial underway to investigate the addition of an anti-TIGIT agent, tiragolumab, to first-line atezolizumab, carboplatin, plus etoposide.

Other immunomodulatory agents have also been combined with ICIs, for example N-803 and BNT411. N-803, an interleukin-15 superagonist, was studied in combination with nivolumab in metastatic NSCLC [82], and is currently being investigated in combination with PD-1/PD-L1 agents in the setting of advanced solid tumors (including SCLC) that have progressed on or after single-agent checkpoint inhibitor in the QUILT-3.055 trial (NCT03228667). The safety and efficacy of BNT411, a TLR7 agonist, is being explored as monotherapy and in combination with atezolizumab, carboplatin, and etoposide in ES-SCLC (NCT04101357).

The small molecules cyclin-dependent kinases (CDK) 4/6 inhibitors and poly (ADP-ribose) polymerase (PARP) inhibitors have both been applied in combination with an ICI in the treatment of SCLC. The efficacy of trilaciclib, a CDK4/6 inhibitor, administered with first-line atezolizumab, carboplatin, and etoposide in ES-SCLC is being investigated in NCT03041311. Durvalumab in combination with PARP inhibitor, olaparib, was studied in a single-arm phase II study of relapsed SCLC and ultimately did not meet the pre-set bar for efficacy [83], but this strategy of simultaneous ICI and PARP inhibition continues to be explored [84].

Although platinum and etoposide are the most established chemotherapies in the treatment of SCLC, lurbinectedin is an alkylating agent that is being investigated in combination with ICIs including pembrolizumab (NCT04358237), nivolumab and ipilimumab (NCT04610658), and atezolizumab (NCT04253145).

Mechanistically, vaccines may potentiate the effects of ICIs given they both act on the adaptive immune system. Ongoing trials include nivolumab plus ipilimumab with a dendritic p53 vaccine (NCT03406715) and atezolizumab in combination with a dendritic cell vaccine (NCT04487756).

Finally, another novel approach to the treatment of SCLC that has shown evidence of antitumor effect in a phase I trial is combination of lutetium-labeled somatostatin analog in combination with nivolumab [85]. This approach takes advantage of somatostatin receptors that are expressed by some neuroendocrine tumors, including SCLC. As we further our understanding of resistance mechanisms to PD-1/CTLA-4 agents and develop novel therapies, additional combination studies are likely to emerge. Understanding optimal sequencing of treatments and how to take advantage of additive or synergistic effects of drugs will be crucial.

8. Conclusions

The treatment landscape of SCLC has been revolutionized by the integration of immunotherapy. While ICIs have established a clear role in the front line treatment of ES-SCLC, the results of several ongoing trials investigating their efficacy in the curative, limited-stage setting are much anticipated. Ultimately despite the substantial advances made with immunotherapies, the reality of SCLC remains that the majority of patients will eventually relapse and experience a poor prognosis. Continued drug development of novel targeted therapies will be crucial, both for use in combination with immunotherapy and/or as later line therapy in the setting of immunotherapy refractory disease.

Author Contributions: S.K.W. and W.T.I. contributed to manuscript drafting and editing. All authors have read and agreed to the published version of the manuscript.

Funding: This research received no external funding.

Institutional Review Board Statement: Not applicable.

Informed Consent Statement: Not applicable.

Data Availability Statement: No new data were created or analyzed in this study. Data sharing is not applicable to this article.

Acknowledgments: W.T.I. was supported by a National Comprehensive Cancer Network (NCCN) Young Investigator Award.

Conflicts of Interest: W.T.I reports consulting for Genentech, Jazz Pharma, G1 Therapeutics, Outcomes Insights, Cello Health, and Defined Health. S.K.W reports no conflicts of interest.

References

1. Byers, L.; Rudin, C.M. Small cell lung cancer: Where do we go from here? *Cancer* **2015**, *121*, 664–672. [CrossRef] [PubMed]
2. Rudin, C.M.; Ismaila, N.; Hann, C.L.; Malhotra, N.; Movsas, B.; Norris, K.; Pietanza, M.C.; Ramalingam, S.S.; Turrisi, A.T.; Giaccone, G. Treatment of Small-Cell Lung Cancer: American Society of Clinical Oncology Endorsement of the American College of Chest Physicians Guideline. *J. Clin. Oncol.* **2015**, *33*, 4106–4111. [CrossRef] [PubMed]
3. Dómine, M.; Morán, T.; Isla, D.; Martí, J.L.; Sullivan, I.; Provencio, M.; Olmedo, M.E.; Ponce, S.; Blasco, A.; Cobo, M. SEOM clinical guidelines for the treatment of small-cell lung cancer (SCLC) (2019). *Clin. Transl. Oncol.* **2020**, *22*, 245–255. [CrossRef] [PubMed]
4. Van Meerbeeck, J.P.; Fennell, D.A.; De Ruysscher, D. Small-cell lung cancer. *Lancet* **2011**, *378*, 1741–1755. [CrossRef]
5. Lally, B.E.; Urbanic, J.J.; Blackstock, A.W.; Miller, A.A.; Perry, M.C. Small Cell Lung Cancer: Have We Made Any Progress Over the Last 25 Years? *Oncologist* **2007**, *12*, 1096–1104. [CrossRef]
6. Oze, I.; Hotta, K.; Kiura, K.; Ochi, N.; Takigawa, N.; Fujiwara, Y.; Tabata, M.; Tanimoto, M. Twenty-Seven Years of Phase III Trials for Patients with Extensive Disease Small-Cell Lung Cancer: Disappointing Results. *PLoS ONE* **2009**, *4*, e7835. [CrossRef]
7. Horn, L.; Mansfield, A.S.; Szczęsna, A.; Havel, L.; Krzakowski, M.; Hochmair, M.J.; Huemer, F.; Losonczy, G.; Johnson, M.L.; Nishio, M.; et al. First-Line Atezolizumab plus Chemotherapy in Extensive-Stage Small-Cell Lung Cancer. *N. Engl. J. Med.* **2018**, *379*, 2220–2229. [CrossRef]
8. Paz-Ares, L.; Dvorkin, M.; Chen, Y.; Reinmuth, N.; Hotta, K.; Trukhin, D.; Statsenko, G.; Hochmair, M.J.; Özgüroğlu, M.; Ji, J.H.; et al. Durvalumab plus platinum–etoposide versus platinum–etoposide in first-line treatment of extensive-stage small-cell lung cancer (CASPIAN): A randomised, controlled, open-label, phase 3 trial. *Lancet* **2019**, *394*, 1929–1939. [CrossRef]
9. Esposito, G.; Palumbo, G.; Carillio, G.; Manzo, A.; Montanino, A.; Sforza, V.; Costanzo, R.; Sandomenico, C.; La Manna, C.; Martucci, N.; et al. Immunotherapy in Small Cell Lung Cancer. *Cancers* **2020**, *12*, 2522. [CrossRef]
10. Iams, W.T.; Porter, J.; Horn, L. Immunotherapeutic approaches for small-cell lung cancer. *Nat. Rev. Clin. Oncol.* **2020**, *17*, 300–312. [CrossRef]
11. Ragavan, M.; Das, M. Systemic Therapy of Extensive Stage Small Cell Lung Cancer in the Era of Immunotherapy. *Curr. Treat. Options Oncol.* **2020**, *21*, 1–14. [CrossRef] [PubMed]
12. Pujol, J.-L.; Greillier, L.; Audigier-Valette, C.; Moro-Sibilot, D.; Uwer, L.; Hureaux, J.; Guisier, F.; Carmier, D.; Madelaine, J.; Otto, J.; et al. A Randomized Non-Comparative Phase II Study of Anti-Programmed Cell Death-Ligand 1 Atezolizumab or Chemotherapy as Second-Line Therapy in Patients with Small Cell Lung Cancer: Results From the IFCT-1603 Trial. *J. Thorac. Oncol.* **2019**, *14*, 903–913. [CrossRef] [PubMed]

13. Reck, M.; Vicente, D.; Ciuleanu, T.; Gettinger, S.; Peters, S.; Horn, L.; Audigier-Valette, C.; Pardo, N.; Juan-Vidal, O.; Cheng, Y.; et al. Efficacy and safety of nivolumab (nivo) monotherapy versus chemotherapy (chemo) in recurrent small cell lung cancer (SCLC): Results from CheckMate 331. *Ann. Oncol.* **2018**, *29*, x43. [CrossRef]
14. Bristol Myers Squibb. Bristol Myers Squibb Statement on Opdivo (nivolumab) Small Cell Lung Cancer U.S. Indication. Available online: https://news.bms.com/news/details/2020/Bristol-Myers-Squibb-Statement-on-Opdivo-nivolumab-Small-Cell-Lung-Cancer-US-Indication/default.aspx (accessed on 19 January 2021).
15. National Comprehensive Guidelines (NCCN). NCCN Clinical Practice Guidelines in Oncology, Small Cell Lung Cancer, Version 2.2021. Available online: https://www.nccn.org/professionals/physician_gls/pdf/sclc.pdf (accessed on 19 January 2021).
16. Doyle, A.; Martin, W.J.; Funa, K.; Gazdar, A.; Carney, D.; Martin, S.E.; Linnoila, I.; Cuttitta, F.; Mulshine, J.; Bunn, P. Markedly decreased expression of class I histocompatibility antigens, protein, and mRNA in human small-cell lung cancer. *J. Exp. Med.* **1985**, *161*, 1135–1151. [CrossRef]
17. Seliger, B. Strategies of Tumor Immune Evasion. *BioDrugs* **2005**, *19*, 347–354. [CrossRef]
18. Efremova, M.; Finotello, F.; Rieder, D.; Trajanoski, Z. Neoantigens Generated by Individual Mutations and Their Role in Cancer Immunity and Immunotherapy. *Front. Immunol.* **2017**, *8*, 1679. [CrossRef]
19. Sabari, J.K.; Lok, B.H.; Laird, J.H.; Poirier, J.T.; Rudin, J.K.S.J.T.P.C.M. Unravelling the biology of SCLC: Implications for therapy. *Nat. Rev. Clin. Oncol.* **2017**, *14*, 549–561. [CrossRef]
20. Yarchoan, M.; Johnson, B.A.; Lutz, E.R.; Laheru, D.A.; Jaffee, E.M. Targeting neoantigens to augment antitumour immunity. *Nat. Rev. Cancer* **2017**, *17*, 209–222. [CrossRef]
21. George, J.; Lim, J.S.; Jang, S.J.; Cun, Y.; Ozretić, L.; Kong, G.; Leenders, F.; Lu, X.; Fernández-Cuesta, L.; Bosco, G.; et al. Comprehensive genomic profiles of small cell lung cancer. *Nat. Cell Biol.* **2015**, *524*, 47–53. [CrossRef]
22. Peifer, M.; Fernández-Cuesta, L.; Sos, M.L.; George, J.; Seidel, D.; Kasper, L.H.; Plenker, D.; Leenders, F.; Sun, R.; Zander, T.; et al. Integrative genome analyses identify key somatic driver mutations of small-cell lung cancer. *Nat. Genet.* **2012**, *44*, 1104–1110. [CrossRef]
23. Govindan, R.; Page, N.; Morgensztern, D.; Read, W.; Tierney, R.; Vlahiotis, A.; Spitznagel, E.L.; Piccirillo, J. Changing Epidemiology of Small-Cell Lung Cancer in the United States Over the Last 30 Years: Analysis of the Surveillance, Epidemiologic, and End Results Database. *J. Clin. Oncol.* **2006**, *24*, 4539–4544. [CrossRef] [PubMed]
24. Hiura, T.; Kagamu, H.; Miura, S.; Ishida, A.; Tanaka, H.; Tanaka, J.; Gejyo, F.; Yoshizawa, H. Both Regulatory T Cells and Antitumor Effector T Cells Are Primed in the Same Draining Lymph Nodes during Tumor Progression. *J. Immunol.* **2005**, *175*, 5058–5066. [CrossRef] [PubMed]
25. Onizuka, S.; Tawara, I.; Shimizu, J.; Sakaguchi, S.; Fujita, T.; Nakayama, E. Tumor rejection by in vivo administration of an-ti-CD25 (interleukin-2 receptor alpha) monoclonal antibody. *Cancer Res.* **1999**, *59*, 3128–3133. [PubMed]
26. Shimizu, J.; Yamazaki, S.; Sakaguchi, S. Induction of tumor immunity by removing CD25+CD4+ T cells: A common basis be-tween tumor immunity and autoimmunity. *J. Immun.* **1999**, *163*, 5211–5218.
27. Koyama, K.; Kagamu, H.; Miura, S.; Hiura, T.; Miyabayashi, T.; Itoh, R.; Kuriyama, H.; Tanaka, H.; Tanaka, J.; Yoshizawa, H.; et al. Reciprocal CD4+ T-Cell Balance of Effector CD62Llow CD4+ and CD62LhighCD25+ CD4+ Regulatory T Cells in Small Cell Lung Cancer Reflects Disease Stage. *Clin. Cancer Res.* **2008**, *14*, 6770–6779. [CrossRef]
28. Eerola, A.K.; Soini, Y.; Pääkkö, P. A high number of tumor-infiltrating lymphocytes are associated with a small tumor size, low tumor stage, and a favorable prognosis in operated small cell lung carcinoma. *Clin. Cancer Res. Off. J. Am. Assoc. Cancer Res.* **2000**, *6*, 1875–1881.
29. Muppa, P.; Terra, S.B.S.P.; Sharma, A.; Mansfield, A.S.; Aubry, M.-C.; Bhinge, K.; Asiedu, M.K.; De Andrade, M.; Janaki, N.; Murphy, S.J.; et al. Immune Cell Infiltration May Be a Key Determinant of Long-Term Survival in Small Cell Lung Cancer. *J. Thorac. Oncol.* **2019**, *14*, 1286–1295. [CrossRef]
30. Wang, W.; Hodkinson, P.; McLaren, F.; MacKean, M.J.; Williams, L.; Howie, S.E.M.; Wallace, W.A.; Sethi, T. Histologic Assessment of Tumor-Associated CD45 + Cell Numbers Is an Independent Predictor of Prognosis in Small Cell Lung Cancer. *Chest* **2013**, *143*, 146–151. [CrossRef]
31. He, Y.; Rozeboom, L.; Rivard, C.J.; Ellison, K.; Dziadziuszko, R.; Yu, H.; Zhou, C.; Hirsch, F.R. MHC class II expression in lung cancer. *Lung Cancer* **2017**, *112*, 75–80. [CrossRef]
32. Schalper, K.A.; Carvajal-Hausdorf, D.E.; McLaughlin, J.F.; Altan, M.; Chiang, A.C.; Velcheti, V.; Kaftan, E.; Zhang, J.; Lu, L.; Rimm, D.L.; et al. Objective measurement and significance of PD-L1, B7-H3, B7-H4 and TILs in small cell lung cancer (SCLC). *J. Clin. Oncol.* **2016**, *34*, 8566. [CrossRef]
33. Maddison, P.; Newsom-Davis, J.; Mills, K.R.; Souhami, R.L. Favourable prognosis in Lambert-Eaton myasthenic syndrome and small-cell lung carcinoma. *Lancet* **1999**, *353*, 117–118. [CrossRef]
34. Iams, W.T.; Shiuan, E.; Meador, C.B.; Roth, M.; Bordeaux, J.; Vaupel, C.; Boyd, K.L.; Summitt, I.B.; Wang, L.L.; Schneider, J.T.; et al. Improved Prognosis and Increased Tumor-Infiltrating Lymphocytes in Patients Who Have SCLC With Neurologic Paraneoplastic Syndromes. *J. Thorac. Oncol.* **2019**, *14*, 1970–1981. [CrossRef] [PubMed]
35. Fife, B.T.; Bluestone, J.A. Control of peripheral T-cell tolerance and autoimmunity via the CTLA-4 and PD-1 pathways. *Immunol. Rev.* **2008**, *224*, 166–182. [CrossRef] [PubMed]
36. Iwai, Y.; Ishida, M.; Tanaka, Y.; Okazaki, T.; Honjo, T.; Minato, N. Involvement of PD-L1 on tumor cells in the escape from host immune system and tumor immunotherapy by PD-L1 blockade. *Proc. Natl. Acad. Sci. USA* **2002**, *99*, 12293–12297. [CrossRef]

47. Reck, M.; Liu, S.; Mansfield, A.; Mok, T.; Scherpereel, A.; Reinmuth, N.; Garassino, M.; De Carpeno, J.; Califano, R.; Nishio, M.; et al. IMpower133: Updated overall survival (OS) analysis of first-line (1L) atezolizumab (atezo) + carboplatin + etoposide in extensive-stage SCLC (ES-SCLC). *Ann. Oncol.* **2019**, *30*, v710–v711. [CrossRef]
48. Paz-Ares, L.G.; Dvorkin, M.; Chen, Y.; Reinmuth, N.; Hotta, K.; Trukhin, D.; Statsenko, G.; Hochmair, M.; Özgüroğlu, M.; Ji, J.H.; et al. Durvalumab ± tremelimumab + platinum-etoposide in first-line extensive-stage SCLC (ES-SCLC): Updated results from the phase III CASPIAN study. *J. Clin. Oncol.* **2020**, *38*, 9002. [CrossRef]
49. Leal, T.; Wang, Y.; Dowlati, A.; Lewis, D.A.; Chen, Y.; Mohindra, A.R.; Razaq, M.; Ahuja, H.G.; Liu, J.; King, D.M.; et al. Randomized phase II clinical trial of cisplatin/carboplatin and etoposide (CE) alone or in combination with nivolumab as frontline therapy for extensive-stage small cell lung cancer (ES-SCLC): ECOG-ACRIN EA5161. *J. Clin. Oncol.* **2020**, *38*, 9000. [CrossRef]
50. Rudin, C.M.; Awad, M.M.; Navarro, A.; Gottfried, M.; Peters, S.; Csőszi, T.; Cheema, P.K.; Rodriguez-Abreu, D.; Wollner, M.; Yang, J.C.-H.; et al. Pembrolizumab or Placebo Plus Etoposide and Platinum as First-Line Therapy for Extensive-Stage Small-Cell Lung Cancer: Randomized, Double-Blind, Phase III KEYNOTE-604 Study. *J. Clin. Oncol.* **2020**, *38*, 2369–2379. [CrossRef]
51. Reck, M.; Bondarenko, I.; Luft, A.; Serwatowski, P.; Barlesi, F.; Chacko, R.; Sebastian, M.; Lu, H.; Cuillerot, J.-M.; Lynch, T.J. Ipilimumab in combination with paclitaxel and carboplatin as first-line therapy in extensive-disease-small-cell lung cancer: Results from a randomized, double-blind, multicenter phase 2 trial. *Ann. Oncol.* **2012**, *24*, 75–83. [CrossRef]
52. Reck, M.; Luft, A.; Szczesna, A.; Havel, L.; Kim, S.-W.; Akerley, W.; Pietanza, M.C.; Wu, Y.-L.; Zielinski, C.; Thomas, M.; et al. Phase III Randomized Trial of Ipilimumab Plus Etoposide and Platinum Versus Placebo Plus Etoposide and Platinum in Extensive-Stage Small-Cell Lung Cancer. *J. Clin. Oncol.* **2016**, *34*, 3740–3748. [CrossRef]
53. Faivre-Finn, C.; Snee, M.; Ashcroft, L.; Appel, W.; Barlesi, F.; Bhatnagar, A.; Bezjak, A.; Cardenal, F.; Fournel, P.; Harden, S.; et al. Concurrent once-daily versus twice-daily chemoradiotherapy in patients with limited-stage small-cell lung cancer (CONVERT): An open-label, phase 3, randomised, superiority trial. *Lancet Oncol.* **2017**, *18*, 1116–1125. [CrossRef]
54. Pignon, J.-P.; Arriagada, R.; Ihde, D.C.; Johnson, D.H.; Perry, M.C.; Souhami, R.L.; Brodin, O.; Joss, R.A.; Kies, M.S.; Lebeau, B.; et al. A meta-analysis of thoracic radiotherapy for small-cell lung cancer. *N. Engl. J. Med.* **1992**, *327*, 1618–1624. [CrossRef] [PubMed]
55. Warde, P.; Payne, D. Does thoracic irradiation improve survival and local control in limited-stage small-cell carcinoma of the lung? A meta-analysis. *J. Clin. Oncol.* **1992**, *10*, 890–895. [CrossRef] [PubMed]
56. Welsh, J.W.; Heymach, J.V.; Guo, C.; Menon, H.; Klein, K.; Cushman, T.R.; Verma, V.; Hess, K.R.; Shroff, G.; Tang, C.; et al. Phase 1/2 Trial of Pembrolizumab and Concurrent Chemoradiation Therapy for Limited-Stage SCLC. *J. Thorac. Oncol.* **2020**, *15*, 1919–1927. [CrossRef] [PubMed]
57. Antonia, S.J.; Villegas, A.; Daniel, D.; Vicente, D.; Murakami, S.; Hui, R.; Kurata, T.; Chiappori, A.; Lee, K.H.; De Wit, M.; et al. Overall survival with durvalumab after chemoradiotherapy in stage III NSCLC. *N. Engl. J. Med.* **2018**, *379*, 2342–2350. [CrossRef] [PubMed]
58. Antonia, S.J.; Villegas, A.; Daniel, D.; Vicente, D.; Murakami, S.; Hui, R.; Yokoi, T.; Chiappori, A.; Lee, K.H.; De Wit, M.; et al. Durvalumab after Chemoradiotherapy in Stage III Non–Small-Cell Lung Cancer. *N. Engl. J. Med.* **2017**, *377*, 1919–1929. [CrossRef] [PubMed]
59. Reck, M.; Rodríguez-Abreu, D.; Robinson, A.G.; Hui, R.; Csőszi, T.; Fülöp, A.; Gottfried, M.; Peled, N.; Tafreshi, A.; Cuffe, S.; et al. Pembrolizumab versus Chemotherapy for PD-L1–Positive Non–Small-Cell Lung Cancer. *N. Engl. J. Med.* **2016**, *375*, 1823–1833. [CrossRef]
60. Lantuejoul, S.; Sound-Tsao, M.; Cooper, W.A.; Girard, N.; Hirsch, F.R.; Roden, A.C.; Lopez-Rios, F.; Jain, D.; Chou, T.-Y.; Motoi, N.; et al. PD-L1 Testing for Lung Cancer in 2019: Perspective From the IASLC Pathology Committee. *J. Thorac. Oncol.* **2020**, *15*, 499–519. [CrossRef]
61. Ilie, M.; Long-Mira, E.; Bence, C.; Butori, C.; Lassalle, S.; Bouhlel, L.; Fazzalari, L.; Zahaf, K.; Lalvée, S.; Washetine, K.; et al. Comparative study of the PD-L1 status between surgically resected specimens and matched biopsies of NSCLC patients reveal major discordances: A potential issue for anti-PD-L1 therapeutic strategies. *Ann. Oncol.* **2015**, *27*, 147–153. [CrossRef]
62. Mansfield, A.S.; Aubry, M.C.; Moser, J.C.; Harrington, S.M.; Dronca, R.S.; Park, S.S.; Dong, H. Temporal and spatial discordance of programmed cell death-ligand 1 expression and lymphocyte tumor infiltration between paired primary lesions and brain metastases in lung cancer. *Ann. Oncol.* **2016**, *27*, 1953–1958. [CrossRef]
63. McLaughlin, J.K.; Han, G.; Schalper, K.A.; Carvajal-Hausdorf, D.; Pelekanou, V.; Rehman, J.; Velcheti, V.; Herbst, R.S.; Lorusso, P.M.; Rimm, D.L. Quantitative Assessment of the Heterogeneity of PD-L1 Expression in Non–Small-Cell Lung Cancer. *JAMA Oncol.* **2016**, *2*, 46–54. [CrossRef] [PubMed]
64. Paz-Ares, L.; Goldman, J.; Garassino, M.; Dvorkin, M.; Trukhin, D.; Statsenko, G.; Hotta, K.; Ji, J.; Hochmair, M.; Voitko, O.; et al. PD-L1 expression, patterns of progression and patient-reported outcomes (PROs) with durvalumab plus platinum-etoposide in ES-SCLC: Results from CASPIAN. *Ann. Oncol.* **2019**, *30*, v928–v929. [CrossRef]
65. Lin, H.; Wei, S.; Hurt, E.M.; Green, M.D.; Zhao, L.; Vatan, L.; Szeliga, W.; Herbst, R.; Harms, P.W.; Fecher, L.A.; et al. Host expression of PD-L1 determines efficacy of PD-L1 pathway blockade–mediated tumor regression. *J. Clin. Investig.* **2018**, *128*, 805–815. [CrossRef] [PubMed]
66. Tang, H.; Liang, Y.; Anders, R.A.; Taube, J.M.; Qiu, X.; Mulgaonkar, A.; Liu, X.; Harrington, S.M.; Guo, J.; Xin, Y.; et al. PD-L1 on host cells is essential for PD-L1 blockade–mediated tumor regression. *J. Clin. Investig.* **2018**, *128*, 580–588. [CrossRef] [PubMed]

57. Schultheis, A.M.; Scheel, A.H.; Ozretić, L.; George, J.; Thomas, R.K.; Hagemann, T.; Zander, T.; Wolf, J.; Buettner, R. PD-L1 expression in small cell neuroendocrine carcinomas. *Eur. J. Cancer* **2015**, *51*, 421–426. [CrossRef]
58. Kim, H.S.; Lee, J.H.; Nam, S.J.; Ock, C.-Y.; Moon, J.-W.; Yoo, C.W.; Lee, G.K.; Han, J.-Y. Association of PD-L1 Expression with Tumor-Infiltrating Immune Cells and Mutation Burden in High-Grade Neuroendocrine Carcinoma of the Lung. *J. Thorac. Oncol.* **2018**, *13*, 636–648. [CrossRef]
59. Samstein, R.M.; Lee, C.-H.; Shoushtari, A.N.; Hellmann, M.D.; Shen, R.; Janjigian, Y.Y.; Barron, D.A.; Zehir, A.; Jordan, E.J.; Omuro, A.; et al. Tumor mutational load predicts survival after immunotherapy across multiple cancer types. *Nat. Genet.* **2019**, *51*, 202–206. [CrossRef]
60. Gubin, M.M.; Zhang, X.; Schuster, H.; Caron, E.; Ward, J.P.; Noguchi, T.; Ivanova, Y.; Hundal, J.; Arthur, C.D.; Krebber, W.J.; et al. Checkpoint blockade cancer immunotherapy targets tumour-specific mutant antigens. *Nature* **2014**, *515*, 577–581. [CrossRef]
61. Ricciuti, B.; Kravets, S.; Dahlberg, S.E.; Umeton, R.; Albayrak, A.; Subegdjo, S.J.; Johnson, B.E.; Nishino, M.; Sholl, L.M.; Awad, M.M. Use of targeted next generation sequencing to characterize tumor mutational burden and efficacy of immune checkpoint inhibition in small cell lung cancer. *J. Immunother. Cancer* **2019**, *7*, 87. [CrossRef]
62. Gandara, D.R.; Paul, S.M.; Kowanetz, M.; Schleifman, E.; Zou, W.; Li, Y.; Rittmeyer, A.; Fehrenbacher, L.; Otto, G.; Malboeuf, C.; et al. Blood-based tumor mutational burden as a predictor of clinical benefit in non-small-cell lung cancer patients treated with atezolizumab. *Nat. Med.* **2018**, *24*, 1441–1448. [CrossRef]
63. Sadelain, M.; Brentjens, R.; Rivière, I. The Basic Principles of Chimeric Antigen Receptor Design. *Cancer Discov.* **2013**, *3*, 388–398. [CrossRef] [PubMed]
64. Crossland, D.L.; Denning, W.L.; Ang, S.; Olivares, S.; Mi, T.; Switzer, K.; Singh, H.; Huls, H.; Gold, K.S.; Glisson, B.S.; et al. Antitumor activity of CD56-chimeric antigen receptor T cells in neuroblastoma and SCLC models. *Oncogene* **2018**, *37*, 3686–3697. [CrossRef] [PubMed]
65. Weiskopf, K.; Jahchan, N.S.; Schnorr, P.J.; Cristea, S.; Ring, A.M.; Maute, R.L.; Volkmer, A.K.; Volkmer, J.-P.; Liu, J.; Lim, J.S.; et al. CD47-blocking immunotherapies stimulate macrophage-mediated destruction of small-cell lung cancer. *J. Clin. Investig.* **2016**, *126*, 2610–2620. [CrossRef] [PubMed]
66. Owen, D.H.; Giffin, M.J.; Bailis, J.M.; Smit, M.-A.D.; Carbone, D.P.; He, K. DLL3: An emerging target in small cell lung cancer. *J. Hematol. Oncol.* **2019**, *12*, 1–8. [CrossRef]
67. Leonetti, A.; Facchinetti, F.; Minari, R.; Cortellini, A.; Rolfo, C.D.; Giovannetti, E.; Tiseo, M. Notch pathway in small-cell lung cancer: From preclinical evidence to therapeutic challenges. *Cell. Oncol.* **2019**, *42*, 261–273. [CrossRef]
68. Tanaka, K.; Isse, K.; Fujihira, T.; Takenoyama, M.; Saunders, L.; Bheddah, S.; Nakanishi, Y.; Okamoto, I. Prevalence of Delta-like protein 3 expression in patients with small cell lung cancer. *Lung Cancer* **2018**, *115*, 116–120. [CrossRef]
69. Slaney, C.Y.; Wang, P.; Darcy, P.K.; Kershaw, M.H. CARs versus BiTEs: A Comparison between T Cell–Redirection Strategies for Cancer Treatment. *Cancer Discov.* **2018**, *8*, 924–934. [CrossRef]
70. Saunders, L.R.; Bankovich, A.J.; Anderson, W.C.; Aujay, M.A.; Bheddah, S.; Black, K.; Desai, R.; Escarpe, P.A.; Hampl, J.; Laysang, A.; et al. A DLL3-targeted antibody-drug conjugate eradicates high-grade pulmonary neuroendocrine tumor-initiating cells in vivo. *Sci. Transl. Med.* **2015**, *7*, 302ra136. [CrossRef]
71. Morgensztern, D.; Besse, B.; Greillier, L.; Santana-Davila, R.; Ready, N.; Hann, C.L.; Glisson, B.S.; Farago, A.F.; Dowlati, A.; Rudin, C.M.; et al. Efficacy and Safety of Rovalpituzumab Tesirine in Third-Line and Beyond Patients with DLL3-Expressing, Relapsed/Refractory Small-Cell Lung Cancer: Results From the Phase II TRINITY Study. *Clin. Cancer Res.* **2019**, *25*, 6958–6966. [CrossRef]
72. Serzan, M.T.; Farid, S.; Liu, S.V. Drugs in development for small cell lung cancer. *J. Thorac. Dis.* **2020**, *12*, 6298–6307. [CrossRef]
73. Calles, A.; Aguado, G.; Sandoval, C.; Álvarez, R. The role of immunotherapy in small cell lung cancer. *Clin. Transl. Oncol.* **2019**, *21*, 961–976. [CrossRef] [PubMed]
74. Saltos, A.; Shafique, M.; Chiappori, A.A. Update on the Biology, Management, and Treatment of Small Cell Lung Cancer (SCLC). *Front. Oncol.* **2020**, *10*, 1074. [CrossRef] [PubMed]
75. Schmidt, M.; Hagner, N.; Marco, A.; König-Merediz, S.A.; Schroff, M.; Wittig, B. Design and Structural Requirements of the Potent and Safe TLR-9 Agonistic Immunomodulator MGN1703. *Nucleic Acid Ther.* **2015**, *25*, 130–140. [CrossRef] [PubMed]
76. Thomas, M.; Ponce-Aix, S.; Navarro, A.; Riera-Knorrenschild, J.; Schmidt, M.; Wiegert, E.; Kapp, K.; Wittig, B.; Mauri, C.; Gómez, M.D.; et al. Immunotherapeutic maintenance treatment with toll-like receptor 9 agonist lefitolimod in patients with extensive-stage small-cell lung cancer: Results from the exploratory, controlled, randomized, international phase II IMPULSE study. *Ann. Oncol.* **2018**, *29*, 2076–2084. [CrossRef]
77. Koyama, S.; Akbay, E.A.; Li, Y.Y.; Herter-Sprie, G.S.; Buczkowski, K.A.; Richards, W.G.; Gandhi, L.; Redig, A.J.; Rodig, S.J.; Asahina, H.; et al. Adaptive resistance to therapeutic PD-1 blockade is associated with upregulation of alternative immune checkpoints. *Nat. Commun.* **2016**, *7*, 10501. [CrossRef] [PubMed]
78. Qin, S.; Xu, L.; Yi, M.; Yu, S.; Wu, K.; Luo, S. Novel immune checkpoint targets: Moving beyond PD-1 and CTLA-4. *Mol. Cancer* **2019**, *18*, 1–14. [CrossRef]
79. Friedlaender, A.; Addeo, A.; Banna, G. New emerging targets in cancer immunotherapy: The role of TIM3. *ESMO Open* **2019**, *4*, e000497. [CrossRef]
80. Uboha, N.V.; Milhem, M.M.; Kovacs, C.; Amin, A.; Magley, A.; Das Purkayastha, D.; Piha-Paul, S.A. Phase II study of spartalizumab (PDR001) and LAG525 in advanced solid tumors and hematologic malignancies. *J. Clin. Oncol.* **2019**, *37*, 2553. [CrossRef]

31. Chauvin, J.-M.; Zarour, H.M. TIGIT in cancer immunotherapy. *J. Immunother. Cancer* **2020**, *8*, e000957. [CrossRef]
32. Wrangle, J.M.; Velcheti, V.; Patel, M.R.; Garrett-Mayer, E.; Hill, E.G.; Ravenel, J.G.; Miller, J.S.; Farhad, M.; Anderton, K.; Lindsey, K.; et al. ALT-803, an IL-15 superagonist, in combination with nivolumab in patients with metastatic non-small cell lung cancer: A non-randomised, open-label, phase 1b trial. *Lancet Oncol.* **2018**, *19*, 694–704. [CrossRef]
33. Thomas, A.; Vilimas, R.; Trindade, C.; Erwin-Cohen, R.; Roper, N.; Xi, L.; Krishnasamy, V.; Levy, E.; Mammen, A.; Nichols, S.; et al. Durvalumab in Combination with Olaparib in Patients with Relapsed SCLC: Results from a Phase II Study. *J. Thorac. Oncol.* **2019**, *14*, 1447–1457. [CrossRef] [PubMed]
34. Cummings, A.L.; Kim, D.D.-Y.; Rosen, L.S.; Garon, E.B.; Wainberg, Z.A.; Slamon, D.J.; Goldman, J.W. A phase Ib/II study of niraparib plus temozolomide plus atezolizumab versus atezolizumab as maintenance therapy in extensive-stage small cell lung cancer (TRIO-US L-06). *J. Clin. Oncol.* **2020**, *38*, TPS9084. [CrossRef]
35. Kim, C.; Liu, S.V.; Subramaniam, D.S.; Torres, T.; Loda, M.; Esposito, G.; Giaccone, G. Phase I study of the 177Lu-DOTA0-Tyr3-Octreotate (lutathera) in combination with nivolumab in patients with neuroendocrine tumors of the lung. *J. Immunother. Cancer* **2020**, *8*, e000980. [CrossRef] [PubMed]

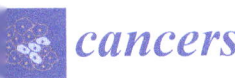

Review

Surgery in Small-Cell Lung Cancer

Nicola Martucci [1,*], Alessandro Morabito [2], Antonello La Rocca [1], Giuseppe De Luca [1], Rossella De Cecio [3], Gerardo Botti [4], Giuseppe Totaro [5], Paolo Muto [5], Carmine Picone [6], Giovanna Esposito [2], Nicola Normanno [7] and Carmine La Manna [1]

1. Thoracic Surgery, Istituto Nazionale Tumori, "Fondazione G. Pascale"—IRCCS, 80131 Naples, Italy; a.larocca@istitutotumori.na.it (A.L.R.); g.deluca@istitutotumori.na.it (G.D.L.); c.lamanna@istitutotumori.na.it (C.L.M.)
2. Thoracic Medical Oncology, Istituto Nazionale Tumori, IRCCS "Fondazione G. Pascale", 80131 Naples, Italy; a.morabito@istitutotumori.na.it (A.M.); espositogiovanna87@gmail.com (G.E.)
3. Pathology, Istituto Nazionale Tumori, "Fondazione G. Pascale"–IRCCS, 80131 Naples, Italy; r.dececio@istitutotumori.na.it
4. Scientific Directorate, Istituto Nazionale Tumori, "Fondazione G. Pascale"–IRCCS, 80131 Naples, Italy; g.botti@istitutotumori.na.it
5. Radiotherapy, Istituto Nazionale Tumori "Fondazione G. Pascale"–IRCCS, 80131 Naples, Italy; g.totaro@istitutotumori.na.it (G.T.); p.muto@istitutotumori.na.it (P.M.)
6. Radiology, Istituto Nazionale Tumori, "Fondazione G. Pascale"–IRCCS, 80131 Naples, Italy; c.picone@istitutotumori.na.it
7. Cellular Biology and Biotherapy, Istituto Nazionale Tumori, "Fondazione G. Pascale"—IRCCS, 80131 Naples, Italy; n.normanno@istitutotumori.na.it
* Correspondence: n.martucci@istitutotumori.na.it; Tel.: +39-08-1590-3262

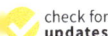

Citation: Martucci, N.; Morabito, A.; La Rocca, A.; De Luca, G.; De Cecio, R.; Botti, G.; Totaro, G.; Muto, P.; Picone, C.; Esposito, G.; et al. Surgery in Small-Cell Lung Cancer. *Cancers* 2021, *13*, 390. https://doi.org/10.3390/cancers13030390

Academic Editor: David Wong
Received: 23 December 2020
Accepted: 18 January 2021
Published: 21 January 2021

Publisher's Note: MDPI stays neutral with regard to jurisdictional claims in published maps and institutional affiliations.

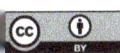

Copyright: © 2021 by the authors. Licensee MDPI, Basel, Switzerland. This article is an open access article distributed under the terms and conditions of the Creative Commons Attribution (CC BY) license (https://creativecommons.org/licenses/by/4.0/).

Simple Summary: Small-cell lung cancer (SCLC) accounts for approximately 15% of all lung cancers and is one of the most aggressive tumors, with poor prognosis and limited therapeutic options. This review summarizes the main results observed with surgery in SCLC, discussing the critical issues related to the use of this approach. Following two old randomized clinical trials showing no benefit with surgery, several prospective, retrospective, and population-based studies have demonstrated the feasibility of a multimodality approach including surgery in addition to chemotherapy and radiotherapy in patients with selected stage I SCLC. Currently, the International Guidelines recommend a surgical approach in selected stage I SCLC patients, after adequate staging within a multimodal approach and after a multidisciplinary evaluation.

Abstract: Small-cell lung cancer (SCLC) is one of the most aggressive tumors, with a rapid growth and early metastases. Approximately 5% of SCLC patients present with early-stage disease (T1,2 N0M0): these patients have a better prognosis, with a 5-year survival up to 50%. Two randomized phase III studies conducted in the 1960s and the 1980s reported negative results with surgery in SCLC patients with early-stage disease and, thereafter, surgery has been largely discouraged. Instead, several subsequent prospective studies have demonstrated the feasibility of a multimodality approach including surgery before or after chemotherapy and followed in most studies by thoracic radiotherapy, with a 5-year survival probability of 36–63% for patients with completely resected stage I SCLC. These results were substantially confirmed by retrospective studies and by large, population-based studies, conducted in the last 40 years, showing the benefit of surgery, particularly lobectomy, in selected patients with early-stage SCLC. On these bases, the International Guidelines recommend a surgical approach in selected stage I SCLC patients, after adequate staging: in these cases, lobectomy with mediastinal lymphadenectomy is considered the standard approach. In all cases, surgery can be offered only as part of a multimodal treatment, which includes chemotherapy with or without radiotherapy and after a proper multidisciplinary evaluation.

Keywords: small-cell lung cancer; lobectomy; pneumonectomy; radiotherapy; chemotherapy; multimodal treatment

1. Introduction

Small-cell lung cancer (SCLC) accounts for approximately 15% of all lung cancers and it is one of the most aggressive tumors, with a rapid growth and early metastases [1,2]. It is typically associated with tobacco use (90% of cases): the risk of developing the disease increases with the duration of smoking and the number of cigarettes smoked each day. The traditional staging system has been developed by the Veteran's Administration Lung Cancer Study Group (VALSG) in the '50s in the United States and it classifies SCLC according to the extent of disease into two stages, extensive and limited [3]. Extensive stage (ES)-SCLC extends one radiation portal, including distant metastases and malignant pleural effusions: it is diagnosed in approximately 70% of patients and has a poor prognosis, with a median survival of about 10–12 months and only about 2% of patients surviving for 5 years [4]. Limited-stage (LS)-SCLC is confined within one radiation portal, defined as a single hemithorax with ipsilateral and supraclavicular nodes: it is diagnosed in approximately 30% of patients and presents a more favorable outcome, with a median survival of 15–20 months, 2- and 5-year survival rates of 20–40% and 12–25%, respectively [5,6]. Moreover, approximately 5% of patients present with early-stage SCLC (T1,2 N0,M0): these patients have a better prognosis, with a 5-year survival up to 50% [7–9]. In this group of patients, a surgical approach can be proposed as part of a multidisciplinary treatment after excluding mediastinal lymph nodes involvement, according to the National Comprehensive Cancer Network (NCCN) guidelines [10]. This review summarizes the main results observed with surgery as single treatment or as part of a multimodality treatment of SCLC, discussing the critical issues related to the use of this approach. We proceeded to a revision of the Medline PUBMED English literature (from January 1959 to December 2020) and we grouped the studies found according to the design (randomized, prospective non-randomized, retrospective and cancer data-based review), with the objective to verify the impact of surgery on survival (reported as median survival and 5-year survival) of patients with SCLC.

2. Surgery as Single Treatment for SCLC

Before the 1960s, surgery has been the treatment of choice for resectable SCLC cases. In 1959, Belcher et al. reported a 5-year survival of 37% in 42 SCLC patients treated with pulmonary lobectomy [11]. In 1962, in a large series of 386 SCLC patients of the Memorial Hospital for Cancer and Allied Diseases of New York, N.Y., USA Watson et al. reported that surgical resections were performed in 7% of SCLC patients, including pneumonectomy in 67%, lobectomy in 22% and wedge resection in 11% of cases [12]. However, only 11% of resected patients have survived for more than 4 years. An exploratory thoracotomy revealed a non-resectable tumors in 84 cases (22% of patients), treated subsequently with different palliative therapies. With radiation therapy alone, only 1 patient survived more than 2 years; 90% of patients died in less than 1 year. In 1960s, the Medical Research Council conducted a randomized trial comparing surgery versus radical radiotherapy in patients with SCLC, without extrathoracic metastases, considered to be operable and fit enough for radical radiotherapy (Table 1) [13]. Overall, 144 patients were admitted to the trial from 29 thoracic centers throughout Great Britain: 71 patients were randomized to surgery arm and 73 to radiotherapy arm. Among patients randomized to the surgical arm, only 48% underwent a complete resection: an explorative thoracotomy was performed in 34% of cases and surgery was definitively excluded in 18% of patients. Among patients randomized to radiotherapy arm, 85% of patients received a curative treatment, while 11% of patients received only a palliative treatment and 4% no radiotherapy at all. The ten-year follow-up of this trial was published in 1973 and showed that the median survival for the surgical arm was 199 days versus 300 days of the radiotherapy arm ($p = 0.04$). Patients who received curative radiotherapy had a higher survival rate than those undergoing surgery over the 2-year (11% vs. 6%) and 5-year (5% vs. 0) period. Moreover, there were no 10-year survivors in the surgical series, while 3 patients remained alive in the radiotherapy group. These results reinforced the previous conclusions of the 2- and 5-year reports of this trial, suggesting that radical radiotherapy was superior to surgery in terms of overall survival in patients with limited SCLC judged to be operable [14,15]. On the basis on these data, the role of surgery alone in limited SCLC gradually decreased and a combined modality of treatment including chemotherapy and radiotherapy (better if starting within 30 days after the beginning of chemotherapy) became the cornerstone of treatment of patients with limited-stage SCLC [16–20]. The combined treatment reduced, in particular, the risk of a thoracic recurrence, while brain metastases became one of the main types of relapse, leading to several trials that evaluated the role of prophylactic cranial irradiation in patients with SCLC with contrasting results [21–23]. In 1999, the meta-analysis of Auperin A. et al. confirmed the role of prophylactic cranial irradiation in reducing the risk of brain metastases and improving overall and disease-free survival of SCLC patients with limited disease [24]. Therefore, the combination of chemotherapy (cisplatin and etoposide) plus chest radiotherapy followed by prophylactic cranial irradiation has been considered the standard treatment for patients with limited-stage SCLC and good performance status, with an objective response rate of approximately 80%, a median overall survival of about 17 months and 12–25% of patient cancer-free at 5 year [4,25].

Table 1. Randomized trials evaluating the role of surgery.

Author	Patients	Treatment	Complete Resection Rate (%)	Median OS (Months)	2-Year OS	5-Year OS
Fox W. et al., 1973 [13]	144	Surgery vs. radiotherapy	48%	6.5 vs. 9.8, $p = 0.04$	4 vs. 10%	1 vs. 5%
Lad T. et al., 1994 [26]	146	Chemotherapy * followed by radiotherapy or surgery plus radiotherapy	77%	18.6 vs. 15.4, $p = 0.78$	20% vs. 20%	n.r.

* cyclophosphamide, doxorubicin, and vincristine for five cycles; OS: overall survival; n.r.: not reported.

3. Surgery Plus Chemotherapy/Radiotherapy in SCLC

3.1. Randomized Studies

The role of surgery to the multimodality management of SCLC has been evaluated by a large multicenter randomized phase III trial, promoted in 1983 by the Lung Cancer Study Group (LCSG), that became an intergroup study with the participation of the Eastern Cooperative Oncology Group (ECOG) and the European organization for Research and Treatment of Cancer (EORTC) (Table 1) [26]. Overall, 328 patients with LS-SCLC were enrolled into the study and treated with cyclophosphamide, doxorubicin, and vincristine for five cycles. Patients who achieved at least a partial response and who were fit enough for surgery were randomized to undergo or not to undergo pulmonary resection and all randomized patients were treated with chest and brain radiotherapy. Among 217 responders, only 146 patients (66%) were randomized to surgery (70 patients) and to no surgery (76 patients). The resection rate was 83%: a complete resection was feasible in 77% of patients and 19% patients had a pathologic complete response. No difference in overall survival was observed between the surgical and no surgical arms (median OS: 15.4 vs. 18.6 months, respectively; $p = 0.78$). Two-year survival was 20% in both groups. Therefore, this trial does not support the efficacy of the addition of pulmonary resection to the multimodality treatment of SCLC. Limits of the trial are the number of incomplete resection (23%), the lack of platinum-based chemotherapy in the neoadjuvant phase of treatment, the possible understadiation of patients due to the unavailability of positron emission tomography (PET)scan. However, based on the results of this trial, surgery has been largely discouraged, also as part of a multimodality strategy of treatment of patients with limited SCLC.

3.2. Prospectives Studies

In the following years, several prospective non-randomized trials have reevaluated the role of surgery in selected LS-SCLC patients (Table 2). A prospective study of adjuvant surgical resection after chemotherapy for patients with LS-SCLC has been conducted by the University of Toronto Lung Oncology Group and published by Shepherd F. et al., on 1989 [27]. Overall, 72 patients received preoperative chemotherapy (cyclophosphamide, doxorubicin and vincristine or cisplatin and etoposide): 80% of patients had an objective response, 79.1% were considerate eligible for surgery, but only 38 patients underwent thoracotomy. The median survival for the resected patients was 21 months and the 5-year survival rate was 36%. A larger experience of the same group on the multimodality treatment of SCLC with surgery and chemotherapy was reported by Shepherd F. et al., on 1991 and it included 119 patients with LS-SCLC [28]. Seventy-nine patients had surgery first followed in 67 cases by adjuvant chemotherapy, while 40 patients had chemotherapy first, followed by surgery. The 5-year survival rate for the whole population was 39%; no difference in terms of overall survival was seen between the two groups of patients ($p = 0.756$). Patients with pathologic stage I had a 5-year survival rate of 51%, significantly better than patients in stage II (28%, $p = 0.001$) and III (19%, $p = 0.001$), supporting the evidence in favor of surgery for patients with stage I disease. Similar results were reported on 1995 by Karrer K. et al., for the LCSG of the International Society of Chemotherapy, in a prospective trial for patients with early-stage SCLC (T1,2,N0,M0) [29]. A total of 183 patients received surgery, followed by 8 cycles of standard chemotherapy (cyclophosphamide, doxorubicin and vincristine) or 6 intermittent cycles of alternating chemotherapy with 3 different drug combinations, and thereafter by prophylactic cranial irradiation. Overall, 152 patients (83%) had a complete resection, resulting in a 3-year survival rate of 44%, while it was 19% for patients with incompletely resected. The 4-year survival probability was 57% for 68 patients with stage pT1-2N0M0R0 after complete resection and it was 37% for patients with stage pT1-2N2M0R0 after surgery. In 1997, another pilot phase II study evaluated the feasibility and activity of a multimodality approach based on neoadjuvant chemotherapy followed by surgical resection in 22 Japanese SCLC patients with stage I–IIIA [30]. All patients received 2–4 cycles of neoadjuvant CAV II (cisplatin, doxorubicin, etoposide), with a response rate of 95.5%, and 21 patients underwent a surgical resection. Median survival was 61.9 months, and the 3-year survival probability was 66.7%, higher for patients with stage I and II than for patients with stage III (73.3% versus 42.9%, respectively, $p = 0.018$). One operation-related death occurred. In 1998 Rea F. et al. reported the results of a large Italian prospective study on 104 patients with SCLC (49% in stage I–II and 51% in stage III) treated at the University of Padua, Italy from 1981 to 1995 with surgery followed by adjuvant chemotherapy and radiotherapy (stage I–II) or with induction chemotherapy followed by surgery and radiotherapy (stage III) [31]. The 30-day mortality was 2%. Median overall survival was 28 months, and the 5-year survival rate was 32%: according to the pathologic stage, 5-year survival was 52.2%, 30% and 15.3% for stage I, II, and III, respectively ($p < 0.001$). In patients without residual tumor after chemotherapy and surgery, the 5-year survival rate was 41%.

Table 2. Prospective non-randomized trials evaluating the role of surgery.

Author	Patients	Treatment	Complete Resection Rate (%)	Median OS (Months)	5-Year OS
Shepherd F. et al., 1989 [27]	72	Chemotherapy * followed by surgery	52.7%	21	36%
Shepherd F. et al., 1991 [28]	119	Surgery (79 pts) followed by chemotherapy ** (69 pts) Chemotherapy ** (40 pts) followed by surgery	87.5%	25	39%
Karrer K. et al., 1995 [29]	183	Surgery followed by Chemotherapy ***	83%	30	n.r.
Fujimori K. et al., 1997 [30]	22	Chemotherapy followed by surgery ****	95.5%	61.9	50%

Table 2. Cont.

Author	Patients	Treatment	Complete Resection Rate (%)	Median OS (Months)	5-Year OS
Rea F. et al., 1998 [31]	104	Surgery followed by chemotherapy + radiotherapy (51 pts) Chemotherapy followed by surgery + radiotherapy (53 pts)	100%	28	32%
Eberhardt W. et al., 1999 [32]	46	Chemotherapy ^ ± RT followed by surgery	72%	36	46%
Tsuchiya R. et al., 2005 [33]	61	Surgery followed by chemotherapy ^	100%	Not reached	57%

OS: overall survival; n.r.: not reported; pts: patients; RT: radiotherapy; * CAV (cyclophosphamide, doxorubicin and vincristine) or cisplatin + etoposide; ** CAV or CAV + etoposide or CAV + methotrexate; *** CAV or cyclophaosphamide, lomustine, methotrexate/CAV/ifosfamide + mesna + etoposide; **** CAV II (cyclophosphamide, doxorubicin and etoposide) or PE (cisplatin + etoposide); ^ PE (cisplatin + etoposide).

In 1999 Eberhardt W. et al. reported the results of multimodality approach including surgery, chemotherapy and radiotherapy in German patients with stage IA–IIIB SCLC [32]. In stage IB/IIA patients received four cycles of cisplatin and etoposide followed by surgery; in stage IIB/IIIA patients received three cycles of cisplatin and etoposide followed by a concurrent chemoradiation cycle including hyperfractionated accelerated radiotherapy and surgery. Forty-six consecutive SCLC patients were enrolled in this study: 6 in stage IB, 2 in stage IIA, 22 in stage IIB/IIIA and 16 in stage IIIB. Forty-three patients (94%) showed an objective response and 23 (72%) underwent radical surgery (R0): 6 patients in stage IB, 2 in stage IIA, 13 in stage IIB/IIIA and 2 in stage IIIB. No perioperative deaths occurred, but a patient died of septicemia. Median survival was 36 months for all patients and 68 months in R0 patients. The 5-year survival rate was 46% and 63% for all patients and for R0 patients, respectively. The authors concluded that this multimodality treatment including surgery, chemotherapy, and radiotherapy proved highly effective with high local control and remarkable long-term survival after complete resection, even in SCLC patients with stages IIB/IIIA. In 2005, the Japan Clinical Oncology LCSG published the results of a phase II trial to determine the feasibility and activity of lung resection followed by adjuvant chemotherapy for SCLC patients with stage I–IIIa [33]. Sixty-two patients with completely resected SCLC entered in the trial and 69% received 4 cycles of cisplatin and etoposide. No treatment associated mortality was observed. Three-year survival was 68% in patients with stage I, 56% in stage II, and 13% in stage IIIa ($p = 0.02$). Local failure was observed in 10% of patients, less frequently in patients with stage IA (4%) and more frequently in patients with stage IIIA (22%). Therefore, also this trial confirmed the feasibility and the good outcome of a surgical approach followed by adjuvant chemotherapy: however, considering that nodal metastases are a major prognostic factor, the authors highlighted the importance of a preoperative evaluation of mediastinal nodal status.

3.3. Retrospective Studies

The evidence coming from prospective non-randomized studies have been confirmed by retrospective studies that have evaluated the role of surgery in LS-SCLC patients (Table 3). The role of initial surgical resection in patients in patients with SCLC has been retrospectively evaluated by the Veterans Administration Surgical Oncology Group and published by Shields et al., on 1982 [34]. The potentially "curative" resections represented 4.7% of all "curative" resections carried out in four prospective adjuvant chemotherapy trials. In the 132 patients included in the analysis, the 5-year survival was 23%, but it was 60%, 31% and 28% in patients with stage pT1N0, pT1N1, and pT2N0, respectively. They concluded that resection is indicated in patients with early disease pT1NO, probably indicated for those with pT2N0 or pT1N1 and contraindicated in patients with any other TNM category.

Table 3. Retrospective trials evaluating the role of surgery.

Author	Patients	Treatment	Complete Resection Rate (%)	Median OS (Months)	5-Year OS
Shields T.W. et al., 1982 [34]	132	Surgery followed by adjuvant chemotherapy	100%	n.r.	23% (59.9% T1N0)
Osterlind K. et al., 1986 [35]	52	Surgery followed by adjuvant chemotherapy	69.2%	30	16% (at 30 months)
Hara N. et al., 1991 [36]	36	Surgery followed by chemotherapy (19 pts) Chemotherapy followed by surgery (17 pts)	44.4%	33	38%
Inoue M. et al., 2000 [37]	91	Surgery followed by chemotherapy (71 pts) or radiotherapy (17 pts)	89%	26	37.1%
Badzio A. et al., 2004 [38]	67	Surgery followed by adjuvant chemotherapy	100%	22	27%
Brock M.V. et al., 2005 [39]	82	Surgery alone (9 pts) Chemotherapy followed by surgery (18 pts) Surgery followed by chemotherapy (45 pts) or other therapy (10 pts)	96.3%	24	42%
Takenaka T. et al., 2015 [40]	88	Surgery alone (16 pts) Surgery + chemotherapy (63 pts) Surgery + chemoradiotherapy (9 pts)	n.r.	18	59% Stage I 39% Stage II 14% Stage III
Zhong L. et al., 2020 [41]	50	Surgery followed by chemotherapy and radiotherapy (30 pts) Chemotherapy followed by surgery, chemotherapy ± radiotherapy (20 pts)	n.r.	79	28%
Casiraghi M. et al., 2020 [42]	65	Surgery upfront (39 pts) followed by chemotherapy Chemotherapy followed by surgery (26 pts)	100%	36	42% (76.6% Stage I)

OS: overall survival; n.r.: not reported; pts: patients.

The long-term benefit of a multimodality strategy based on surgery followed by adjuvant chemotherapy has been reported by Osterlind K. et al., in 1986, analyzing a consecutive series of 874 SCLC patients treated with chemotherapy with or without radiotherapy at the Finsen Institute, Copenhagen, Denmark, between 1973 and 1981 [35]. Among 437 patients with limited disease, 150 were considered operable: 52 patients underwent a radical resection, 44 were considered non-resectable at the thoracotomy and 54 operable patients were not operated due to the treatment policy at the hospitals from which they were referred that excluded surgery for SCLC. Overall, 36 patients received a radical resection, while 16 patients had microscopic (9 cases) or macroscopic (7 cases) residual tumor. The 30-month disease-free-survival (DFS) rate was 33% for completely resected patients, 12.5% for those with residual disease and 13% for patients operable but not operated, suggesting a possible role for surgery in limited SCLC patients with early disease.

The role of surgery in the treatment of 81 Japanese patients with clinically localized SCLC was evaluated by Hara N. et al. [36]. Overall, 36 patients underwent surgical resection: the surgery was done upfront in 19 cases followed by adjuvant chemotherapy and after neoadjuvant chemotherapy in 17 cases. The remaining 45 patients received chemotherapy plus radiotherapy. Median OS was 33 months, and the 5-year survival was 38% for the 36 surgical patients. Patients with stage I and II showed a 5-year survival of 25% and a median OS of 33 months.

Similar findings were reported in 2000 in another Japanese study by Inoue M. et al., on 91 SCLC patients treated with a multimodality strategy including pulmonary resection [37]. The five-year survival probability was 37.1%: it was 56.1% for stage IA, 30% for stage IB, 57.1% for stage IIA and 42.9% for stage IIB. Patients treated with surgery plus chemotherapy had a better 5-year probability of survival than that of those treated with surgery alone (54.9% versus 22.2%, respectively; $p = 0.015$). Moreover, the 5-year survival rate of patients treated with four or more cycles of chemotherapy was 80.0%. The authors concluded that thoracic resection in combination with chemotherapy treatment offers the best results in patients with stage IA-IIB SCLC. In 2004, Badzio A. et al. reported a retrospective comparative analysis of survival in 134 patients with LS-SCLC treated between 1984 and 1996 with either complete surgical resection followed by chemotherapy (67 patients), or with conventional non-surgical management (67 patients) [38]. The control group was selected using the methodology of "pair-matched case-control", among 176 patients with LS-SCLC treated without surgery, but potentially eligible for resection. The two groups were balanced for prognostic factors. Patients treated with surgery and adjuvant chemotherapy had a better median survival than those treated without surgery (22 versus 11 months, $p < 0.001$) and a lower incidence of local relapse (15% versus 55%, respectively, $p < 0.001$). The 5-year survival probabilities were 27% and 4% in the surgical and non-surgical group, respectively, suggesting a possible role of surgery in limited-stage SCLC.

These positive findings were confirmed by a large retrospective study of Brock V et al. conducted on 1415 patients with SCLC treated from 1976 to 2002 at the Johns Hopkins Medical Institutions, Baltimore, Md (USA): 82 patients (6%) had undergone curative surgery and had a 5-year survival of 42% [39]. In particular, 9/82 patients (11%) received surgery alone, 18/82 neoadjuvant chemotherapy followed by surgery (22%) and 45/82 surgery followed by adjuvant chemotherapy (55%). Prophylactic cranial irradiation was given to 23% of patients. The 5-year survival was better for patients receiving platinum versus non-platinum regimens (68% versus 32.2%, $p = 0.04$) and for patients undergoing lobectomies than limited resections (50% versus 20%, $p = 0.03$). Furthermore, the 5-year survivals for patients with stage I disease who received adjuvant platinum versus non-platinum chemotherapy were 86% versus 42%, respectively ($p = 0.02$), supporting a reconsideration of the role of surgery in the multimodality strategy of treatment for selected patients with LS-SCLC. More recently, Takenaka T. et al. compared the outcomes of surgical resections to other conventional non-surgical treatments in 277 Japanese patients who received treatment for LD-SCLC (18% with stage I) from 1974 through 2011 [40]. Surgery was performed in 31.7% of cases and included pneumonectomy in 11.1% of cases, lobectomy in 84.1% of cases and limited resections in 4.5% of cases. The 5-year survival rates for all patients according to stage were 58% in stage I, 29% in stage II and 18% in stage III. The 5-year survival rates of the patients with and without surgery were 62% and 25% in stage I ($p < 0.01$), 33% and 24% in stage II ($p = 0.95$), 18% and 18% in stage III ($p = 0.35$), respectively. Moreover, the study showed that the 5-year survival rates according to the treatment period were 20% in the 1970/1980s, 21% in the 1990s and 40% in the 2000s ($p < 0.01$). Therefore, also this study suggest that surgery is effective for patients with stage I SCLC. A Chinese retrospective study has been recently published on 2020 to analyze the effects of radical surgery and concurrent chemoradiotherapy on the prognosis of 157 patients with LS-SCLC, treated in a single Institution from 2011 to 2018 [41]. Overall, 50 patients received surgery after neoadjuvant chemotherapy or followed by adjuvant chemotherapy, while 102 patients received concurrent chemoradiotherapy. Median progression-free survival (73 versus 10.5 months, $p < 0.0001$) and overall survival (79 versus 23 months, $p < 0.0001$) were significantly longer in the surgical group than non-surgical group, respectively. Finally, a retrospective analysis has been recently published by Casiraghi M et al., reporting the outcomes of Italian patients with SCLC undergoing surgery at the European Institute of Oncology of Milan [42]. Among 324 patients treated between 1998 and 2018, 65 patients (20%) underwent surgical resection with curative intent: upfront in 60% of cases, after chemotherapy (36.9%) and after chemotherapy plus radiotherapy (3.1%). Forty-four patients (67.7%) underwent adjuvant treatment and 23.1% patients prophylactic cranial irradiation. Median overall survival after resection was 36 months, while 5 and 10-year OS was 42% and 25.4%, respectively. At multivariate analysis pathological stage was the strongest prognostic factor: in particular, *p*-stage I patients had a 5-year OS of 76.6 % (log-rank $p < 0.0001$).

4. Cancer Database Review

Data on larger populations with SCLC treated with surgery have been reported by studies that analyzed different national cancer data base (Table 4). One of the first cancer data base review has been published by Rostad et al., on 2004 and it was conducted on the Norway Cancer Registry, evaluating all patients with SCLC diagnosed between 1993–1999 in Norway [43]. The purpose of the study was to identify the proportion of patients with operable SCLC and to compare the resection specimens from operated patients with more than 5-year survival with those with shorter survival. Overall, 2442 patients with SCLC were identified: 697 patients were considered to have limited disease and 180 patients were classified as stage I. For stage I, 96 patients were considered potentially operable and 38 patients were effectively resected (39%): the 5-year survival rate was 11.3% in conventionally treated patients compared to 44.9% for those who underwent surgical resection. Therefore, the authors concluded that patients with SCLC in stage I could be referred to surgery as long-time survival is good. A large U.S population-based database, the Surveillance, Epidemiology, and End Results (SEER) registry, was used by Schreiber et al. to determine survival outcomes of SCLC patients who underwent surgery between 1988 and 2002, coded as localized disease (T1-T2Nx-N0) or regional disease (T3-T4Nx-N0) [8]. In total, 14,179 patients were identified in SEER registry and 863 underwent surgery. Surgery was more commonly associated with early-stage (T1T2) disease ($p < 0.001$) and with improved survival for the whole cohort (28 versus 13 months for no surgery; 5-year OS rate 34.6 versus 9.9%, $p < 0.001$), and for patients with early (42 versus 15 months; 5-year OS rate 44.8 versus 13,7%, respectively, $p < 0.001$) and regional disease (22 versus 12 months; 5-year OS rate 26.3% versus 9.3%, respectively, $p < 0.001$). Patients with early disease who underwent lobectomy had a median survival of 65 months and a 5-year OS rate of 52.6%. The multivariate analysis confirmed the benefit of lobectomy across all time intervals ($p = 0.002$). In conclusion, this population-based study confirmed the role of surgery, particularly lobectomy, in selected patients with early-stage SCLC. The same SEER database was then used by Yu et al. to better characterize outcomes of patients with SCLC in stage I treated from 1988 to 2004 [7]. A total of 1560 patients were identified: 15.8% underwent lobectomy, 7.8% a surgical resection less extensive than a lobectomy and 0.6% a pneumonectomy. Among the patients who underwent a lobectomy, 17% received chest radiotherapy. For all patients, 3- and 5-year OS was 31% and 21.1%, respectively. The 3- and 5-year OS probability was 58% and 50%, respectively, for all patients who had a lobectomy (64.9% and 57.1% for those who did also receive radiotherapy). Therefore, based on this analysis on a large series of stage I SCLC patients, surgery without radiotherapy seemed to offer good outcome in selected patients who undergo lobectomy and who are node-negative. Similar findings were reported also by Varlotto et al. who evaluated the incidence of stage I-II SCLC and defined the optimal local therapy through an analysis of 2214 early-stage SCLC patients identified in the SEER database from 1988 to 2005 [44]. Early-stage SCLC represented a 3–5% of all SCLC until 2003 and, by 2005, increased to 7%. Surgery for early-stage SCLC achieved a peak at 47% in 1990, but then progressively declined to 16% by 2005. The median OS for all patients was 20 months. Patients treated with lobectomy had longer median survival than those treated with radiotherapy alone (50 vs. 20 months, $p < 0.0001$). The use of radiotherapy did not affect prognosis after limited resection (30 vs. 28 months, $p = 0.585$). Results of multivariate analysis demonstrated that survival was independently related to age, year of diagnosis, tumor size, stage, and treatment (lobectomy versus sub-lobar resection versus radiotherapy alone). Therefore, the authors concluded that in patients with early-stage SCLC lobectomy provided superior survival, but the addition of radiotherapy to resection was associated with no additional benefit. Weksler

B. et al. queried the SEER database for patients with SCLC from 1988 to 2007 and they identified 3566 patients with stage I (75.3%) o II (24.7%) [45]. Overall median survival for all patients was 18.0 months. Lung resection was performed in 25.1% of cases: median OS was 34 versus 16 months for surgical versus non-surgical patients, respectively ($p < 0.001$). Median survival was longer after lobectomy or pneumonectomy than after wedge resection (39 versus 28 months, respectively, $p = 0.0001$). Radiotherapy was performed in 49.6% of cases and in 22.6% of resected patients. The multivariate analysis showed that female, younger age, stage I, treatment with radiotherapy, lymph node staging, and lung resection were significantly associated with survival. The analysis of the largest database on SCLC has been published by Gaspar et al., on 2012 [46]. Overall, 68,611 patients with SCLC in the National Cancer Data Base (NCDB) were analyzed to describe demographic characteristics, treatment strategies and survival changes between 1992 and 2007: 25,499 cases presented LS-SCLC. Four patient cohorts of patients diagnosed in 1992, 1997, 2002, and 2007 were examined. Median OS for patients with ES-SCLC and LS-SCLC was 6.1 and 12.9 months, respectively, and it was not significantly improved between 1992 and 2002, despite changes in demographics and treatments. Surgery alone or in combination with chemotherapy or radiotherapy was performed in 5.5% of cases and was associated with improved survival: median OS for patients with early-stage SCLC undergoing surgery or no surgery was 30.8 versus 15 months ($p < 0.01$). If surgery was performed, patients with early-stage disease benefited from the addition of chemotherapy. The multivariate analysis confirmed that female sex, age <70 years, and receipt of surgery were associated with improved survival for LS-SCLC. Radiotherapy decreased the hazard ratio for stage III SCLC patients, but not for those with earlier disease. Chemotherapy decreased the Hazard ratio (HR) for all patients with LS-CLC. Patients with ES-SCLC treated with radiation in addition to chemotherapy had better survival than those who received only chemotherapy. A retrospective analysis of 243 patients from Japanese Lung Cancer Registry who underwent surgery in 2004 has been reported by Takei H. et al., on 2014 [47]. The authors found that of the 11,663 resected patients, 243 patients had a SCLC (2.1%): the 5-year survival rate for all cases was 52.6% (64.3% in patients with stage IA). The multivariate analysis showed that the age, gender, c-stage, and surgical curability were significant prognostic factors. More recently, the NCDB was reviewed for patients with clinical T1–3 N1 M0 SCLC who underwent concurrent chemoradiation versus surgery and adjuvant therapy from 2003 to 2011 [48]. Overall, 1041 patients met the inclusion criteria: 96 patients (9%) underwent surgery and adjuvant chemotherapy with or without radiotherapy, while 945 patients (91%) underwent chemoradiotherapy alone. The 5-year survival was 31.4% for the surgery group and 26.3% for the chemoradiation group ($p = 0.03$). The multivariate analysis demonstrated that surgery plus adjuvant chemotherapy with or without radiotherapy was associated with improved survival compared with chemoradiotherapy (HR 0.74, 95%CI: 0.56 to 0.97). An improved long-term survival was observed for surgery and adjuvant chemotherapy compared with chemoradiotherapy also when the analysis was limited to 2301 node-negative SCLC patients of the same (NCDB) data base, with a 5-year OS of 47.6% versus 29.8%, $p < 0.001$ [49]. Similar findings were reported on a larger number of patients of the NCDB reviewed from 1998 to 2011. Surgery was performed in 9% of patients with potentially resectable SCLC: 5-year OS was 51%, 25%, and 18% for resected patients with stages I, II, and IIIA, respectively [50]. Addition of surgery to chemotherapy was associated with improved survival, independently of age, stage, and comorbidity score (HR: 0.57; 95%CI: 0.47–0.68). Therefore, all these studies supported the re-evaluation of the role of surgery in the multimodality treatment of early-stage SCLC patients.

Table 4. Cancer database review.

Author	Database	All SCLC Patients	Stage I SCLC	Treatment	Resection Rate (%)	Median OS (Months)	5-Year OS
Rostad H. et al., 2004 [43]	Norway Cancer Registry	2442	180	Surgery (38 pts) followed by chemotherapy or radiotherapy (25 pts)	21%	54	44.9%
Schreiber D. et al., 2010 [8]	SEER	14,179	2382	Surgery (863 pts) followed by radiotherapy (241 pts)	36%	28	34.6%
Yu JB. et al., 2010 [7]	SEER	1560	1560	Surgery (378 pts) followed by radiotherapy (38 pts)	24.2%	58	50.3% (surgery alone) 57.1 (surgery + RT)
Varlotto JM et al., 2011 [44]	SEER	2214	1690	Surgery (448 pts) followed by radiotherapy (59 pts)	26.5%	50	47.4% (surgery alone)
Weksler B. et al., 2012 [45]	SEER	3566	2686	Surgery (683 pts) followed by radiotherapy (202 pts)	25.4%	34	29.6%
Gaspar LE. et al., 2012 [46]	NCDB	68,611	4103	Surgery (1395 pts)	34%	30.8	9.7% (LS-SCLC)
Takei H. et al., 2014 [47]	Japanese Lung Cancer Registry	243	168	Surgery (168 pts) followed by chemotherapy (158 pts)	88.1% *	Not reached	52.6%
Yang CGJ. et al., 2017 [48]	NCDB	4490	1041 °	Surgery (96 pts) followed by chemotherapy ± radiotherapy	9.2%	33.3	31.4%
Combs SE. et al., 2015 [50]	NCDB	203,229	4893	Surgery (1009 pts) followed by chemotherapy	20.6%	Not reached	51%

SEER: Surveillance, Epidemiology, and End Results database; NCDB: National Cancer Data Base; n.r.: not reported; RT: radiotherapy; pts: patients; LS-SCLC: limited-stage Small-Cell Lung Cancer; * Complete resection rate (R0); ° Stage I–II; pts: patients.

5. Discussion and Conclusions

The scenario of treatment of SCLC is changed in the last few years, after decades of no progress. Immunotherapy with atezolizumab or durvalumab has been approved in combination with platinum and etoposide in the first line therapy of patients with ES-SCLC, while nivolumab and pembrolizumab as single agents showed anti-tumor activity and were approved in patients with ES-SCLC after platinum-based therapy and at least one prior line of therapy [51]. Moreover, recently the Food and Drug Administration granted accelerated approval to lurbinectedin, a selective inhibitor of oncogenic transcription, for patients with metastatic SCLC in progression on or after platinum-based chemotherapy, based on the positive result of a phase 2 study [52]. For patients with LS-SCLC several phase 3 studies are evaluating the role of immunotherapy in combination with chemotherapy and radiotherapy. Is there still a role for surgery in selected patients with limited-stage disease? Unfortunately, clinical evidence coming from literature is quite weak. Only two randomized clinical trials have evaluated the role of surgery in patients with SCLC, but they were both old studies, including a limited number of patients (about 150). Most evidence comes from prospective non-randomized studies and retrospective analysis, but they were generally conducted in one Institution and once again on few patients (in most cases less than one hundred). The greater evidence is derived from large cancer data base review that reported results observed in national, large series of patients (thousands or tens of thousands). The randomized trials of the MRC in the 1960s and of the LCSG in the 1980s showed the inferiority of surgery versus curative radiotherapy in terms of overall survival in patients with limited SCLC judged to be operable, previously not treated or treated with neoadjuvant chemotherapy, according to the design of MRC and LCSG study, respectively. However, limits of these old studies are the lack of chemotherapy in the MRC or the lack of a platinum-based chemotherapy in LCSG in the neoadjuvant phase, the low power and the high rate of incomplete resection of both studies, the unavailability of

PET scan, with possible under-staging of patients. Several subsequent prospective studies have confirmed the feasibility of a multimodality approach including surgery before or after chemotherapy and followed in most studies by thoracic radiotherapy, with a 5-year survival probability of 36–63% for patients with completely resected stage I. These results were substantially confirmed by the retrospective studies conducted in the last 40 years: notwithstanding the limits of all these studies (retrospective evaluation, selection bias, heterogeneity of patients and treatments), the best outcome was observed for patients with limited disease who underwent surgical resection in addition to chemotherapy and radiotherapy, with a 5-year survival probability of 27–86%. Large, population-base studies, conducted from the 1990s in Europe, U.S and Japan confirmed the benefit of surgery, particularly lobectomy, in selected patients with early-stage SCLC: the resection rate was 5–9% in the different series and the 5-year survival rate was 31–51% for patients with stage I who underwent to surgical resection within a multimodality treatment strategy. Multivariate analyses confirmed, in particular, the benefit of lobectomy in early-stage SCLC, while for radiotherapy the benefit was mainly limited to stage III. In 2015 Stish et al. reviewed the outcomes and patterns of failure for 54 patients with SCLC treated with definitive surgical resection at Majo Clinic (Rochester, USA). Patients undergoing wedge resection or segmentectomy had an increased risk of intrathoracic recurrence compared with those who received a lobectomy or pneumonectomy (HR:3.5; $p = 0.01$) [53]. Moreover, the 5-year overall survival was significantly longer after lobectomy or pneumonectomy versus wedge resection or segmentectomy (48% versus 15%, respectively; $p = 0.03$).

The role of surgery in stage I-III SCLC has been also evaluated by a recent meta-analysis including two randomized trials and 13 retrospective studies for a total of 41,483 eligible patients [54]. The results of this meta-analysis confirmed that surgery significantly improved overall survival when compared to non-surgical treatments in the retrospective studies (HR: 0.56; 95%CI: 0.49–0.64, $p < 0.001$), but not in the 2 "older" randomized clinical trials (HR: 0.77; 95%CI: 0.32–1.84, $p = 0.55$). Moreover, sub-lobar resections resulted in a worse survival than lobectomy (HR: 0.64; 95%CI: 0.56–0.74, $p < 0.001$). Based on this evidence, the NCCN Guidelines Version 1.2021, the ACCP, ASCO and ESMO guidelines highlight that surgery is justified for selected stage I (T1-2,N0M0) SCLC patients [10,55–57]. The preferred surgical approach is lobectomy with mediastinal lymph node dissection that can be proposed after excluding a mediastinal lymph node involvement (with CT scan, PET-CT scan, or EBUS and/or mediastinoscopy if enlarged). Pathologic mediastinal staging is not required if the patient is not a candidate for surgical resection. In patients potentially eligible for surgery, staging procedures should be completed quickly, without significantly delaying the treatment, due to the aggressiveness of the disease. After surgery, adjuvant chemotherapy with platinum and etoposide for four cycles should be administered. In case of unforeseen nodal mediastinal involvement (N1 or N2) or in those patients without a systematic nodal dissection, thoracic radiotherapy after surgery should be considered. On the contrary, there is no role for surgery after induction chemotherapy in patients with N2 disease. Alternatively, due to the lack of randomized trials, combined concurrent chemoradiotherapy can be offered to patients with T1,2N0M0 and it is the first option for patients with significant concomitant medical illnesses who are at increased risk of perioperative complications. All patients with T1-2N0M0 should be considered for prophylactic cranial irradiation (PCI) after surgery and adjuvant chemotherapy.

In conclusion, the role of surgery in SCLC has been much debated and the International Guidelines recommend a surgical approach only in selected stage I patients, after adequate staging. For patient candidates for surgery, lobectomy with mediastinal lymphadenectomy is considered the standard approach, while sub-lobar resections are not considered appropriate. In all cases, surgery can be offered only as part of a multimodal treatment, which includes chemotherapy with or without radiotherapy and after a proper multidisciplinary evaluation.

Author Contributions: Conceptualization, N.M., A.M. and C.L.M.; writing-original draft preparation, N.M. and A.M.; writing-review and editing, N.M., A.M., A.L.R., G.D.L., R.D.C., G.B., G.T., P.M.,

C.P., G.E., N.N., C.L.M.: supervision, N.M., A.M., G.E. All authors have read and agreed to the published version of the manuscript.

Funding: This research received no external funding.

Acknowledgments: The authors are grateful to Alessandra Trocino, Librarian at IRCCS "G. Pascale" of Naples, Italy, for the bibliographic assistance.

Conflicts of Interest: Alessandro Morabito declares the following conflicts of interest: Speaker's fee: MSD, BMS, Boehringer, Pfizer, Roche, AstraZeneca; Advisory Board: Takeda, Eli-Lilly. Nicola Normanno declares the following personal financial interests (speaker's fee and/or advisory boards): MSD, Qiagen, Bayer, Biocartis, Incyte, Roche, BMS, MERCK, Thermofisher, Boehringer Ingelheim, Astrazeneca, Sanofi, Eli-Lilly; Institutional financial interests (financial support to research projects): MERCK, Sysmex, Thermofisher, QIAGEN, Roche, Astrazeneca, Biocartis. Non-financial interests: President, International Quality Network for Pathology (IQN Path); President, Italian Cancer Society (SIC). All the other Author declare no conflict of interest.

References

1. Van Meerbeeck, J.P.; Fennell, D.A.; De Ruysscher, D.K. Small-cell lung cancer. *Lancet* **2011**, *378*, 1741–1755. [CrossRef]
2. Byers, L.A.; Rudin, C.M. Small cell lung cancer: Where do we go from here? *Cancer* **2015**, *121*, 664–672. [CrossRef] [PubMed]
3. Mountain, C.F. The international system for staging lung cancer. *Semin. Surg. Oncol.* **2000**, *18*, 106–115. [CrossRef]
4. Jackman, D.M.; Johnson, B.E. Small-cell lung cancer. *Lancet* **2005**, *366*, 1385–1396. [CrossRef]
5. Bernhardt, E.B.; Jalal, S.I. Small Cell Lung Cancer. *Cancer Treat. Res.* **2016**, *170*, 301–322. [CrossRef]
6. Turrisi, A.T.; Kim, K.; Blum, R.; Sause, W.T.; Livingston, R.B.; Komaki, R.; Wagner, H.; Aisner, S.; Johnson, D.H. Twice-Daily Compared with Once-Daily Thoracic Radiotherapy in Limited Small-Cell Lung Cancer Treated Concurrently with Cisplatin and Etoposide. *N. Engl. J. Med.* **1999**, *340*, 265–271. [CrossRef]
7. Yu, J.B.; Decker, R.H.; Detterbeck, F.C.; Wilson, L.D. Surveillance Epidemiology and End Results Evaluation of the Role of Surgery for Stage I Small Cell Lung Cancer. *J. Thorac. Oncol.* **2010**, *5*, 215–219. [CrossRef]
8. Schreiber, D.; Rineer, J.; Weedon, J.; Vongtama, D.; Wortham, A.; Kim, A.; Han, P.; Choi, K.; Rotman, M. Survival outcomes with the use of surgery in limited-stage small cell lung cancer: Should its role be re-evaluated? *Cancer* **2010**, *116*, 1350–1357. [CrossRef]
9. Shepherd, F.A.; Crowley, J.J.; Van Houtte, P.; Postmus, P.E.; Carney, D.; Chansky, K.; Shaikh, Z.; Goldstraw, P. The International Association for the Study of Lung Cancer Lung Cancer Staging Project: Proposals Regarding the Clinical Staging of Small Cell Lung Cancer in the Forthcoming (Seventh) Edition of the Tumor, Node, Metastasis Classification for Lung Cancer. *J. Thorac. Oncol.* **2007**, *2*, 1067–1077. [CrossRef]
10. National Comprehensive Cancer Network. NCCN Guidelines Version 1.2021. Small Cell Lung Cancer. Available online: https://www.nccn.org/professionals/physician_gls/pdf/sclc.pdf (accessed on 23 December 2020).
11. Belcher, J.R. Lobectomy for bronchial carcinoma. *Lancet* **1959**, *274*, 639–642. [CrossRef]
12. Watson, W.L.; Berg, J.W. Oat cell lung cancer. *Cancer* **1962**, *15*, 759–768. [CrossRef]
13. Fox, W.; Scadding, J. Medical research council comparative trial of surgery and radiotherapy for primary treatment of small-celled or oat-celled carcinoma of bronchus: Ten-year follow-up. *Lancet* **1973**, *302*, 63–65. [CrossRef]
14. Scadding, J.G. Comparative trial of surgery and radiotherapy for the primary treatment of small-celled or oat-celled carcinoma of the bronchus. First report to the Medical Research Council by the working-party on the evaluation of different methods of therapy in carcinoma of the bronchus. *Lancet* **1966**, *2*, 979–986.
15. Miller, A.B.; Fox, W.; Tall, R. Five-year follow-up of the medical research council comparative trial of surgery and radiotherapy for the primary treatment of small-celled or oat-celled carcinoma of the bronchus: A report to the medical research council working party on the evaluation of different methods of therapy in carcinoma of the bronchus. *Lancet* **1969**, *294*, 501–505.
16. Medical Research Council Lung Cancer Working Party. Radiotherapy alone or with chemotherapy in the treatment of small-cell carcinoma of the lung. *Br. J. Cancer* **1979**, *40*, 1–10. [CrossRef]
17. Perry, M.C.; Eaton, W.L.; Propert, K.J.; Ware, J.H.; Zimmer, B.; Chahinian, A.P.; Skarin, A.; Carey, R.W.; Kreisman, H.; Faulkner, C.; et al. Chemotherapy with or without Radiation Therapy in Limited Small-Cell Carcinoma of the Lung. *N. Engl. J. Med.* **1987**, *316*, 912–918. [CrossRef]
18. Pignon, J.-P.; Arriagada, R.; Ihde, D.C.; Johnson, D.H.; Perry, M.C.; Souhami, R.L.; Brodin, O.; Joss, R.A.; Kies, M.S.; Lebeau, B.; et al. A meta-analysis of thoracic radiotherapy for small-cell lung cancer. *N. Engl. J. Med.* **1992**, *327*, 1618–1624. [CrossRef]
19. Warde, P.; Payne, D. Does thoracic irradiation improve survival and local control in limited-stage small-cell carcinoma of the lung? A meta-analysis. *J. Clin. Oncol.* **1992**, *10*, 890–895. [CrossRef]
20. De Ruysscher, D.; Pijls-Johannesma, M.; Vansteenkiste, J.; Kester, A.; Rutten, I.; Lambin, P. Systematic review and meta-analysis of randomised, controlled trials of the timing of chest radiotherapy in patients with limited-stage, small-cell lung cancer. *Ann. Oncol.* **2005**, *17*, 543–552. [CrossRef]
21. Hirsch, F.R.; Paulson, O.B.; Hansen, H.H.; Vraa-Jensen, J. Intracranial metastases in small cell carcinoma of the lung: Correlation of clinical and autopsy findings. *Cancer* **1982**, *50*, 2433–2437. [CrossRef]

22. Arriagada, R.; Le Chevalier, T.; Borie, F.; Riviere, A.; Chomy, P.; Monnet, I.; Tardivon, A.; Viader, F.; Tarayre, M.; Benhamou, S. Prophylactic Cranial Irradiation for Patients with Small-Cell Lung Cancer in Complete Remission. *J. Natl. Cancer Inst.* **1995**, *87*, 183–190. [CrossRef]
23. Gregor, A.; Cull, A.; Stephens, R.; Kirkpatrick, J.; Yarnold, J.; Girling, D.; Macbeth, F.; Stout, R.; Machin, D. Prophylactic cranial irradiation is indicated following complete response to induction therapy in small cell lung cancer: Results of a multicentre randomised trial. United Kingdom Coordinating Committee for Cancer Research (UKCCCR) and the European Organization for Research and Treatment of Cancer (EORTC). *Eur. J. Cancer* **1997**, *33*, 1752–1758. [CrossRef]
24. Aupérin, A.; Arriagada, R.; Pignon, J.-P.; Le Péchoux, C.; Gregor, A.; Stephens, R.J.; Kristjansen, P.E.; Johnson, B.E.; Ueoka, H.; Wagner, H.; et al. Prophylactic Cranial Irradiation for Patients with Small-Cell Lung Cancer in Complete Remission. *N. Engl. J. Med.* **1999**, *341*, 476–484. [CrossRef]
25. Stahel, R.; Thatcher, N.; Früh, M.; Le Péchoux, C.; Postmus, P.E.; Sorensen, J.B.; Felip, E.; Panel Members. 1st ESMO Consensus Conference in lung cancer; Lugano 2010: Small-cell lung cancer. *Ann. Oncol.* **2011**, *22*, 1973–1980. [CrossRef]
26. Lad, T.; Piantadosi, S.; Thomas, P.; Payne, D.; Ruckdeschel, J.; Giaccone, G. A Prospective Randomized Trial to Determine the Benefit of Surgical Resection of Residual Disease Following Response of Small Cell Lung Cancer to Combination Chemotherapy. *Chest* **1994**, *106*, 320S–323S. [CrossRef]
27. Shepherd, F.A.; Ginsberg, R.J.; Patterson, G.A.; Evans, W.K.; Feld, R. A prospective study of adjuvant surgical re-section after chemotherapy for limited small cell lung cancer. A University of Toronto Lung Oncology Group study. *J. Thorac. Cardiovasc. Surg.* **1989**, *97*, 177–186. [CrossRef]
28. Shepherd, F.A.; Ginsberg, R.J.; Feld, R.; Evans, W.K.; Johansen, E. Surgical treatment for limited small-cell lung cancer: The University of Toronto Lung Oncology Group experience. *J. Thorac. Cardiovasc. Surg.* **1991**, *101*, 385–393. [CrossRef]
29. Karrer, K.; Ulsperger, E. Surgery for Cure Followed by Chemotherapy in Small Cell Carcinoma of the Lung: For the Isc-Lung Cancer Study Group. *Acta Oncol.* **1995**, *34*, 899–906. [CrossRef]
30. Fujimori, K.; Yokoyama, A.; Kurita, Y.; Terashima, M. A Pilot Phase 2 Study of Surgical Treatment After Induction Chemotherapy for Resectable Stage I to IIIA Small Cell Lung Cancer. *Chest* **1997**, *111*, 1089–1093. [CrossRef]
31. Rea, F.; Callegaro, D.; Favaretto, A.; Loy, M.; Paccagnella, A.; Fantoni, U.; Festi, G.; Sartori, F. Long term results of surgery and chemotherapy in small cell lung cancer1. *Eur. J. Cardio-Thorac. Surg.* **1998**, *14*, 398–402. [CrossRef]
32. Eberhardt, W.; Stamatis, G.; Stuschke, M.; Wilke, H.; Müller, M.R.; Kolks, S.; Flasshove, M.; Schütte, J.; Stahl, M.; Schlenger, L.; et al. Prognostically orientated multimodality treatment including surgery for selected patients of small-cell lung cancer patients stages IB to IIIB: Long-term results of a phase II trial. *Br. J. Cancer* **1999**, *81*, 1206–1212. [CrossRef]
33. Tsuchiya, R.; Suzuki, K.; Ichinose, Y.; Watanabe, Y.; Yasumitsu, T.; Ishizuka, N.; Kato, H. Phase II trial of postoperative adjuvant cisplatin and etoposide in patients with completely resected stage I-IIIa small cell lung cancer: The Japan Clinical Oncology Lung Cancer Study Group Trial (JCOG9101). *J. Thorac. Cardiovasc. Surg.* **2005**, *129*, 977–983. [CrossRef]
34. Shields, T.W.; Higgins, G.A., Jr.; Mathews, M.J.; Keehn, R.J. Surgical resection in the management of small cell car-cinoma of the lung. *J. Thorac. Cardiovasc. Surg.* **1982**, *84*, 481–488. [CrossRef]
35. Østerlind, K.; Hansen, M.; Hansen, H.H.; Dombernowsky, P. Influence of surgical resection prior to chemotherapy on the long-term results in small cell lung cancer. A study of 150 operable patients. *Eur. J. Cancer Clin. Oncol.* **1986**, *22*, 589–593. [CrossRef]
36. Hara, N.; Ohta, M.; Ichinose, Y.; Motohiro, A.; Kuda, T.; Asoh, H.; Kawasaki, M. Influence of surgical resection before and after chemotherapy on survival in small cell lung cancer. *J. Surg. Oncol.* **1991**, *47*, 53–61. [CrossRef]
37. Inoue, M.; Miyoshi, S.; Yasumitsu, T.; Mori, T.; Iuchi, K.; Maeda, H.; Matsuda, H. Surgical results for small cell lung cancer based on the new TNM staging system. *Ann. Thorac. Surg.* **2000**, *70*, 1615–1619. [CrossRef]
38. Badzio, A.; Kurowski, K.; Karnicka-Mlodkowska, H.; Jassem, J. A retrospective comparative study of surgery followed by chemotherapy vs. non-surgical management in limited-disease small cell lung cancer. *Eur. J. Cardio-Thorac. Surg.* **2004**, *26*, 183–188. [CrossRef]
39. Brock, M.V.; Hooker, C.M.; Syphard, J.E.; Westra, W.; Xu, L.; Alberg, A.J.; Mason, D.; Baylin, S.B.; Herman, J.G.; Yung, R.C.; et al. Surgical resection of limited disease small cell lung cancer in the new era of platinum chemotherapy: Its time has come. *J. Thorac. Cardiovasc. Surg.* **2005**, *129*, 64–72. [CrossRef]
40. Takenaka, T.; Takenoyama, M.; Inamasu, E.; Yoshida, T.; Toyokawa, G.; Nosaki, K.; Hirai, F.; Yamaguchi, M.; Shimokawa, M.; Seto, T.; et al. Role of surgical resection for patients with limited disease-small cell lung cancer. *Lung Cancer* **2015**, *88*, 52–56. [CrossRef]
41. Zhong, L.; Suo, J.; Wang, Y.; Han, J.; Zhou, H.; Wei, H.; Zhu, J. Prognosis of limited-stage small cell lung cancer with comprehensive treatment including radical resection. *World J. Surg. Oncol.* **2020**, *18*, 1–7. [CrossRef]
42. Casiraghi, M.; Sedda, G.; Del Signore, E.; Piperno, G.; Maisonneuve, P.; Petrella, F.; De Marinis, F.; Spaggiari, L. Surgery for small cell lung cancer: When and how. *Lung Cancer* **2020**, *152*, 71–77. [CrossRef]
43. Rostad, H.; Naalsund, A.; Bertelsen, R.J.; Strand, T.-E.; Scott, H.; Strøm, E.H.; Norstein, J. Small cell lung cancer in Norway. Should more patients have been offered surgical therapy? *Eur. J. Cardio-Thorac. Surg.* **2004**, *26*, 782–786. [CrossRef]
44. Varlotto, J.M.; Medford-Davis, L.N.; Recht, A.; Flickinger, J.C.; Schaefer, E.; Zander, D.S.; DeCamp, M.M. Should Large Cell Neuroendocrine Lung Carcinoma be Classified and Treated as a Small Cell Lung Cancer or with Other Large Cell Carcinomas? *J. Thorac. Oncol.* **2011**, *6*, 1050–1058. [CrossRef]

45. Weksler, B.; Nason, K.S.; Shende, M.; Landreneau, R.J.; Pennathur, A. Surgical Resection Should Be Considered for Stage I and II Small Cell Carcinoma of the Lung. *Ann. Thorac. Surg.* **2012**, *94*, 889–893. [CrossRef]
46. Gaspar, L.E.; McNamara, E.J.; Gay, E.G.; Putnam, J.B.; Crawford, J.; Herbst, R.S.; Bonner, J.A. Small-Cell Lung Cancer: Prognostic Factors and Changing Treatment Over 15 Years. *Clin. Lung Cancer* **2012**, *13*, 115–122. [CrossRef]
47. Takei, H.; Kondo, H.; Miyaoka, E.; Asamura, H.; Yoshino, I.; Date, H.; Okumura, M.; Tada, H.; Fujii, Y.; Nakanishi, Y.; et al. Surgery for Small Cell Lung Cancer: A Retrospective Analysis of 243 Patients from Japanese Lung Cancer Registry in 2004. *J. Thorac. Oncol.* **2014**, *9*, 1140–1145. [CrossRef]
48. Yang, C.-F.J.; Chan, D.Y.; Speicher, P.J.; Gulack, B.C.; Tong, B.C.; Hartwig, M.G.; Kelsey, C.R.; D'Amico, T.A.; Berry, M.F.; Harpole, D.H. Surgery Versus Optimal Medical Management for N1 Small Cell Lung Cancer. *Ann. Thorac. Surg.* **2017**, *103*, 1767–1772. [CrossRef]
49. Yang, C.-F.J.; Chan, D.Y.; Shah, S.A.; Yerokun, B.A.; Wang, X.F.; D'Amico, T.A.; Berry, M.F.; Harpole, D.H., Jr. Long-term Survival After Surgery Compared with Concurrent Chemoradiation for Node-negative Small Cell Lung Cancer. *Ann. Surg.* **2018**, *268*, 1105–1112. [CrossRef]
50. Combs, S.E.; Hancock, J.G.; Boffa, D.J.; Decker, R.H.; Detterbeck, F.C.; Kim, A.W. Bolstering the Case for Lobectomy in Stages I, II, and IIIA Small-Cell Lung Cancer Using the National Cancer Data Base. *J. Thorac. Oncol.* **2015**, *10*, 316–323. [CrossRef]
51. Esposito, G.; Palumbo, G.; Carillio, G.; Manzo, A.; Montanino, A.; Sforza, V.; Costanzo, R.; Sandomenico, C.; La Manna, C.; Martucci, N.; et al. Immunotherapy in Small Cell Lung Cancer. *Cancers* **2020**, *12*, 2522. [CrossRef]
52. Trigo, J.M.; Subbiah, V.; Besse, B.; Moreno, V.; López, R.; Sala, M.A.; Peters, S.; Ponce, S.; Fernández, C.; Alfaro, V.; et al. Lurbinectedin as second-line treatment for patients with small-cell lung cancer: A single-arm, open-label, phase 2 basket trial. *Lancet Oncol.* **2020**, *21*, 645–654. [CrossRef]
53. Stish, B.J.; Hallemeier, C.L.; Olivier, K.R.; Harmsen, W.S.; Allen, M.S.; Garces, Y.I. Long-Term Outcomes and Patterns of Failure After Surgical Resection of Small-Cell Lung Cancer. *Clin. Lung Cancer* **2015**, *16*, e67–e73. [CrossRef] [PubMed]
54. Liu, T.; Chen, Z.; Dang, J.; Li, G. The role of surgery in stage I to III small cell lung cancer: A systematic review and meta-analysis. *PLoS ONE* **2018**, *13*, e0210001. [CrossRef]
55. Rudin, C.M.; Ismaila, N.; Hann, C.L.; Malhotra, N.; Movsas, B.; Norris, K.; Pietanza, M.C.; Ramalingam, S.S.; Turrisi, A.T.; Giaccone, G. Treatment of Small-Cell Lung Cancer: American Society of Clinical Oncology Endorsement of the American College of Chest Physicians Guideline. *J. Clin. Oncol.* **2015**, *33*, 4106–4111. [CrossRef] [PubMed]
56. Jett, J.R.; Schild, S.E.; Kesler, K.A.; Kalemkerian, G.P. Treatment of Small Cell Lung Cancer: Diagnosis and manage-ment of lung cancer, 3rd ed: American College of Chest Physicians evidence-based clinical practice guidelines. *Chest* **2013**, *143*, e400S–e419S. [CrossRef] [PubMed]
57. Früh, M.; De Ruysscher, D.; Popat, S.; Crinò, L.; Peters, S.; Felip, E.; ESMO Guidelines Working Group. Small-cell lung cancer (SCLC): ESMO Clinical Practice Guidelines for diagnosis, treatment and follow-up. *Ann. Oncol.* **2013**, *24*, vi99–vi105. [CrossRef] [PubMed]

MDPI
St. Alban-Anlage 66
4052 Basel
Switzerland
Tel. +41 61 683 77 34
Fax +41 61 302 89 18
www.mdpi.com

Cancers Editorial Office
E-mail: cancers@mdpi.com
www.mdpi.com/journal/cancers

www.ingramcontent.com/pod-product-compliance
Lightning Source LLC
LaVergne TN
LVHW070611100526
838202LV00012B/620